Praise for *Where Two Worlds Touch*

Very few writers possess the wit and spunk of Jade Angelica, especially combined with an uncanny insight into the art of giving care. Information about the science and medical treatment of Alzheimer's disease is readily available, but caregivers searching for spiritual guidance have largely been left on their own. Angelica offers much-needed guidance on topics like "Healing When There Is No Cure," "Redefining Survival," and "Forgetting, Forgiving, and Reconciling." Angelica's life story as an estranged daughter, a Harvard theological student, and eventually the primary caregiver for her mom has led her to a place where she can hold the hands of other caregivers and share her hopeful credo, that two worlds can indeed touch, even if one world is altered by distance and disease.

— Joanne Koenig Coste, author of *Learning to Speak Alzheimer's*, on the first edition

Jade Angelica takes us on a journey through the veils of life in her book about Alzheimer's and caregiving, *Where Two Worlds Touch*. Her hand reaches out, lifts us up, and guides our flight through the cloud cover. She leads us through the crisp blue tunnel where the bright light beams through.

Softly and subtly, her storytelling instills new perceptions of what is before us and what is possible. How situations we felt made no sense and were frustrating and exhausting are given a new view.

Jade's authentic voice shifts our beliefs. She shows how our souls never disconnect; even though communication may be delivered differently and quietly. She shows us there are different levels of unconditional love and compassion which can flip a sad negative narrative into one of peace, joy, and contentment. Thank you, Jade, for amplifying how small acts of kindness benefit all of us.

— Lori La Bey, founder of Alzheimer's Speaks and Dementia Map

Every chaplain, theologian, caregiver, and healthcare professional can find profound truth captured on each page of *Where Two Worlds Touch*. Jade Angelica builds from the narrative of her experience as a caregiver, and invites the reader to journey with her into the highly significant theo-philosophical literature that has arisen in the last decade around the experience of the deeply forgetful and those who care for them. The reader will find that there is a place for love and hope and continuing selfhood in an experience that is more than just half-full if we can see it rightly. This is a beautiful book and the deepest I have read on the topic.

— Dr. Stephen G. Post, author of *Dignity for Deeply Forgetful People: How Caregivers Can Meet the Challenges of Alzheimer's Disease*

I am so very impressed by this exceptionally well-written and well-researched book. Jade Angelica deserves rave reviews for her unique balance of compassion, insight, and scientific support on a very complex issue. I strongly recommend *Where Two Worlds Touch* for caregivers of individuals with Alzheimer's dementia.

— Dr. Robert A. Stern, former Clinical Core Director, Alzheimer's Disease Center, Boston University School of Medicine

Where Two Worlds Touch is an accessible and compassionate guide to understanding and loving someone with Alzheimer's. Through her own personal experience and spiritual training, Jade Angelica offers a shift in perspective about Alzheimer's that shines a loving light on what is still there instead of what is lost. This is the book I wished for when my grandmother had Alzheimer's.

— Dr. Lisa Genova, *New York Times* best-selling author of *Still Alice* and *Remember: The Science of Memory and the Art of Forgetting*

Jade Angelica has written an engaging and reflective book that is both personal and political. The commandment to honor your parent is not always easy. Angelica's focus on the care of people with Alzheimer's highlights this and brings out the often unspoken challenges of the practical, emotional, moral, and spiritual work we need to do to protect the most vulnerable members of our society.

— Rabbi Sara Paasche-Orlow, Spiritual Care Director, Hebrew SeniorLife, Boston

Where Two Worlds Touch is a timely manifesto that will forever change the way our society cares for individuals with dementia. This is a must-read book for all caretakers of patients with Alzheimer's disease. Angelica is a prescient observer of the human condition and has done a wonderful job of providing rich anecdotes, clear prose, and novel strategies that really work. Given that there is currently no cure for Alzheimer's disease, it is imperative that our society develop and follow a humane standard of care for these individuals. *Where Two Worlds Touch* provides a blueprint for how we can ameliorate the suffering of and dramatically improve the quality of life for Alzheimer's patients.

— Dr. Justin Feinstein, President and Director, Float Research Collective, Laureate Institute for Brain Research, Tulsa

Jade Angelica is a sojourner from the land of Alzheimer's bearing witness that all there is not lost. Her testimony is even more outrageous: We can experience in that far country depths of being alive, and in love, that the worlds of perfect health may never understand. *Where Two Worlds Touch* is a treasure chest of spiritual gems, the boon of an adventure into and out of the valley of the shadow of death. If you or someone you love are in the land of Alzheimer's, read this spirited-inspired travel log and find your way home.

— Michael Verde, Founder and Director, Memory Bridge

Where Two Worlds Touch is the best book on caring for a loved one with Alzheimer's that I have ever read. Jade C. Angelica knows what she is talking about. Her voice is warm, authentic, and loving. She offers wisdom, comfort, and assurance, revealing how this journey can be an experience of surprising grace and spiritual growth."

— Michael Leach, editor of "Soul Seeing" in *National Catholic Reporter*; author of *Soul Seeing: Light, Love, Forgiveness*; and caregiver to wife Vickie for twenty years

Where Two Worlds Touch is a deeply moving and insightful exploration of Alzheimer's caregiving that seamlessly blends personal experience, scientific research, and spiritual wisdom. Jade Angelica offers a compassionate and empowering perspective, revealing the profound connections and moments of grace that are possible even in the face of cognitive decline. Through her heartfelt narrative and nuanced understanding, Angelica illuminates the enduring value and beauty of every person, regardless of their cognitive state. This book is an invaluable resource for anyone touched by Alzheimer's, providing both practical guidance and spiritual nourishment for the caregiving journey. Angelica's work stands as a testament to the power of love, hope, and the enduring human spirit.

— Rev. Professor John Swinton, Professor in Practical Theology and Pastoral Care, King's College, University of Aberdeen

From my experience both as a neurologist treating people who are living with dementia and a care partner for my parents who had Alzheimer's disease, I have learned that the deepest losses associated with dementia are in the realm of relationships. Some of the greatest gifts care partners can receive are the belief and hope that meaningful relationships can be maintained with people who are advancing in dementia and guidance on ways to foster those relationships and shore up selfhood in the process. In her beautiful book, *Where Two Worlds Touch*, as well as in her educational presentations and workshops, Jade Angelica offers these gifts with insight, intelligence, honest, and compassion, lightening the burdens of many in the process. I consider Jade's book an essential part of my library.

— Dr. Daniel C. Potts, neurologist, Tuscaloosa VA Medical Center

Jade Angelica's *Where Two Worlds Touch* provides an insightful and poignant journey into caring for a loved one living with dementia. It invites the reader to enter into a compassionate and dignified world that connects the latest in Alzheimer's research while invoking person-centered approaches through meaningful improvisation. A heartfelt reality that many can resonate with while embarking upon a world of caregiving.

— Dr. Angel C. Duncan, Executive Arts Director, Cognitive Dynamic Foundation

In *Where Two Worlds Touch: The Spirit and Science of Alzheimer's Caregiving*, Jade Angelica masterfully weaves her personal journey as a caregiver with scientific insights and spiritual reflections, offering readers a profound guide to finding meaning, connection, and even grace in the face of caring for someone with Alzheimer's disease. Her beautifully written narrative, enriched with practical advice, coping strategies, and meditative practices, is both insightful and deeply compassionate. This book not only acknowledges the immense challenges of caregiving but also reveals how we can discover purpose and forge a deeper bond with our loved ones, even in the most difficult and lonely moments. I hope every caregiver of a loved one with dementia has the opportunity to read this wonderful book.

— Dr. Edmarie Guzmán-Vélez, Postdoctoral Fellow, Multicultural Alzheimer's Prevention Program (MAPP)

www.skinnerhouse.org
Printed in the United States
Cover design by Carol Chu
Author photo by Coleen Hein

The cover image is of a gingko leaf. In many cultures around the world, ginkgo leaves are symbolically rich, representing strength, endurance, vitality, transformation, spirituality, resilience, hope, peace, enlightenment, memory, longevity in relationships, and eternal life.

Print ISBN: 978-1-55896-930-8
Ebook ISBN: 978-1-55896-931-5
Audiobook ISBN: 978-1-55896-933-9

4 3 2 1 / 26 25 24

Library of Congress Cataloging-in-Publication Data

Names: Angelica, Jade C. (Jade Christine), 1952- author.
Title: Where two worlds touch : the spirit and science of Alzheimer's
    caregiving / Jade C. Angelica.
Description: Boston : Skinner House Books, [2024] | Includes
    bibliographical references. | Summary: "Challenging the predominant
    beliefs about people with Alzheimer's, Angelica weaves a spiritual
    memoir and pastoral guide for those who love someone with Alzheimer's"--
    Provided by publisher.
Identifiers: LCCN 2024005956 (print) | LCCN 2024005957 (ebook) | ISBN
    9781558969308 (print) | ISBN 9781558969315 (ebook)
Subjects: LCSH: Alzheimer's disease--Patients--Care. | Alzheimer's
    disease--Patients--Biography. | Aging parents--Care--Religious aspects.
Classification: LCC RC523 .A545 2024 (print) | LCC RC523 (ebook) | DDC
    616.8/311--dc23/eng/20240708
LC record available at https://lccn.loc.gov/2024005956
LC ebook record available at https://lccn.loc.gov/2024005957

We are grateful for permission to reprint the following copyrighted material:
"Facts and Figures about Alzheimer's and Dementia," adapted from Alzheimer's Association website, alz.org. Used with permission of the Alzheimer's Association.
Adaptation of "Yes, Virginia, There Is a Santa Claus," by Jade Angelica, in *The Journal of Pastoral Care and Counseling*, Vol. 65, No. 2 (2011), 10:1-2. Used with permission of *The Journal of Pastoral Care and Counseling*.
Adaptation of "Elephant and the Blind Men" from *Jain World*, www.jainworld.com/education/stories25.asp. Used with permission of Jain World.
"The Wind of the Spirit" by Myra Scovel. Used with permission of the poet's heirs.
"How Shall I?" by Libbie Deverich Stoddard. Used with permission of the author.
"Absolutely Clear," from the Penguin publication *The Subject Tonight Is Love: Sixty Wild and Sweet Poems of Hafiz* by Daniel Ladinsky, 2003 © with permission. www.danielladinsky.com.
Letter to the Alzheimer's Association by Sol Rogers. Used with permission of the author.
"Theses on Healing (and Cure)" by Fred Reklau, from *Partners in Care: Medicine and Ministry Together,* used by permission of the author and Wipf and Stock Publishers, www.wipfand-stock.com
Gott spricht zu jedem.../God speaks to each of us..." from RILKE'S BOOK OF HOURS: LOVE POEMS TO GOD by Rainer Maria Rilke, translated by Anita Barrows and Joanna Macy, translation copyright © 1996 by Anita Barrows and Joanna Macy. Used by permission of Riverhead, an imprint of Penguin Publishing Group, a division of Penguin Random House LLC. All rights reserved.
Reading 698, by Wayne B. Arnason, in *Singing the Living Tradition* (Unitarian Universalist Association, 1993). Reprinted by permission of the author.

WHERE TWO WORLDS TOUCH

THE SPIRIT AND SCIENCE OF ALZHEIMER'S CAREGIVING

JADE C. ANGELICA

Skinner House Books
Boston

Contents

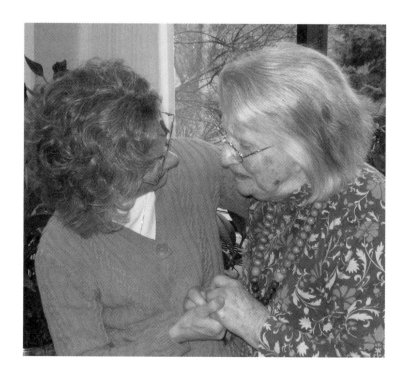

All the stories in this book about Alzheimer's are true and are based either on my own observations and recollections or on caregiver interviews and conversations, all of which are shared with permission. In some cases, names and certain details have been changed according to family members' requests for privacy.

In honor and memory of my mom, Jeanne, this work is dedicated to the beautiful, enlivened souls who have Alzheimer's disease and to all those who love and care for them. You are my inspiration.

—JA

Foreword

Rev. Jade C. Angelica is a sought-after leader in thought, word, and action when it comes to making and holding a place in our hearts and lives for deeply forgetful people. For a book to ring true with so much astonishing insight, its author has to be personally steeped in caregiving experience and to have gained the immense wisdom that can only come from navigating its many challenges. But the author also needs to have a compelling background in the meaning and significance of human vulnerability, dependence, and caregiving, and an ability to convey this with narrative beauty and depth of heart. Jade Angelica does this with words that jump right off the page into the inner being of the reader, who feels a sense of immense *expectancy* with each turning of the page.

In 2001, I had been invited to Andover Newton Theological School in the Boston area to devote an annual lecture there to what it might really mean to include people with dementia under the fully open umbrella of loving kindness within an inclusive spirituality that resisted the implicit and explicit bias of the "hypercognitive values" that so badly undermine their moral status. I first met Jade years later as a result of this lecture when she was pursuing a doctor of ministry degree in Faith, Health and Spirituality. A Unitarian Universalist, a graduate of Harvard Divinity School, and a very active leader at the closely related

Andover-Newton Theological School, Jade learned about my work through her advisor, Professor Brita Gill-Austern. It was my great delight and honor to talk with Jade, and to learn of her commitment to people with dementia, generated in large part by her visionary inclusive spirituality and also by the developing narrative of her mother, who seemed to be developing dementia secondary to Alzheimer's back home in Iowa. Already Jade had started to articulate what was to become perhaps the most recognized humanistic, philosophic, loving, inclusive, and practical approach to caring for these beloved individuals, who are indeed more deeply forgetful and often more behaviorally challenged than those who are spared dementia.

Jade covers all the positive capacities of deeply forgetful people that caregivers need to be reminded of and learn to work with: creativity, symbolism, emotion, relationality, mirth, movement and dance, song, beauty, smell/taste, spirituality, touch, consciousness, continuity of self-identity, and hope.

The subtitle of this book is worth paying attention to: "The Spirit and Science of Alzheimer's Caregiving." There is really no way to address caregiving fully other than at this tremendously important interface. As Jade points out, Alzheimer's and other forms of dementia are not matters for doctors alone. Indeed, while there is a certain value in what modern medical science can contribute, there are as of yet no "magic bullets" to prevent, slow progression of, or reverse dementia in all its variations. Jade does a splendid and even nuanced job of bringing the caregiver up to date on many aspects of the science involved in providing optimal care as the challenges arise, and the fact remains that, for the most part, it is the movement beyond the biomedical model that is essential to well-being. She carefully and caringly writes of the embodied self, the emotional self, the cognitive self, the relational self, and the spiritual self.

Very quickly, the reader notices how important the giving and receiving of pure love is between the caregiver and the one cared for, who can also be learned from. Jade develops a model of caregiving that has some discernible roots in her engagement with the great Jewish spiritual thinker Martin Buber in his classic work *I and Thou*, which the author studied extensively and formatively in her early years as a student in Boston. She is able to bring reality to the idea that, while caregiving is indeed an action of devoted presence, empathy, listening, and giving, it is a relational dynamic in which the caregiver learns, finds degrees of joy, finds hope in surprising episodes of lucidity, and certainly reaches deeper perspectives on healing at virtually every level. In other words, this book, while realistic, is not another one-sided discussion of "the burdens of caregiving," but rather leans toward all that can be gained from providing care.

Certainly, Jade describes her life journey as profoundly deepened and transformed by her having had the chance to care for her mother in her years of vulnerability and dependence. While we humans tend to think of ourselves as invulnerable and independent, this is a deception foisted upon us by certain dominant social myths. The fact is that when we enter this world, we are completely vulnerable, frail, and entirely dependent on others for love and protection. At various points along the journey of life, illness or injury will come along, and we will realize the truth that vulnerability and dependence are our ultimate human realities, especially as we grow old and inevitably frail.

Jade's life has been blessed, on the one hand, by her innate or perhaps infused capacity for compassionate love and, on the other hand, by a mother who despite human imperfections became in a very special way Jade's teacher until her final moments and even remains so now for all of us who open the pages of this unique, uplifting, challenging, and elegant book. Read these pages because you will learn that the ultimate human reality is by necessity love, and that the test for love is provided when we encounter deeply forgetful people who look to us to sing an old familiar song, to be present in a way that brings them back into the human community, and to recognize meaning in their lives. Indeed, on a very practical note, Jade's book is about techniques of communication and presence that she has developed over the years as her life's calling, knowing that nothing can separate anyone from the ways and power of pure love.

Stephen G. Post, PhD
Stony Brook University Renaissance School of Medicine
Director of the Center for Medical Humanities,
Compassionate Care & Bioethics

Introduction

Dear Readers,

Welcome to the second edition of *Where Two Worlds Touch*. I'm honored to be invited into your experience of Alzheimer's learning and caring, and grateful for the opportunity to share many of the discoveries I made about life and love during the years of caring for my mom, Jeanne. My hope is that some of what I've learned will resonate with your minds and hearts, and make a difference for you and people living with Alzheimer's or other diseases of dementia.

The original manuscript for this book was crafted during the first two years after Mom died from Alzheimer's. Writing it was a catharsis for me while I processed the experience of being her faithful companion, as well as an opportunity to enlighten and inspire others who are curious about Alzheimer's disease and care. Now, ten years later, I'm grateful for the renewed opportunity to enhance the book with additional experiences and discoveries from the world of Alzheimer's. This edition includes updates based on research since the book was first published, with expanded discussion of medications, emotional memory, and caregiver experiences, as well as more information and stories about the particular impacts of Alzheimer's on oppressed populations. During these years, I have also learned more about different spiritualities and theologies that have valuable insights for Alzheimer's caregiving, and I hope that you will find them personally meaningful as well.

Where Two Worlds Touch is crafted like a tapestry, woven together by poetry and stories drawn from my experiences and those of other Alzheimer's caregivers, informed by literature in the Alzheimer's field of research, and grounded by spiritual, theological, and scientific resources. The personal stories about Mom and me, and other caregivers and their loved ones, anchor the universal aspects of my message within individual lives. Unless otherwise cited in the endnotes, stories about others come from personal conversations, interviews, and correspondence. One of my intentions is to remind everyone of the inherent dignity and worth of all people—even people with cognitive decline—and to reinforce the reality that interconnectedness is a central aspect of being human. We are not separate from people with Alzheimer's. Our lives are woven together in the tapestry of life, and we are on this journey together.

Although this book is the culmination of many years of academic study in a unique doctoral program called "Faith, Health, and Spirituality," the information is presented in a style designed to open hearts and engage the spiritual imagination of readers, as well as to be intellectually stimulating. The writing style is intended to be accessible for a general audience of family and professional Alzheimer's caregivers, with the goal of sharing forward the wisdom and comfort I received from my many teachers and companions. For those interested in the more academic aspects of my study of Alzheimer's care, including brain science, current research, and theological ideas, detailed references are located in the notes at the end of the book.

The topics and issues I present are discussed in the context of spirituality, since this is my main area of interest and education, and my primary source of comfort and guidance—especially during life's hardest times. The words *God* and *spirit,* which have deep meaning for me, are used often. Understanding that these words have different meanings for different people, I aspire to use them in an inclusive way. According to theologian Marcus Borg, words from various traditions used to name the sacred—such as *God, Yahweh, Brahman, Atman, Allah, the Tao,* and *Great Spirit*—are "understood as that nonmaterial reality or presence that is experienced in extraordinary moments .... *The sacred (or numinous)* refers to the other reality that is encountered in these experiences."[1] Borg's understanding of these sacred words resonates with my own.

Early in my ministry education, I was given the opportunity to enroll in an upper-level course called "Healing Is Meeting: The Vision of Martin Buber," taught by Professor Brita Gill-Austern. Brita became one of my professional and life mentors over the next many decades, and she was an important guide as I developed my work in the Alzheimer's world. Her course on Martin Buber informed my worldview and planted seeds for transformation that have blossomed in various manifestations ever since. Almost fifteen years after taking this course, with Buber's insights about deep spiritual meetings between people still imprinted in my mind and heart, I encountered Alzheimer's disease. It was then that enrolling in this course felt more like Destiny than mere opportunity.

Like many people are, I was frightened to engage with Alzheimer's. However, my mother's diagnosis in 2001 beckoned me across the threshold of her mysterious world. I said "Yes" and was led into surprising connection with her. There, seeds of transformation sprouted, and in many ways, Mom and I met each other for the first time. Inspired by Martin Buber, one important message in *Where Two Worlds Touch* is about the power and potential of true encounter. Although this message is relayed partially through the tender and enlightening "meetings" I experienced with Mom, this book is about more than the relationship between Mom and me. It's about meeting people with Alzheimer's and falling into love and respect for them. It's about meeting caregivers who have learned to bear the unbearable, who demonstrate that it's okay—even desirable—to commit to caregiving even if it means our own lives must change. It's about recognizing our limitations as individuals and the inability of science and medicine to so far delay or cure this disease. It's about accepting our frustrations and suffering and then opening our hearts to hope and healing as we encounter a degenerative terminal disease. It's about the tender responsibility of becoming the legal guardian for a person who is completely helpless, and then struggling with awesome decisions about life and death. It's about grappling with the realities of Alzheimer's disease and the impact of these realities on individuals, families, communities, and whole societies. It's about caregivers telling our stories and meeting scientists who will heed them, and help us change the world of Alzheimer's care. It's about understanding ourselves and our humanity— our feelings, thoughts, reactions, and beliefs—as we view life through the lens of Alzheimer's. And it's about discovering life-giving possibilities in every corner of life. All of these represent the "true encounters" Buber names as healing.

Much that happens in the world of Alzheimer's is about loss. And so it may surprise you that my story is not about losing my mother while she was living with Alzheimer's; in many ways it's about finding her. Accordingly, my reflections on our experiences don't focus only on the inevitable losses and grief that accompany cognitive decline; they focus also on what remains, what can be found, and what's possible.

One caregiving setting I specifically address is the often-dreaded nursing home, more recently rebranded as care centers and/or memory care units, or also known as skilled nursing facilities As the time nears when it may be necessary for caregivers to move their loved ones to assisted living or nursing home facilities, it's important to appreciate the difficulties of this life change for everyone involved. It's an environment that we caregivers may need to return to again and again in order to fully understand and accept that this is now our loved one's home, and to be comfortable there. It's important to be gentle with ourselves during this transition, but also to be committed and disciplined in our efforts to overcome any resistance. Self-awareness, a critical component in the lives of Alzheimer's caregivers, will aid us in noticing resistance and moving toward accepting what is—including the need for help.

The "Spiritual Practices" section offers some ideas for enhancing self-care, which is another component of successful, satisfying caregiving. Self-care includes practices such as relaxation, exercise, and seeking support, in addition to self-awareness and acceptance, and is essential because family caregivers, especially, are at heightened risk for health problems and depression due to stress. Caregivers are strongly encouraged to give themselves permission to care for themselves as well as their loved ones . . . since self-care may just be our saving grace.

As part of my research for the book, I interviewed Mary Anne, a family caregiver. After this book was first published, Mary Anne and I met for lunch. The day before, she had read the story I wrote about her relationship with her mother, Ione, to her husband. He asked if what I wrote were my words or Mary Anne's. They were her words, of course. He expressed some surprise about Mary Anne's self-awareness and her depth of feeling about her mother's illness and decline. Mary Anne replied, "It was really helpful to talk to Jade about what I was feeling. No one had asked me these questions, so I hadn't actually thought about it before." Since pondering these questions increased Mary Anne's self-awareness and was so helpful to her,

I have included them in the section "Reflection Questions." If other caregivers feel inclined to explore your own hearts and minds, you may choose to use these questions as a guide.

For more than twenty years, I have been immersed in rich learning about Alzheimer's disease and caregiving. Combining my academic inquiry, my experience as a spiritual director, and my personal encounters with people with Alzheimer's and their caregivers, I write as a spiritual companion for family caregivers and anyone who loves someone with Alzheimer's. *Where Two Worlds Touch* is unique among Alzheimer's resources in that it describes the experience of caregiving through the lens of a spiritual journey—my journey—revealing how this challenging experience has the potential to lead us through Alzheimer's into healing and wholeness, revealing how this journey invites us to recognize various worlds touching: the worlds of science and spirit, the worlds of healing and the arts, the worlds of loss and gratitude, the worlds of suffering and meaning, and most importantly our personal worlds touching the alternate but very real worlds of our loved ones. By embracing people with Alzheimer's with open hearts, compassionate presence, and holy vision, it's possible that caregivers on this sacred journey will bear witness to the transforming power of Alzheimer's, as I did. It's also possible that caregivers will notice and receive unexpected gifts and experience awe and gratitude for the ways that Alzheimer's can touch our hearts and transform our lives.

My purpose for sharing my story and my discoveries is to reassure caregivers that they and their loved ones with Alzheimer's need not suffer in isolation or be overwhelmed by fear, loss, or responsibility. A blessing written by a ministry colleague has been a travelling companion of mine for many years through many perils. As you begin this book, dear readers, I share this blessing:

Take courage friends. The way is often hard, the path is never clear, and the stakes are very high. Take courage. For deep down, there is another truth: You are not alone.

—Wayne Arnason[2]

As you journey on through life, dear readers, I wish you abundant blessings, rich learnings, and supportive, loving guides.

Yours in companionship,
Jade Angelica
September 2024

I

In the Beginning

God speaks to each of us as he makes us, then walks with us silently out of the night.

These are the words we dimly hear:

You, sent out beyond your recall, go to the limits of your longing. Embody me.

Flare up like a flame and make big shadows I can move in.

Let everything happen to you: beauty and terror. Just keep going. No feeling is final. Don't let yourself lose me.

Nearby is the country they call life. You will know it by its seriousness.

Give me your hand.

—Rainer Maria Rilke

Three months after having hip replacement surgery, my mother Jeanne, then eighty-two, walked by herself to an appointment with her primary care doctor. That day she revealed a concern she was having about her memory. Indicating that memory loss was an early sign of Alzheimer's, the doctor prescribed a trial of Aricept.

Then Mom took what must have been a lonely walk home. About a mile in distance, this walk marked Mom's first steps on what became a ten-year journey through Alzheimer's disease.

Years later, reading about this appointment in Mom's medical file, my heart was overcome by emotion. Aware of her lifelong aversion to doctors, I felt compassion for the humility it took for her to be open and vulnerable about her decline and to ask for help. I also felt admiration for her bravery in self-reporting this symptom, because she surely knew what it meant. Mom had cared for her older sister, Milly, who died from Alzheimer's nine years earlier. As I visualized Mom taking those first, solitary steps into Alzheimer's, the rightness of my decision to change my life and be beside her during the final years and months, weeks and days—moments—of her life was reinforced yet again.

Every person's and every family's journey into Alzheimer's will begin, unfold, and end uniquely—because it will be ours and we are unique. Our histories, circumstances, fears, needs, and longings cohere into what our experience with Alzheimer's will become for us. I know that some caregivers will face many of the same challenges I did; I also know that some caregivers will face challenges that are even more—or possibly less—daunting. We are embarking on the path from starting points determined by different family backgrounds and current circumstances, different races, cultures, and sexual orientations and genders; different relationships with our loved ones; different financial circumstances; different knowledge about the disease; different interactions with the world of health care; different faith understandings. Different everything. And so it's important to acknowledge that our identities, backgrounds, and present circumstances matter in caregiving as well as in life.

Although there are infinite differences in the practicalities and emotions of caregiver experiences, the similarities of our sorrows and joys, the consistency of our struggles and victories, and those tiny unforgettable, forever cherished moments of connection with our loved ones are what will bind caregivers together as we find our way along this mysterious path.

As Mom's spirit and I become your companions on this journey, we hope that our story and our discoveries will bring comfort and inspiration to people with Alzheimer's and their caregivers. We hope our story will help families, health care professionals, and communities develop a deeper understanding of dementia and nurture the belief that meaningful relationships remain possible throughout all the stages and diminishments of Alzheimer's.

Take my hand as we cross the threshold together into the world of Alzheimer's . . . .

1 Awakening

Oblivion was my first companion on the Alzheimer's journey. I simply wasn't there to witness the beginning of Mom's decline. We were separated geographically by twelve hundred miles. I lived in Portland, Maine, and Mom lived in Dubuque, Iowa— our hometown. Complicated circumstances in both of our lives had prevented us from seeing each other for a few years. When we spoke on the phone, I didn't register any decline because I had always attributed oddities in Mom's memory, speech, or mood to drinking.

Twenty-five years earlier, I had begun separating emotionally from Mom. Before this, we had been very close, perhaps too close. As a child, I was her shadow, trying desperately to win her attention and approval. As a young adult, I had trouble identifying my own opinions, preferences, and needs, particularly if they seemed contrary to hers. In order to become my own person, I needed both geographic and emotional distance.

I also needed to protect myself from Mom's judgmental nature, alcoholic lifestyle, and limited worldview, which didn't allow me to choose sobriety or my own religious beliefs, to express vegetarian or sugar-free dietary preferences, or to speak my truth about what it was like for me growing up in an alcoholic, abusive home. Alcohol was the centerpiece of our family life and social gatherings, and my relationship with Mom became especially strained when I stopped drinking.

After Mom moved to what her generation referred to as a nursing home, and I moved to Iowa to be her advocate, companion, and comforter, a relative criticized me for not spending more time with Mom during the years before Alzheimer's when she "could have appreciated" my presence. Although this criticism was hurtful to me, I realized that there was much this relative didn't understand about me, my family, my relationship with Mom, or my healing journey. Mom might have appreciated more visits from me during the years of separation, but possibly not. I was such a disappointment to her.

When I was in Iowa for my twenty-fifth high school reunion, the local paper wrote a story about my book on the moral emergency of child sexual abuse. Although neither book nor article revealed my personal history of familial sexual abuse, Mom was shamed and threatened by what she perceived as public exposure. After reading the article in the morning paper, she flew into an alcohol-fueled rage. Her critical rants, echoing off the walls of her small house, culminated with the pronouncement, "I am not proud of you."

I was devastated.

By this time of my life, I had been sober for over fifteen years, overcoming addictions to alcohol, drugs, and food; I had graduated from Harvard Divinity School; I was an ordained minister (albeit not in Mom's religious tradition); I was doing a meaningful ministry on behalf of abused children and had published books and articles in the hopes of protecting them; I had received professional recognition and achieved a modest amount of financial security. By social standards, I had achieved some success. Although I had tried to please Mom by making deliberate and specific efforts to connect with her, in Mom's eyes and heart, I was a disappointment.

If modern theologian Richard Rohr is accurate in his belief that on the spiritual journey, we have to leave home in order to actually find our way home,[1] it was precisely those years of geographic and emotional separation that allowed me to come home to Mom during her time of greatest need. In her book *Fierce Love*, activist, preacher, and public theologian Jacqui Lewis informed my understanding of how and why those years of separation made such a difference in my caring for my mother. It wasn't just about the distance, although that did provide a layer of protection for me. It was about the efforts I had made to heal the wounds from my childhood by addressing the addictions that were masking my truth; it was about uncovering and healing the shame and self-criticism that permeated my being; it was about looking at my story with empathy and finding wisdom from the journey that was/is my life.

Lewis describes the childhood experiences of many of us:

> In the classroom, on the playground, in houses of worship, or at home, too many children feel unsafe, undervalued, unlovable. They are taught— overtly or implicitly—that they are unworthy of love, which makes loving others difficult, if not impossible."[2]

The fierce love Lewis refers to so eloquently and personally is grounded first and foremost in self-love. It's not an easy task, developing this self-love. I know from personal experience; and Lewis takes us along on her own winding and arduous journey, ultimately leading us by example to the awareness that loving ourselves will help us to be "curious about others, compassionate toward others, as gracious to your neighbor [or mother with Alzheimer's] as you are to yourself."[3] One of my teachers from the Hindu Vedic tradition, Acharya Shunya, echoes Lewis' message, revealing the ancient universality and necessity of self-love. "Those that wish to serve others need to begin by practicing loving kindness to themselves."

By the time my sibling placed Mom in the nursing home and moved away, leaving no one in Iowa to look after Mom, I had developed enough self-love to know that being alone in a nursing home in the midst of diminishments from Alzheimer's disease was not how my heart wanted my mother—or anyone—to live the last years of her life. And I was ready to serve.

I don't know if Mom ever did feel proud of me. But her whole-souled smiles, her hugs and kisses, and her expressive sounds and admiring looks during the three and a half years we had together at the end of her life communicated to me that my presence as her daily companion in the nursing home was definitely appreciated.

In 2002, when I learned from a cousin who saw Mom occasionally that signs of Alzheimer's were definitely present, avoidance became my next companion on the journey. Not denial, which is common for Alzheimer's family members, but avoidance. I knew Alzheimer's was among us. I knew because Alzheimer's had been a cloud over our family for nearly thirty years: Both of Mom's older sisters had some form of dementia, probably Alzheimer's. I still vividly remember the day in 1973 when dear Aunt Milly wandered off during a family picnic in the picturesque river town of Guttenberg, Iowa. She had gone to the restroom and never returned. In my photo collection there's a picture of her on that day, wearing my royal blue "Brothers III" volleyball jacket and a bewildered smile. We had no idea, in this moment, what was happening.

That was the beginning for our family; and now, Milly's daughter was telling me that Mom was showing signs of this disease. She encouraged me to read books about Alzheimer's, to watch videos and movies, and to explore the Alzheimer's Association website. I politely listened to her while consciously disguising my impatience, thanked her, and chose to avoid the entire subject. Fear, of course, was the foundation of my avoidance. David Shenk, a journalist who researched Alzheimer's disease and wrote *The Forgetting—Alzheimer's: Portrait of an Epidemic*, had also once been an avoider. He helped me to feel forgiven for my avoidance and explained why this is a common reaction.

> Opening the book, one fears, is tantamount to looking straight into the face of Alzheimer's—and perhaps one's own dark future.... So we avoid it. We don't read the books; we don't ask the questions; we don't visit our newly diagnosed neighbor.... It's only natural to not want to explore such awful thoughts.[4]

Because Shenk and I have travelled through the valley of Alzheimer's avoidance, we wouldn't dare to judge others who are also following this path.

Avoidance was an effective companion for me—until 2003. Milly's daughter made the thoughtful and generous offer to bring Mom to Maine to visit me. Her offer was accompanied by the foreboding, "Before it's too late." Meaning before Mom forgot me—which she never did, by the way. I accepted this offer and agreed to the visit. Mom was thrilled, as demonstrated by her packed suitcase ready and waiting by the front door of her house for two weeks before the trip. Still feeling the need to protect myself from my alcoholic family, I was apprehensive.

To prepare myself for this visit from my mother and what I considered to be my first conscious, face-to-face meeting with

Alzheimer's, I attended a personal growth workshop, one of many such experiences I had sought out during my twenty-plus years of healing. Influenced by Episcopal priest Alan Jones to believe that the journey of our souls often presents itself in the form of a story,[5] I was especially intrigued when the workshop leader, who had a Jungian perspective, suggested that we could learn about our unconscious drives and longings by writing our life stories on one page.

I did this creative writing assignment eagerly and was impressed by my own poetic conciseness and my understanding of my life. Over dinner the night before Mom arrived, I told a friend about the workshop. Convinced that my one-page life story was well written and accurate, I read it to my friend with pride. It was a story of being vulnerable—as a child and as a woman—and being abused, abandoned, and betrayed by the very people who were entrusted with my care and safety. My friend looked at me across the dinner table with astonished eyes. Expecting praise, I was shocked by her reply. "You've done so much with your life, Jade. Why do you keep telling *that* story?"

The wisdom of my soul instantly knew the answer to her question: Because almost every part of my being, including my imagination, had been severely wounded by abusers in my childhood and my adult intimate relationships. Parts of me had healed, and other parts were continuing to heal. But my friend's question made me realize that I had closed down my imagination and shut myself off from seeing any new possibilities in my life story. Fortunately, this conversation raised my awareness about this pattern just in time. A new possibility—in the form of my mother in decline from Alzheimer's disease—was about to step off a plane and awaken my soul to an unimagined future.

Mom and her travelling companion, Milly's daughter, arrived for a three-day visit in May. It's a breathtakingly beautiful time of year along Maine's southern coast, but Mom seemed to have eyes only for me. When she walked off the plane and caught sight of me, her face erupted into joy that radiated throughout her entire visit. She took my hand at the airport, and she didn't let go.

The changes in Mom were poignant, touching my heart in unexpected ways. One surprising change was that her judgmental nature seemed to be replaced by a kind of sweetness. It seemed that she had forgotten what a disappointment I had previously been to her. She called me "my girl," smiled genuinely at me, and reached out to connect with me physically whenever possible.

Mom seemed curious about herself and her environment. There was a full-length mirror in the hallway of my apartment, and every time she passed the mirror, she paused at length to examine her reflection and comb her hair. Almost every picture from that trip shows Mom holding her comb in one hand. When I served our first lunch together, she was more interested in the silverware than in the food. She picked up her fork and looked closely at the handle. She turned it over, stroked it, and touched it to her cheek. In order to turn her attention away from the fork, I had to coax her into tasting the food. Not until much later did I realize the source of her fork fascination. When I first moved out on my own, Mom gave me this set of silver-plated flatware, which had belonged to her mother. This silverware, engraved with the initial T—the first letter of Mom's maiden name—was familiar from childhood. Unquestionably, some kind of recognition was happening for her.

Mom's surprising behaviors opened my heart and riveted my attention. I wanted to connect with her, to be supportive and caring, but it was clear that I didn't know what to do or how to be in her presence. I didn't know how to communicate with this transforming being, how to meet her needs, how to keep her safe, or how to navigate social practices such as dinner in a restaurant or attending a concert with someone who no longer understood—or practiced—conventional behaviors. One evening at a concert by a group of local a cappella singers, I had a flashback to a movie experience with my nephew when he was five. After fidgeting for a while, Mom started talking out loud. "Shhhh" didn't help. Finally, Mom stood up, just as my nephew had, and shouted, just as my nephew had, "This is taking too long!" It was time to go.

My mom with Alzheimer's equaled a mystery to me, and the growing collection of things I didn't know resulted in me feeling inadequate and afraid. My brief encounter with Mom during this phase of her disease opened my heart and informed my mind to the helplessness that often overwhelms both those living with Alzheimer's and their caregivers. None of us knows what's happening, but whatever it is, we're not in control. And we don't know what to do about any of it.

During our time together in Maine, Mom and I were unconsciously planting the seeds for a new bond that would grow between us. Reading a letter that Mom wrote after returning to Iowa, it seemed as if my lifelong desire, to be noticed and appreciated by her, was being fulfilled: "I'm more lonesome for you since visiting you," she wrote, "because you were especially nice to me. I never realized how caring you were." It was as if my mother were seeing me for the first time. I knew this was somehow a profound experience; but I didn't understand the significance, or why it felt so profound, until years later when I heard Jacqui Lewis speak at a spiritual care conference. She introduced me to the concept of ubuntu which comes from the Zulu phrase, *Umuntu ngumuntu ngabant.*[6] According to theologian and Anglican Bishop Desmond Tutu, "Ubuntu speaks particularly about the fact that you can't exist as a human being in isolation. It speaks about our inter-connectedness. You can't be human all by yourself."[7] What

Lewis said next brought me back to that moment reading Mom's letter and feeling recognized. When members of the Zulu Nation of South Africa meet each other, they offer, as a greeting, the word, *Sawubona*. It means *I see you*. The person greeted could respond with *Sikhona*, which means, *I am here; I exist.*[8] Another response is *Yebo Sawubona*, which means *I see you seeing me.*[9] This tells us that being recognized by another brings us more fully into existence, more fully into relationship, more fully into understanding that we are not human alone.[10] Feeling seen in an ubuntu moment with her own mother as she was nearing death, Lewis said she felt blessed and her heart sang out, "*Yebo sawubona*, Mommy,"[11] Just like it was with my Mom! She saw me; I noticed; and like Lewis, I felt the blessings that arise from the deeply human experience of being recognized as our authentic selves.

Over the next several months, Mom and I talked on the phone and wrote to each other regularly. I began noticing that my efforts to connect with her, which had previously been mostly obligatory and dreaded, were now expressed with enthusiasm and tenderness. Being seen by Mom seemingly marked a turning point in our relationship. Who I was with her, who she was with me and to me became a reflection of ubuntu. We were experiencing what Jacqui Lewis calls a "love revolution." We were rising up "out of the ashes" of our previous relational reality because we were seeing each other at last.[12]

This relational shift paired with the damage to Mom's rational thinking somehow freed her to engage and communicate with me differently. Our phone interactions were uncomplicated yet sweetly sincere. We talked about day-to-day activities. She was playing cribbage, walking the dog, feeding the birds, and planting flowers. I was learning to cook, walking alone by the ocean, and studying spiritual direction. A most significant change was that Mom listened to what I was saying; she really listened—without changing the subject in the middle of my sentences as she had throughout my life.

As we talked and wrote about plans to get together again, Mom even offered creative solutions for meeting my complex health needs regarding travelling instead of criticizing me as she had in the past. This highlighted how much she wanted to be with me. Every precious interaction encouraged me, opened my heart further, and nourished our relationship.

Mom's letters, written on the teeniest stationery I'd ever seen (smaller than an index card), were simple and sweet. Using few words, she encouraged my endeavors and communicated honestly about her feelings. She was thrilled that I was studying spiritual direction. She probably didn't know what this was exactly, but she knew it was about getting closer to God. "I'm all for that!" she wrote repeatedly. She asked me to teach her how to concentrate when she prayed and how to deepen her relationship with God. She even expressed interest in my writing and asked me to send my articles to her. She had never done this before. She apologized for making mistakes in her handwriting and sometimes wrote the same letter twice, copying it over to correct the mistakes and then sending both copies. Her awareness of her failing abilities and her efforts to send a nicely written letter touched me deeply. It seemed that Mom was building a home in my soul.

In Mom's letters, she repeatedly thanked me for gifts I had sent, and I felt so grateful for her desire to appreciate me. She offered to send money to me for rent, probably recalling my financial troubles after my engagement had ended three years earlier. Although I didn't need the money at this time, her thoughtful effort to take care of me woke me up, and I began recognizing many more of Mom's thoughtful efforts. The ubuntu moments between us were multiplying and seemingly weaving us together in a blanket of shared warmth and caring.

Having grown up on a farm, Mom loved plants and was a gifted gardener. She searched her seed books and found a special flower called Jade Eyes. She ordered the bulbs from a catalog, and when they arrived, she sent me the two biggest ones—presumably the heartiest, she said—to plant in my landlord's yard. She also planted two bulbs in her yard, so we would have "twins." The gorgeous blooms, puffs of tiny white flowers with very tiny jade green centers, came up in the spring in our yards in Maine and Iowa. Reaching across the miles that separated us, these blooms symbolized our deepening sense of connection.

Then Mom had a car accident and lost her driver's license. She was studying so hard, and taking and retaking the driver's test to get her license back. She wrote about this in every letter. The final failure—the doctor's statement that she was not competent to drive—was so painful for her. The compassion I felt for Mom's lost sense of freedom moved me to tears. It was the thorny threshold of her transformation from independence to dependence. She was beginning to understand that dependent people must often wait for their needs to be met, if they are met at all. She cried because she couldn't go to the grocery store when she wanted to. I cried too, wishing I were there to take her.

As Mom's letters arrived less frequently, our phone conversations awakened concerns within me for her welfare. For example, learning that she was taking Alzheimer's medication and still drinking heavily caused some worry. But I didn't realize exactly how dangerous this was because I had consistently and successfully avoided learning anything specific about Alzheimer's. Later, when I accompanied Mom to doctors' appointments, I became enlightened about the potential hazards of alcohol use by people with Alzheimer's and other forms of dementia.

Almost exactly a year after Mom's visit to Maine, I was startled awake in the night by a frightening dream about her failing health. I was sure something serious had happened to her. When I called in the morning, my sibling, who was living with Mom, answered the phone and told me a story that resurrected my panicked memories of that day in 1973 when Aunt Milly had wandered away from the family picnic. My sibling had taken Mom on a camping trip to Minnesota. Mom had gone to use the restroom and, not wanting to be there, she departed from the campground with intention. She wasn't wandering aimlessly, as one might expect. State troopers found her walking on an interstate highway and she told them she was going "home to Dubuque." The next stop had been the hospital emergency room, where Mom was given antipsychotic drugs to calm her out-of-control emotions. The hospital report documents the anger and despair of a frightened, confused, and extremely vulnerable person.

Learning from this experience, my sibling realized that taking Mom on camping trips wasn't such a good idea. Since there was a similar trip planned later in the summer, I was asked to stay with Mom for those two weeks. Eager to spend time with her, I enthusiastically said, "Yes, of course I'll come!"

Then my sibling said that Mom had become uncooperative, describing her as angry and her behavior as volatile and combative. According to my sibling, Mom had no appetite and refused her medication as well as her meals. My sibling coached me to be stern if I wanted Mom to obey, suggesting that I raise my voice, threaten to take her to the mental hospital, or give her the antipsychotic medication prescribed by her doctor. Alarmingly, my sibling added that after Mom took the meds to calm down, she was kind of out of it for a few weeks. My enthusiasm drained away, and I was terrified. What had I said yes to?

In my heart, I knew there had to be a way to care for my vulnerable mother that didn't involve yelling, threatening, or giving medication that wasn't even recommended for use by people with dementia. There *had* to be a better way, and my desire to find it catapulted me out of avoidance.

Intellectually and emotionally unprepared, and terrified by the mystery before me, I was nonetheless about to take my first steps on the journey through Alzheimer's.

2 Accepting and Improvising

To prepare myself for my upcoming trip into the unknown waiting for me in Iowa, I undertook a thorough search of the Alzheimer's Association website. I was specifically looking for information about how to interact with and care for Mom in ways that were gentler, more compassionate, and more effective than what my sibling was suggesting. I didn't find anything particularly helpful—it was 2004 and there wasn't much to find about compassionate caregiving—but I did encounter the terrifying details and statistics I had been carefully avoiding. The importance of my quest, however, motivated me to soldier on through my rising terror.

One night, as I talked on the phone to a colleague, my distress and confusion about Alzheimer's disease and being with Mom were highly evident. Offering understanding and concrete caring for my heightened emotional state, my colleague recommended a new book, first published about six months earlier: *Learning to Speak Alzheimer's,* by Joanne Koenig Coste.

When we ended our call, I immediately ordered the book online. It arrived just in time for me to toss it into my carry-on bag, and I began reading it on the plane en route to Iowa. I had stepped onto American Airlines flight #409 in Portland, terrified about the mysterious world I was about to enter. But when I stepped off that airplane three hours later at O'Hare, my connector airport to Dubuque, I felt informed, inspired, and prepared to try out what seemed to be a much better way.

Shortly after the birth of her fourth child, Joanne Koenig Coste found herself also caring for her husband, who was diagnosed with progressive dementia in his mid-forties. With so little information available at the time, Coste had learned how to be an Alzheimer's caregiver through trial and error. And she learned well! By sharing what she had discovered through her own experiences, Coste became a renowned and innovative teacher known for implementing positive methods of caring for people living with Alzheimer's. And she had now become my first guide on this journey.

One reason that I recognized and resonated with Coste's wisdom was something that happened after my engagement ended a few years earlier. I was so sad all the time, and a friend wondered if having some fun might be helpful for my healing. She suggested that I take a class in improvisational theater. Why I ever followed up on this idea is still a mystery to me because I was not the improvisation type! I much preferred to plan and then have things unfold according to the plan; I preferred logic and order and knowing what to expect. But I took the class anyway, and as my friend predicted, it was so much fun. Once I overcame my fear of not knowing what in the world was going on, I fell in love with the craft of improvisation, which I then studied and practiced for several years in Maine and in Boston.

Almost instantly, I noticed that improvisation, when practiced not as comedy but as an intentional method for increasing self-awareness and being present in the moment, possessed tremendous potential for healing and transformation.

It was through this lens of improvisation that I read a section from *Learning to Speak Alzheimer's* that changed my life—and Mom's:

> The staff was busily opening draperies, letting the first beams of morning light into the rooms inhabited by the forty-five residents on floor two of the nursing center.
>
> "I want to see my mother," Mary said softly to no one in particular as she shuffled from her room, holding on to the wall.
>
> Claire, a young nurse's aide who happened to pass by at that moment, took Mary's hand. Then she said, sympathetically, "Mary, your mother has been dead a long time."
>
> "Don't be so fresh," Mary said, pulling her hand away, "You don't know what you're talking about."
>
> "Try to remember, Mary. You haven't seen your mother in years. She died when you were in your forties. You're eighty-seven now."
>
> Mary shoved Claire out of her path. "My mother was right here this morning. We had breakfast together like always. Now get out of my way."
>
> Gently, Claire took Mary's arm and began to guide her to the large-print calendar hanging in the nurses' station.
>
> "No. I'm not going with you."
>
> Claire tightened her grip. "I want to show you the date. Your mother died a long time ago."
>
> Mary sputtered, "You—you—you—*hussy.*" Then, swinging her free arm, Mary caught the aide with a backhand slap to the face. Claire called for help.
>
> Her colleagues responded and quickly subdued Mary, injecting her with an antipsychotic medication. For the rest of the morning, the staff kept Mary restrained to a

chair in front of the nurses' station, where they could see her.[13]

Reading this scenario caused my breathing to freeze in a moment of fear, wondering if this was the kind of volatile behavior my sibling was experiencing with Mom. I started to breathe again as Coste analyzed the reasons for the conflict. The aide's response, she explained, was a form of "reality orientation," which attempts to bring a seemingly confused person back to the current time and place. Although still taught in nursing schools and recommended as an intervention for elders who are forgetful from time to time, Paul Raia, dementia specialist and Vice President with the Alzheimer's Association in Massachusetts, does not recommend reality orientation for people of any age with any kind of dementia. The cognitive decline that accompanies Alzheimer's increasingly limits the ability of people with this disease to process information that contradicts their own mental understanding. Ignoring and/or dismissing their experiences and their emotions could lead to catastrophic behavior.[14] Thirty-five years later, Raia's approach remains state-of-the-art thinking that, unfortunately, a lot of people, including physicians, have a hard time accepting.

Coste and Raia, colleagues in this work, taught and recommended an alternative approach, which they called "habilitation therapy."[15] "The aim of habilitation therapy is not to restore people with a dementia such as Alzheimer's disease to what they once were," Raia writes, "but to maximize their functional independence and morale." This approach is "defined as a proactive environmental therapy characterized by creating and maintaining positive emotions." Raia identifies the goal of habilitation therapy as to "bring about a positive emotion and maintain that emotional state throughout the day." He also describes communication as the most critical area for eliciting positive emotions.[16]

Continuing my reading in *Learning to Speak Alzheimer's*, I was intrigued to learn how the earlier scene might have unfolded with a staff member trained in the habilitation model of communicating.

> When Mary expressed her wish to see her mother, the nursing aide said simply, "Tell me about her."
> "She's a great cook," Mary said.
> "What does she make that you especially like?"
> "Oh, her pies are the best. I can never match 'em. Oh, dear, now I'm getting hungry."
> Claire took Mary's hand and guided her toward the dining room. "Me, too," she said. "You have a cup of coffee while I go get your friend Pat—we'll be right back."
> Dignity intact, free from medical or chemical restraint, Mary sat back with her coffee and awaited her friend's arrival. Thoughts of her mother faded, replaced by the positive experience of Claire's smiling face and extended hand.[17]

Somewhere over Michigan while reading this revised scene, it was as if a lightbulb appeared over my head. "Oh my God!" I heard myself exclaim out loud, "This woman is doing improv!" This was a moment of exceptional awareness, and I was thrilled to discover a way for communicating and connecting with Mom that was already familiar to me: meeting her in her improvised reality. I could do that!

I wondered if the author realized that she had described a beautifully crafted improv scene. Probably not, I concluded. It's more likely that Coste is a natural yes-sayer to the twists and turns of life. Acknowledging and accepting the uncontrollable changes perpetuated by her husband's dementia, she recognized that she had to "deal with the reality of today." "I vowed," she writes, "to learn to live with this person who was inhabiting the body of the man I cherished. I had to detach myself emotionally from the man my husband used to be and live now with the man he had become."[18]

Coste recommends that caregivers meet people with Alzheimer's in their current place or time, in their world—wherever, whenever, whatever that might be—and find joy with them there. She encourages caregivers to be ready for anything to happen, therefore being alert and more able to respond appropriately to emotions that are being expressed beneath failing words. Describing her own attitudes toward her husband and her interactions with him, she models for caregivers how to be *willing*. Coste didn't instigate conflict, but she welcomed every conflict as an opportunity to ease her husband's suffering and to return from discord to peace.

Through my own clumsy efforts at improvising, I had learned that being ready for anything to happen and being willing to accept anything is easier said than done, especially if a person is naturally inclined to be a no-sayer, as I was at the time. From improvisation teacher Keith Johnstone, I learned more about this attitude and felt encouraged: "There are far more 'No' sayers around than 'Yes' sayers," according to Johnstone. And for good reason, in my opinion. "Those who say 'No' are rewarded by the safety they attain [whereas] those who say 'Yes' are rewarded by the adventures they have."[19]

As an Alzheimer's family caregiver, oh how I wanted to follow a safe path. But I learned from Coste that for people with the disease as well as for engaged caregivers, Alzheimer's is all about adventure. It's all about yes. Fortunately, Johnstone encouraged me by saying no-sayers can be trained to behave like yes-sayers.

According to Richard Rohr, all of life is a yes-saying training camp. He claims that the first half of life, "when we are naturally and rightly preoccupied with establishing our identity—climbing, achieving, and performing—defines itself by 'No.'" We are staying safe. The second half of life takes us on a "further journey," he writes, "one that involves challenges, mistakes, loss of control, broader horizons and necessary suffering that actually shocks us out of our comfort zone."[20] This further journey is defined by "Yes!"

Johnstone's version of saying yes from the perspective of improvisation sounds enticing: "adventure." Rohr's version of saying yes, from the perspective of the spiritual journey, sounds challenging: "shocked out of our comfort zone." From the perspective of a recovering no-sayer, I learned that engagement with both versions requires intention, practice, and the courage to unconditionally choose to say "Yes!" In addition, I learned that saying yes to the challenges, mistakes, loss of control, broader horizons, and necessary suffering that constitute the adventure of Alzheimer's disease also requires compassion, love, and an openness to being transformed.

My efforts to heal from my failed relationship had led me to the broader horizons of improvisation and helped me to see my life pattern of resistance. Prior to this time, when I didn't like or want what was happening, I used will, skill, and effort trying to make situations fit my preferences. This endeavor was exhausting and usually futile. When this willful approach is implemented in an improvised scene, it's called "blocking the offer." This is in the realm of no-saying. Scared improvisers are seeking safety, and this inevitably leads to a very bad scene. My own fear and resistance became crystal clear during a class scene when my partner said, "I've dropped my contact lens on the floor." I blocked this offer and negated her reality when I said, "Oh no. It's probably still in your eye. Let me look." In the real world, if I had moved closer to have a look, I might have stepped on her contact, resulting in all kinds of conflict. My no-saying impulse was so strong that, even in a class during a theater game, I couldn't accept the offer my partner had extended, that she dropped her contact lens. I could have made the obvious response and said, "Yikes? Contact on the floor! I'm afraid to move." Then my partner would have felt validated, and an interesting scene might have evolved. What happened instead was the predictable conflict. "No," she said firmly as she pushed me away. "I dropped it." This was *her* reality.

Improvisation, I learned, is not about being clever or original. It's about being obvious. It's about accepting the offer that has been extended by your scene partner, considering it valid, and then saying or doing the next logical thing. To do improv well, we need to be willing to say yes—to accept what's happening and what's being said as true and valid—even when our scene partner offers a new or surprising direction. As improv coach Katie Goodman explains, our willing yes is "not from a complacent or docile position but from a bouncy 'bring it on' space."[21] From this bouncy place, there is endless freedom and possibility.

The opportunity for me to practice saying a bouncy yes in the context of Alzheimer's arose during my first day alone with Mom. Fortunately, awareness about what was happening dawned on me, and thankfully, inspiration came from somewhere. Drawing from the improv techniques I was studying, I facilitated a turning point that took me onto the road of adventure and discovery.

Mom and I were sitting at the dining room table playing cribbage, a game we had enjoyed playing together for more than forty years. In fact, the story went around our neighborhood that I had learned to count 15-2, 15-4, 15-6 before I learned to count 1-2-3. The game was going along quite well. Mom was playing in a way that didn't reveal her diminishing cognitive abilities. She was winning as usual, but she must have thought I was getting too close for comfort. In the middle of a hand, she stopped playing and said, "You're very good at this game."

"Well, thank you," I replied.

"Who taught you how to play?" Mom asked.

This question caught me completely by surprise because Mom had taught me to play. So I decided to remind her.

"You did," I told her.

"No, I didn't."

Doesn't she remember? I thought. "Yes, you did," I said.

"No, I didn't."

How could she not remember? "Yes, you did," I said emphatically, thinking that my mighty resistance would somehow help her to remember and admit her error.

"NO, I DIDN'T!" Mom resisted my resistance with even greater emphasis, becoming visibly agitated.

We continued like this for several seconds: "Yes, you did." "No, I didn't." As Mom became more and more agitated, I felt more and more anxious. Finally, in an attempt to distract her from our differing recollections, I tried a technique I had heard about, redirecting.

"It's your play," I said, trying to refocus her attention on the game.

It worked! She was redirected, and the game continued. I was relieved, but only briefly. A few minutes later, seeming to remember the earlier conversation, Mom said, "No, really, who taught you how to play?"

I also remembered our agitated discussion and didn't want to repeat it. Calling upon my improv training, I spoke the truth, but a little differently.

"No, really, who taught you how to play?" Mom asked again.

"My mother did," I replied.

"Oh," Mom said with surprise in her voice. "I didn't know Aunt Stella knew how to play cribbage."

Aunt Stella! My mother? What?

A few heartbeats later, I realized that something in Mom's diminishing brain was telling her that I was her cousin, Eileen. I was sitting just two feet away from her, and she didn't recognize me, her daughter. What was going on? I was shocked but decided to follow Coste's suggestion. I put myself into Mom's world at this moment—wherever that was, I had no idea. But I said, "Yes, my mother was a very good cribbage player."

"And she was a very good cook too," Mom added with certainty.

I had never met Mom's Aunt Stella, but I remembered the story about cooking from *Learning to Speak Alzheimer's*, so I borrowed the line.

"What did Aunt Stella make that you liked best?"

"Knepfles!" Mom replied, smiling with enthusiasm.

For a while, we talked about Aunt Stella's cooking and how to make knepfles (noodles from Mom's Alsace heritage). Then the game joyfully continued. Mom won, of course!

Family members often feel hurt and frustrated when loved ones with Alzheimer's don't remember our names, or if and how we're related. In these instances, the losses we experience through Alzheimer's are heightened and the pain feels so heavy it can become almost unbearable. Through the lens of improvisation, however, families might come to understand that recognizing and playing the roles we've been cast into—instead of demanding to be recognized as ourselves—may enhance our connections with our loved ones. We can create joyful, healing moments for them and ourselves instead of having to endure hurtful, heartbreaking ones.

In the earlier stages, people with Alzheimer's are aware that they are forgetting important things and people. Correcting them about our names and relationships or reminding them they have forgotten could feel demeaning and humiliating to them. Or as I discovered, correcting them could aggravate them because they will relentlessly perceive us to be wrong. There is a subtle point to consider, however. In the early stages, reminding them who we are might actually be helpful. For example, when coming into the room, it can be a good idea to make eye contact and say, "Hi, Mom, it's Jade, your daughter." This is a reminder, not a correction, and is different from saying, "No, Mom. I'm not Eileen, your cousin. Don't you know me? It's me, Jade, your daughter."[22]

When I was younger, and under completely different circumstances, I would feel slighted and very hurt when Mom called me by my sibling's name. So I was surprised not to feel slighted during the confused and confusing conversation that erupted during the cribbage game. Seemingly, my excitement about knowing what to do overcame any potential upset over not being recognized. In a situation simmering with conflict and hurt feelings, I had figured out something to say that resulted in a touching and happy outcome. A true connection had taken place. Being cast as Eileen didn't cause emotional upset because I instinctively knew, in that healing moment and through the rest of Mom's life with Alzheimer's, that she was doing her best. She looked at me and saw her beloved Eileen. I didn't understand *how* this was possible; but I did understand that it *was* possible.

Throughout our time together, Mom seamlessly moved in and out of current reality without any warning. One minute I was her daughter; the next, I was someone else. For Valentine's Day that year, I had sent Mom an amethyst bracelet handmade for her by an artist friend of mine. My sibling told me that it had broken and they threw it away. Imagine my surprise when, one day, Mom and I were looking for her earrings and I came across the bracelet in her jewelry box. Only the clasp was broken.

"Look, Mom," I said, "here's the bracelet I sent you. The clasp is broken, but all the pieces are here. I'll take it all back to Maine with me, and I'll ask the artist to fix it for you."

I picked up the bracelet, and Mom looked very worried. "You can't take that," she said. "My daughter gave that to me."

Who she thought I was, well, I didn't know. And it wasn't exactly clear when she had shifted out of current reality and lost her ability to recognize me. But still, sweet tears welled up in my eyes because six months after receiving this gift, she remembered that it had come from me.

"OK," I said. "I won't take it with me. But what if we mail it to your daughter and ask her to have it fixed."

"That would be good," Mom replied, her worried expression fading. "It's pretty. I'd like to wear it."

"Let's go to the store and get a padded envelope, and then we can go to the post office and mail it."

Mom said, "OK."

And so, we did that. I mailed the bracelet to myself. The mission was accomplished while Mom's beliefs, wishes, and current reality were honored. And I have the ongoing joy of reliving this healing moment of connection every time I wear her bracelet.

At other times, there were people coming and going in Mom's world who remained mysteries to me. In order to stay grounded during this time in Iowa, one morning I attended an Alanon meeting. Still unaware at the time about the perils of leaving Mom alone, I thought she would be fine. When I came home, she was standing in the middle of the den with a puzzled look on her face.

"Hi, Mom," I said tentatively, gently touching her shoulder. "Is everything all right?"

"There was a man here," she said. "He came to the door and told me that my father said he could spend the night here. I don't know where he should sleep."

"Well," I replied, pausing to accept this as valid and to consider the next logical thing to say. "Let's look at the possibilities." We then walked through the house and discussed various options. When we got to the top of the basement steps, Mom said, "I told him he couldn't sleep down there." (It was my sibling's room.) We evaluated other options and finally decided that our guest could sleep on the sofa bed in the living room. A gracious hostess, Mom collected sheets and blankets and a pillow, which she gently laid on the sofa. I suggested we wait to make up the bed until later. After Mom went to bed that night, I put everything away.

The next afternoon, Mom came to me with a man's white shirt, nicely ironed and on a hanger.

"That man must have left this shirt behind," she said.

I had no idea who owned this shirt, but I said, "I'm sure he'll be back for it. Let's hang it in the closet so it doesn't get wrinkled." This we did, and that was the last I heard about my grandfather's mysterious friend or the shirt.

My expectations of Mom began to shift into the realm of realism according to Alzheimer's, and I began to accept that what's happening is what's happening. Making this important shift planted another seed for the healing of our relationship as well as for developing skills for effective Alzheimer's caregiving.

During those weeks with Mom, I welcomed and enjoyed daily opportunities to meet her in her reality and learn more about her world. I practiced recognizing and playing my role, and when I was successful, Mom's behavior didn't remotely resemble what my sibling had described—thankfully.

Given the expectations my sibling and the Alzheimer's Association website had established for me, Mom continually surprised me. Much to my relief, the nonalcoholic beer I gave her was received as an acceptable substitute for the real thing, and she guzzled it with gusto! She even took all of her pills cooperatively.

Not as advertised, Mom's appetite was ravenous. However, her quirky preference that we eat the same things had survived Alzheimer's, and I worried because our diets were vastly different: meat and potatoes versus vegan. When I tried to make a hamburger for Mom as an alternative to the chickpea burger I was making for myself, she adamantly refused. Although I knew she'd like the hamburger better, I followed her lead, and we both ate chickpea burgers that night. Throughout my visit, Mom adapted to my vegetarian diet, pronouncing everything I made for her "delicious." As long as we had the exact same food on our plates, she was happy.

There were some episodes, though, where I missed my cue, and a meaningful yes was either delayed or altogether absent. These experiences helped me to understand more about the moods, behaviors, and challenges my sibling and other caregivers described.

Mom's doctor had prescribed vitamin B-12 because a deficiency can increase memory disorders. We had gone to the kind of funky, kind of dingy health food store in town to buy ingredients for my recipes, and on the supplement shelf, I saw B-12. I showed Mom and headed to the checkout with the bottle. Her face instantly red and her eyes flaring with anger, Mom snatched the bottle from my hand. Through clenched teeth she said, "I'm not getting this."

The Mom I knew was all about appearances, so I was shocked by her angry reaction in a public place. Not welcoming a confusing scene escalating in the store, I didn't try to convince her that the doctor wanted her to take this. I timidly said, "OK," and put the bottle back on the shelf. We bought our food and left the store.

Although I was rattled by Mom's public anger, I was equally curious about what had happened. As soon as I regained my composure, I was able to shift into improv mode and inquire about Mom's world. "Why didn't you want the B-12? Your doctor thinks it might be helpful for you. He prescribed it."

"Well," Mom said, her posture huffy and her tone arrogant, "I'm not getting it there. I want to get it at Hartig's" (her drugstore).

Ohhhh. It was the funky, dingy store she was resisting! It never would have occurred to me that this was the source of her resistance. We went to Hartig's, bought the B-12, and went home. Mom took it right away.

I was grateful that my curiosity carried me back into Mom's moment where I was able to meet her and to learn more about her reasons for resisting. I assumed that people with Alzheimer's couldn't think or decide—and that we needed to think and decide for them. I learned from Mom that this presumption could make people with Alzheimer's justifiably angry. Without the curiosity that led to a healing moment of connection, I might have reported Mom to her doctor as being angry, uncooperative, and refusing her prescribed medications. The result for her could have been weeks of being out of it from the antipsychotic medication the doctor was prescribing to make her more cooperative. In essence, this medication was taking away Mom's will.

I later learned from the work of Tom Kitwood and Kathleen Bredin that assertive behavior from a person with Alzheimer's, which is usually in the form of dissent, is a sign of well-being and can be observed even into the later stages of the disease process.[23] By meeting Mom in her moment of resistance instead of trying to convince her to buy the vitamins,

I learned something about the status of her mental abilities, her preferences, and her desire to be heard and taken seriously. I also learned something about the importance of being respectful in the context of cognitive decline, and not assuming that I always knew—more clearly than Mom did—what she wanted or was thinking, or what was best for her.

One afternoon, we were preparing dinner together. Mom's attention to detail and her ability to concentrate on a task were astounding, making her the absolute best assistant cook. Initiating what I thought was idle conversation, I asked her if she liked her primary care doctor. (We had an appointment to see him in a few days.)

"No, I don't," she vehemently replied.

"Really? Why not?" I was surprised by her clarity.

"Because he always speaks to the other adult in the room." Again, I was surprised by her clarity.

Mom still knew that she was a person in the room and should be directly spoken to by her doctor about her own health concerns. And she knew what was in her heart and her mind and could still communicate about this—if asked. I had to learn how to draw her out, then how to listen and hear her. After I became Mom's guardian and had the authority to do so, I changed her doctor.

There was another poignant learning time that helped me to understand my sibling's description of Mom as angry, uncooperative, and combative. At this moment of learning, I felt especially helpless, and "Yes" remained unspoken. When Mom and I met with her neurologist, he suggested that she attend an adult day center in order to maintain her verbal skills through practice and to uplift her emotional state through socialization. After arranging for a social worker from the Alzheimer's Association to accompany us to the local centers for tours, I told Mom about the plan. She adamantly refused to go, accusing me of coming to Iowa to "garage" her away in a nursing home. As I rationally refuted this, explaining that the neurologist thought the adult day program would be beneficial, Mom became frustrated and upset because I wasn't hearing her, and she slapped my forearm. This ended the scene instantly. Startled and upset, I started to cry. Mom fled the house by the side door and stomped furiously through her backyard. As if restrained by an invisible fence, she stopped right at the edge of her yard and looked out over the expanse of neighboring backyards. She stood there for a long time, seeming bewildered and frightened. Watching her from inside the house, ensuring that she was safe, my heart recognized her diminishing independence and just knew how much she hated that. Without effort or conscious thought, my tears of surprise and hurt transformed to tears of compassion.

Although I didn't know what to do next, I didn't want to leave Mom alone. As soon as I felt calm enough, I took some birdseed outside and stood next to her. I took her hand and said, "Here's your birdseed, Mom. Let's feed your birds." This was Mom's favorite activity. She took the seed from me and fed her birds. The adult day center was not mentioned again.

My study of Alzheimer's on the plane had informed me that Mom's behavior did not include an intention to be uncooperative or willful. She was trying to preserve her dignity and to communicate her needs and desires, using her remaining, although limited, cognitive abilities. She was marching to her own tune. With the help of improvisation, I was able to get into step with her, and with only a few glitches, our time together went very well. We became close and compatible companions.

In her own way, Mom was able to tell me that my efforts to learn about Alzheimer's, my attempts to communicate creatively, my compassionate attention, and my curiosity had made an impression on her. The day before I was leaving to return to Maine, Mom looked up at me from her chair in the living room and said, "Will you stay and take care of me? You're so kind to me."

To my recollection, my fiercely independent, highly competent mother had never before asked me—or anyone—for help. So unexpected and stunning was this moment that it remains etched in my memory even now, twenty years later. The experience of hearing this request from Mom and seeing the sincere pleading in her eyes opened my heart. Although I quietly explained to her that I would do my best to return and be her "guardian angel," my heart shouted out, "Yes!"

3 Waiting and Preparing

My own dawning awareness of Mom's obvious decline awakened the mother lion within me. My natural instincts toward Mom became sweetly tender and fiercely protective. During her early years with the disease, I was powerless to care for her in any meaningful way because my sibling had complete control. As is often the case for out-of-town family members, my input was not welcome, and although it was difficult for me, I had to accept this. After Mom noticed my kindness, however, and asked me to stay and take care of her, I made a herculean attempt to become her legal guardian. Unfortunately, the Iowa courts at the time were not favorable toward out-of-state relatives seeking guardianship. Although I was willing to move to Iowa if granted guardianship, I had little hope of success because my sibling was already living with Mom.

Having to accept the fact that family and legal circumstances beyond my control would allow me to care about Mom only from a distance was pure anguish for me. One day, in the midst of my despair, the closing lines from Mary Oliver's poem "The Journey" drifted into my consciousness. I was reminded that the only life I could save was my own. As I wept, I felt held and consoled by this poem. Although I felt truly overwhelmed by my helplessness, I knew that Oliver's words were true. I couldn't "save" Mom. Not now anyway. Amidst an ocean of tears, my herculean effort was temporarily put on hold.

Soon after returning to Maine following my heart-opening time with Mom, I tried to manage my feelings of helplessness by seeking out additional legal opinions. One Iowa lawyer who was particularly insightful and understanding reviewed the case, counseled me in important ways, and then offered the frustrating advice to "sit tight until something significant happens." This advice was hard to hear and harder to abide by, partly because I was standing at a crossroads in my own life, ready to leave Maine. It would have been perfect timing for me to move to Iowa.

I learned through this experience, however, that sometimes it's important to just wait. What some could interpret as caregivers doing nothing might actually be a manifestation of wisdom, spiritual maturity, and what spiritual directors often refer to as "careful, benign neglect." In the world of Alzheimer's, sometimes the most prudent action is to pause patiently, in awareness and readiness, as life and circumstances unfold. When caregivers are caught in these complex situations of family and illness, our embrace of this process and our appropriate response at the appropriate time will make all the difference in the lives of our loved ones.

Saving the only life I could save—my own—was all I could do at that moment. I didn't know it then, but accepting my limitations and focusing on my own health and well-being would benefit both Mom and me in the future. Much later, I realized that maintaining good self-care for myself throughout Mom's journey through Alzheimer's gave me a strong foundation for building a better quality of life for her. At the time, however, I felt that I had failed Mom. Not being able to immediately fulfill her request—to stay with her and to care for her with kindness—remains one of my life's greatest regrets.

Since caring for and about Mom from a distance was my only option, I decided to join her on this journey by learning more about Alzheimer's and the family dynamics associated with Alzheimer's care. With this goal in mind, I contacted Dr. William Berlinger, a psychiatrist who had been the medical director of a nursing home system in Massachusetts for many years and had evaluated thousands of people with Alzheimer's and related disorders. When I told him about discovering the improvisation-Alzheimer's connection, he was overjoyed. To my surprise, he said that years earlier he had tried to hire improvisers from ImprovBoston and Improv Asylum[24] to come to his nursing homes. He wanted them to teach his staff how to communicate effectively with people with dementia using the "Yes, and . . ." improv techniques. Unfortunately, his board of directors, administrators, and nurses resisted this approach, declaring the idea as nonsense.

Indeed, there had been, and likely still is, controversy in the field about this. Often, creative ways of communicating with people with memory loss, particularly those that veer away from reality orientation, are considered by some to be undignified. There is especially prickly resistance, bordering on outrage, if creative communication involves any kind of fantasy interaction that could be interpreted as lying.

Cardiologist Sandeep Jauhar, in an article written in 2023, reports that, during the years of caring for his father who had Alzheimer's, he fought against the practice of "lying" to his father—and his siblings who supported it—as a matter of principle. He said that as a physician, he "had seen how even well-meaning deception, such as withholding bad news, could be damaging." He believed that having a healthy relationship with their father, must be "based only on truth and trust." "Small lies," he claimed, "even if told with the best of intentions, would undermine [Dad's] dignity and erode what little connection we had left with him."[25]

This attitude is likely born from the Ten Commandments of the Judeo-Christian Tradition. We learn as children from the ninth commandment that we "shall not bear false witness against our neighbors,"[26] and that if we do, it's a sin. We learn that lies cause harm and can result in negative consequences for others as well as for ourselves. But as we mature, we are invited to consider the nuances of life and if there are circumstances in which telling a lie is a way to prevent harm. For example, when Nazi soldiers knocked on the doors of Aryan German citizens who harbored Jewish neighbors in their attics, when these soldiers searched their homes, when they demanded to know if any Jews were hiding there, and the homeowners lied and answered "No," their lie was life-giving; it was brave, and morally the right thing to do. So perhaps lying is not prohibited in all circumstances.

The Hindu Vedic tradition also offers a list of ten moral/ethical "observances and restraints." This list includes truthfulness; however, the most important restraint on the list is *Ahimsa*, "non-harming or non-violence in thought, word, and deed." We've learned, from our own and others' attempts at using reality orientation around people with Alzheimer's, that truth-telling can cause harm, and so, in this world of Alzheimer's, causing no harm trumps truth-telling every time. As Rukmini Chaitanya explained in a lecture on the Patanjali Sutras, "It is far better to stay silent than to say a truth that comes from the wrong motivation [in the Alzheimer's context, believing that I/my position and opinion is the only valid one], or will cause pain."[27]

To counter concerns around lying among Alzheimer's families and caregivers, and to relieve intuitive, yes-saying caregivers of any guilt they might harbor about lying, Paul Raia explains, "These are not lies, these are what I call 'therapeutic fiblettes'—inroads into the patient's reality. It is only if we become comfortable and creative in the use of the fiblettes that we become effective [caregivers]."[28]

We enter into fantasy play with children all the time without calling it deception or creating a moral dilemma; so why can't we have the same freedom when communicating with people with dementia? It's not about lying, actually; it's about connection, respect, quality of life, cooperation, staying calm, doing no harm, and dignity. It's also about reviving our imaginations if, in our adult lives, we haven't used much imagination and that internal process is rusty. One caregiver, Sondy, told me that one of the things she discovered about herself while caring for her wife, Liz, who had dementia, was how much she liked to play, to use her imagination to make things up that would enhance the connection with Liz and keep her calm and happy. "It doesn't always have to be brutal honesty," Sondy said. Most importantly, it's about doing our best so people with Alzheimer's feel they have been heard and that they and their concerns are being taken seriously.

The world of improv teaches us to say the next logical thing when our scene partner makes an offer, which the craft requires us to accept as valid. The next logical thing to say when people with Alzheimer's speak from their reality may not seem true or rational in our world, but it will seem just right in theirs. And the reality of their world is where we will and must meet them, even if it feels uncomfortable for us because we are experiencing a different reality, or because we want to control the interaction or situation. "Honesty," remarked American religious leader James Faust, "is more than not lying. It is truth telling, truth speaking, truth living, and truth loving."[29] Fiblettes are truth living and loving in the world of Alzheimer's.

In Jauhar's article, he notes that the approach Paul Raia and Joanne Koenig Coste introduced to me and the U.S. Alzheimer's world originated in England in the 1990s: "A homemaker named Penny Garner, whose mother, Dorothy, had dementia, began to advocate a new approach, one that differed from the traditional reality orientation. Ms. Garner noticed that allowing Dorothy to have her perspective, no matter how absurd, kept her calm and happy." Allowing Dorothy to have her perspective does seem like respect, but labeling her perspective as "absurd" does not. It implies that the caregivers' reality is the only sensible reality. Jauhar writes that Ms. Garner was the "genesis of an approach often known as therapeutic deception."[30] I'd not heard the phrase *therapeutic deception* before reading this article, and it caused me to recoil. It sounds so serious and manipulative. I feel much more resonance with Raia's bouncy, yes-saying "fiblette." But whatever we call this practice—therapeutic deception, therapeutic fiblettes, or my preference, "therapeutic improv," which acknowledges that the practice is relational, the most important word to remember is *therapeutic*.

However, as shown by Coste's story of Mary wanting to see her mother and my cribbage-playing interaction with Mom, the creative, logical thing to say to a person with Alzheimer's when their perspective seems not true to us need not always be a fiblette. But if you need fiblettes to relieve anger or anxiety or sadness, and to return a person with Alzheimer's to a state of calmness, do not hesitate to use them! Even Jauhar, through his experiences with his father and his research for a book, concluded that deception "may uphold a different conception of the patient's dignity—respecting the integrity of his worldview, however askew it may be."[31] From my perspective, I would revise Jauhar's last phrase this way: *respecting the integrity of their worldview by considering it valid.*

The forerunner for the creative deception/fiblette/improv intervention was Validation, a form of therapy developed by social worker Naomi Feil between 1963 and 1980. Feil's first book, published in 1982, is described as a book "for all those who care 'for' and 'about' disoriented old-old people."[32] One of the issues Feil noticed was that "very old people often struggle to resolve unfinished life issues before death,"[33] and Validation was originally offered as a therapeutic counseling approach for elders. Although not specific to communicating and connecting with people with Alzheimer's or dementia, the detailed and complex Validation method has relevance for this population and was revised over the years to meet their needs. It has shown scores of caregivers how to "accept people where *they* are"; how to "help helpers become comfortable with disoriented old-old [and people with cognitive decline] who freely express feelings"; and how to "tell the reason behind the feelings."[34]

Feil's Validation therapy is more than a communication technique; it is a healing technique. At its foundation, Validation requires empathy. From this place of empathy, we can invite the old-old, and people of any age living with Alzheimer's or dementia, to share the truth of their lives, truth that perhaps has been repressed for a lifetime, causing a festering and painful wound.

In her caregiving memoir *Being My Mom's Mom*, Loretta Veney shares a story of such a truth that surfaced during her mom's life with Alzheimer's. It started as a typical scenario that happens often in the lives of people with cognitive decline. Loretta's mother, Doris, who lived in a large retirement community, had been to the laundry room. She put her clothes in the washer and then shifted them to the dryer, being sure to check the time so she knew when to come back and get them. She was an hour late returning to the laundry room, and her clothes were gone. Doris reported this to the front desk receptionist, who reassured her that whatever happened was unintentional and that a sign would be posted. Doris, quite upset and convinced that her clothes would not be returned, shared the details of this incident with Loretta. She was sure this was deliberate, that her belongings were thrown away, and that the person who took her clothes did so because she was Black. Loretta was stunned by this assertation. Although there were only a few Black people living in this retirement community of more than a hundred units, she had never before heard any reports—from her mother or anyone else—about racist comments or behavior. What probably happened was that this incident of missing laundry caused Doris' lifelong wound of being persecuted because of her race to surface and her accusation came from that wounded place.

Loretta, a security professional, launched an investigation into the missing laundry. She talked with staff at the retirement community and asked Doris to describe the missing items. Item by item, Loretta was able to help Doris find her clothes, all neatly folded in her own closet. Of course, Doris had forgotten that she had gone to the laundry room and retrieved and folded and put away her clothes. But she had not forgotten the pain of racial prejudice that had impacted her life.[35] In situations like this, even with those who have cognitive decline, Validation therapy has the potential to draw people out, invite them to talk about and share some of their pain with us, and to feel validated and embraced by us. There is great potential for heart and soul-healing in Validation therapy, and using therapeutic improv techniques is one of the best ways to open the door to the process of Validation in this context

Dr. Berlingeri became a valued guide for me as I explored ways to unravel the mysteries Alzheimer's had brought into my life as I endeavored to effectively communicate with Mom and struggled to understand why and how Alzheimer's was stirring up dormant family dynamics. Through our many discussions, he shared his experience and wisdom and helped me begin to formulate an embodied knowing of how to be a compassionate and effective Alzheimer's caregiver. He introduced me to two necessary concepts for caregivers to grasp and integrate into our way of being with people with Alzheimer's: *phenomenology* and *consensus reality.*

Many people would like medical science to provide absolute guidelines about how to interact and communicate with people with Alzheimer's, but I have come to understand that science doesn't always consider the unique ways human beings experience life, especially when the brain is altered by disease and thought processes and behaviors become unpredictable. Therefore, the *phenomenology* of Alzheimer's— those qualities and practices that can be observed through our senses and intuition in the presence of those afflicted—is the most informative and reliable guide for creating satisfying interpersonal experiences and good quality of life when caring for this population. Because of the decline of cognition and capacity in people with Alzheimer's and their ever-changing, ever-increasing needs, caregivers' observation skills are crucial to the well-being of this population. Having a loved one receive an Alzheimer's diagnosis could be the perfect time for caregivers to take up the practice of mindfulness meditation to enhance their ability to observe. The ten minutes a day this takes could save much time in enlisting cooperation and spare much heartache for everyone.

It is necessary to accept that, as the disease process relentlessly marches on, people with Alzheimer's will not be the most reliable reporters of what's happening for them. Declining verbal abilities will make it difficult for them to report side effects of medications, to be specific about pain, or to clearly express their wants and needs. People with Alzheimer's won't remember if they've eaten meals or taken medication—or folded and put away the laundry. Facial expressions, body language, emotional expression, and sounds are often the caregivers' only signs, especially in the later stages, and being attentive to our loved ones with dementia in new and different ways becomes a critical protocol. Caregiving, therefore, requires vigilance in observing, recognizing, and responding to what needs to be done.

After noticing what our loved ones need, the challenge becomes helping them without negating their remaining autonomy by imposing unnecessary, demeaning assistance. Observation is important at this point as well. Something caregivers will notice is that structure, including a regular schedule, is a beneficial tool for gaining cooperation from people with Alzheimer's because bodies instinctively and readily adapt to routines. Adopting a specific, consistent time for medication, a nap, a walk, an activity, or meals could avert stress and conflict because it will feel right to the person with Alzheimer's when a caregiver says, "It's time to . . . ." This approach is likely not to be received as the imposition of another's will onto them.

It's also important to know that our loved ones with Alzheimer's can only initiate activities to the level of their current capacity, and we shouldn't assume that they can't or don't want to do something because they don't start it or express an interest in it. We may need to draw them out. During a music experience with people with dementia at our local Memory Café, all who were there witnessed the complexity of memory in action, how it remains in people with Alzheimer's, and how it can surprise us. That remaining memory, however, is not necessarily in the cognitive part of the brain. Jim, a resident from the local memory care unit who attended the Memory Café that day, demonstrated body memory for us.

He had lived at the memory care unit for several months and was described as quiet and prone to staying in his room, not talking or engaging with other residents or staff. When the music started, I went around the circle and one by one took each person's hands, made eye contact, and said, "Welcome." From my body language, I guess, Jim thought I was asking him to dance. He stood up, paused for a heartbeat, smiled, and then swept me into a dance hold. "OK!" I thought, "We're dancing." And around the circle we danced. He definitely still had the moves! Jim came to every Memory Café after this, and we danced each time. This inspired other couples to dance at the Café, and I was told that Jim danced through every day at the care center—because they now knew how to engage him. He couldn't tell them he loved to dance, but this music activity coupled with an accidental invitation from me opened the door to pure joy for Jim—and wisdom for all.

Overall, we caregivers need to overcome our resistance to accepting the illness, change the ways we meet the realities of people living with Alzheimer's, and embrace their moments. In order to accomplish all of this, we have to accept that it is impossible to reach *consensus reality*—a general agreement about reality—with people who have lost the ability to gather and analyze new data or to shift their thinking at will. When Dr. Berlingeri first introduced consensus reality, it was a new concept for me, and I wasn't exactly sure how it related to my interactions with Mom or the differences in our perceptions of the present and recollections of the past. As I wondered more about this concept, I vaguely remembered a story about an elephant and six blind men from Indostan that I first heard as a child. I went to the library and found various illustrated versions of the story in the children's section. More research revealed that this ancient parable dates back to about 500 BC and was prevalent in multiple religious traditions of India at the time. Studying this parable helped me to grasp what consensus reality means in relationship to people with Alzheimer's. I share this version of "The Elephant and the Blind Men" from the Jain Tradition, along with the Jain interpretation.

Once upon a time, there lived six blind men in a village. One day the villagers told them, "Hey, there is an elephant in the village today." The blind men had no idea what an elephant was, but they decided, "Even though we would not be able to see it, let us go and feel it anyway." All of them went to where the elephant was, and every one of them touched the elephant.

"Hey, the elephant is like a tree," said the first man, who touched his leg.

"Oh, no! It is like a rope," said the second man, who touched the tail.

"Oh, no! It is like a snake," said the third man, who touched the trunk of the elephant.

"It is like a big hand fan," said the fourth man, who touched the ear of the elephant.

"It is like a huge wall," said the fifth man, who touched the belly of the elephant.

"It is like a spear," said the sixth man, who touched the tusk of the elephant.

They began to argue about the elephant, every one of them insisting that he was right. It looked like they were getting agitated. A wise man was passing by and he saw this.

He stopped and asked them, "What is the matter?"

They said, "We cannot agree to what the elephant is like." Each one of them told what he thought the elephant was like.

The wise man calmly explained to them, "All of you are right. The reason every one of you is telling it differently is because each of you touched a different part of the elephant. Actually, the elephant has all the features you describe."

"Oh!" everyone said.

There was no more fighting. They felt happy that all of them were right.

The moral of the story in the Jain tradition is that there may be some truth in what someone says. Sometimes we can perceive that truth and sometimes not. Others may have a different perspective with which we may not agree, but rather than arguing, we should say, "Maybe you have your reasons." This way we don't get in arguments. This allows us to live in harmony with the people of different thinking.[36]

In the story, each man's position about the elephant is valid because it comes from empirical experience, which is based on observation or experience rather than theory or pure logic, and is really tough to challenge, even in the world of science. It's important to note that blindness is ultimately not the reason for the failure of understanding in this story; rather it's the unwillingness of the men to believe in the experiences of each other. Similarly, Alzheimer's is not the reason for the conflict when the understandings of caregivers and people with Alzheimer's collide. When people with Alzheimer's share their "different thinking" with us, we often fail to grasp their reality. From their perspective, born of cognitive decline, they absolutely cannot grasp our reality. Even though it's not easy to set aside our own truth, that's exactly what we need to do. Trying to convince people with Alzheimer's that we're right or trying to persuade them to do what we want them to do is a sure recipe for conflict—and possibly disaster. Therefore, we need to give them opportunities to show us their realities so we can meet them there. In my life with Mom and Alzheimer's, I discovered that this requires mindful attention, patience, open-mindedness, and a willingness to be surprised.

Other caregivers have discovered this as well. As soon as Leslie's father, Arnold, moved into an assisted-living facility, he created quite a commotion. He refused to get out of bed in the morning and after naps, explaining that there were things on the floor that he didn't want to step on and break. To the staff's eyes or Leslie's, there was nothing on the floor, but Arnold insisted there was. Every morning and at other times during the day, aides struggled to get him out of bed. This generated distress for Arnold and the aides alike.

Observing this situation, most would conclude that Arnold was hallucinating. He has Alzheimer's, after all. But his observant daughter noticed a section of wood paneling on the wall at the end of Arnold's bed that resembled the flooring material. On this wood paneling hung a clock and a thermostat, "things" her father could see while lying in his bed. Leslie enlisted the assistance of a nurse to cover the wood wall paneling with fabric. This simple intervention erased Arnold's concern about the things on the floor. After that, he got out of bed every day without worry or resistance. He wasn't hallucinating after all. Indeed, he had his reasons.

While I was waiting for something significant to happen that would open the door for me to be an active participant in Mom's care, I continued to explore the intersection of Alzheimer's disease and improvisation. Without question, the improv way of being in the world can open doors to spirituality. This discovery manifested into reality for me in the context of Alzheimer's caregiving when I was able to meet Mom in her world—because there, we both experienced healing.

Some of the spiritual elements inherent in the practice of improv that are particularly useful in the Alzheimer's caregiving experience are:

- meeting in true connection
- being present in *this* moment
- expanding awareness of ourselves and others
- increasing observation through the senses
- letting go of the need, and even the desire, to control
- letting go of the need to know what happens next
- accepting what is; saying yes to reality
- finding the gifts in every experience offered in life
- responding in a way that is supportive and promotes self-esteem and dignity
- acknowledging interdependence
- experiencing, embracing, and expressing joy moment by moment

Will Luera, currently the Director of Improvisation at Florida Studio Theatre, was artistic director of ImprovBoston when he came to Maine to teach classes for my improvisation practice group. Impressed by Will's interpersonal sensitivity as a teacher, as well as his talent, I contacted him to explore his interest in helping me develop a workshop for communicating with people with Alzheimer's using improvisation. When I described how the integration of spirituality and improv could provide healing for people with Alzheimer's and their caregivers, Will was intrigued. The potential of such a creative and purposeful application for the craft he loved inspired him. He immediately agreed to help with the workshop and was on the next train to Maine. We ate soup, walked by the ocean, and gave birth to the *Healing Moments for Alzheimer's* programs for Alzheimer's families, friends, and informal and professional caregivers.

Over the winter, the psychiatrist, the improviser, and I (the minister/caregiver) met several times sharing our wisdom about Alzheimer's caregiving and improv from our three different perspectives and areas of expertise. The building blocks from this unique collaboration became the foundation for the unique caregiving techniques that would be life-changing for me, for Mom, and for thousands of others from all around the country who were living with Alzheimer's or other diseases of dementia, and their caregivers.

After completing my spiritual direction training in the summer of 2005, I left Maine and moved back to Boston. I wanted to pursue two programs of study that, to an objective observer, may have seemed completely unrelated: improvisation and a doctorate of ministry in faith, health, and spirituality. To me, these areas of interest had become inseparable.

During my first day of class at ImprovBoston, my teacher said something profound and unforgettable: "The first rule of improvisation is to make your scene partner look good." This rule eventually became my mantra for compassionate, effective Alzheimer's caregiving.

Then the significant something I had been waiting for happened. In September of 2006, my sibling moved Mom to a nursing home. Six months later, my sibling moved away; 1200 miles away. Over the next year, these actions caused me, literally, to emotionally and physically move back and forth across the threshold between Mom's world and my world. And as the Rilke poem invites, I let everything happen to me—the beauty and the terror of this journey—and I just kept going.

II

Into the Heart of Alzheimer's

You do not need to know precisely what is happening, or exactly where it is all going. What you need is to recognize the possibilities and challenges offered by the present moment, and to embrace them with courage, faith, and hope.

—THOMAS MERTON

Relief was my initial reaction when I learned that Mom had moved to a nursing home. I no longer had to worry about her walking into traffic, drinking alcohol and passing out, missing meals, burning herself with hot water, falling and freezing, or cooking and setting herself on fire. She would be "safe." This move also opened the door for me to have more contact with Mom and to be more involved in her life and care.

During my winter break from school, I went to Iowa for several days. Although nursing homes were not among my most desired settings, being reunited with Mom after two and a half years—no matter where—warmed my heart. I was delighted to notice some of Mom's remaining skills, which included recognizing me—I was still her "girl"—and reading her name. Every time we passed by the door to her room, she paused, looked at the name plate on the wall, and read her name aloud. Meeting Mom's social worker, advocate, aides, and nurses helped me to understand her current life and needs. When it was time to return to Boston, it was hard to leave her.

My sibling's move out of town three months later muddied my relief. Mom was alone in a nursing home, "garaged" and abandoned. She was living her worst nightmare. For me, however, it was no longer the perfect time to relocate to Iowa. I was happy being back in Boston after seven years in Maine. My doctor of ministry program, focusing on spirituality and spiritual direction for seminarians, was exactly the study I felt called to pursue. It was my life's work, I was sure. Moving to Dubuque, focusing on Mom's care, would be a detour for me, or so I thought.

At this juncture, the experience of going back and forth across the threshold between Mom's world of Alzheimer's in Iowa and my world of spiritual study in Boston troubled my soul. I *had* to do something, and I considered a variety of options. One possibility included relocating Mom to

Massachusetts. Although I didn't have the legal authority at the time to move her, I investigated and toured nursing homes near my apartment. Another option was to rent small apartments in both Massachusetts and Iowa and be with Mom during school breaks. That summer, I went to Iowa for seven weeks to further explore the possibility of having dual residences.

After being with Mom and much going back and forth emotionally, I moved to Iowa in February 2008. I made the decision with the belief that I would need to discontinue my doctoral studies. However, the professors and school administrators agreed to work with me from a distance, which was a novel teaching method at the time. That first semester, an experimental e-course called "Ministry to the Elderly" was offered. "Ah," I thought, "Since I'm going to be in a nursing home every day, this could be helpful!"

Indeed it was! It also changed the whole course of my doctoral studies, and my life actually. This course opened the door for the practical integration of my academic interests in spirituality and my personal experiences with Alzheimer's. Although I didn't know what would happen or where it would lead, I stayed open to possibilities.

Let's journey together, with courage, faith, and hope, into the unknown . . .

4 Healing When There Is No Cure

One recent afternoon, I was having tea with my friend Janaan. A few years ago, her beloved husband died after a long journey through an Alzheimer's-type dementia. Without question, Janaan and Carl were on the journey together, and she considered each day with him an opportunity for loving. As we shared stories about caring for Carl and Mom, Janaan said, "If I had it to do over, I would, gratefully. And," she added with endearing certainty, "I would do it better." "Oh," I thought, with tears in my eyes. "How I *wish* I could do it over. How I wish I could have known at the beginning of my caregiving journey with Mom what I knew at the end!" Given my rich learning and experience, I would have been an even better caregiver.

After many years of caring for his beloved wife Virginia, Cape Cod writer Elliot Stanley Goldman reached this conclusion: "Alzheimer's is not a doctor's disease. It belongs to the caregivers—family, nurses, aides—who see the patient through the long affliction for which there is no cure and no clear guidelines for what to expect at any stage."[1] More than thirty years after Goldman wrote those words, his conclusion continues to ring true. In fact, it has been true since 1901, when German physician Alois Alzheimer became acquainted with a new patient, Auguste D. During their first meetings, Auguste's observable symptoms included "unexplainable bursts of anger, and then a strange series of memory problems." A skilled diagnostician, Alzheimer followed systematic protocol with Auguste in an effort to exclude certain conditions and discover the cause of her symptoms. But after ruling out all known diseases as the possible cause of an illness that presented as a psychiatric disorder, Alzheimer was left with a mystery. Throughout her illness over the next five years, Auguste remained hospitalized, experiencing a steady decline of her remaining capacities and receiving what would today be identified as palliative care. The treatment goals were to keep her safe, clean, and as comfortable as possible.

Following her death in 1906, Dr. Alzheimer, ever-perplexed about the cause of these symptoms, performed an autopsy and dissected Auguste D.'s brain.[2] The autopsy revealed "peculiar clumps" (now known as *plaques*) and "a tangled bundle of fibrils" (now known as *tangles*) never before observed by medical scientists and, until recently, generally presumed to be the cause of Alzheimer's.[3]

Currently, it's estimated that 6.9 million Americans over the age of 65 are living with Alzheimer's disease, the most common form of dementia. In addition, 5.7 million are experiencing mild cognitive impairment (MCI) due to Alzheimer's disease, and approximately 200,000 people in the U.S. ages 30 to 64 have early-onset Alzheimer's. The number of people with Alzheimer's is projected to reach 8.5 million by 2030 and 13.8 million by 2060.[4] As a result of this relentless trend, Alzheimer's researcher Zaven Khachaturian asserts, "We have to solve this problem, or it's going to overwhelm us .... the numbers are going to double every twenty years . . . . the duration of the illness is going to get much longer. That's the really devastating part." [5]

Contemplating the duration is especially devastating because people with Alzheimer's cannot care for themselves for many years of their lives, sometimes a decade or more. In 2022, it was predicted that care for people with Alzheimer's and other dementias would cost the nation $321 billion. For 2024, it is predicted that care for people with Alzheimer's and other dementias will cost the nation $360 billion. By 2050, these costs could reach nearly $1 trillion annually. For a number of years, Alzheimer's was the sixth leading cause of death across all ages in the United States until COVID-19 became the third leading cause of death in 2020 and pushed Alzheimer's to seventh. Since we all are potentially at the mercy of this disease, particularly as we age, finding cause and cure and identifying preventative methods are urgent priorities.

Although billions of dollars are devoted annually to these critical research efforts—in 2022 alone, the federal budget included $3.7 billion to study Alzheimer's at the National Institutes of Health,[6] Alzheimer's disease continues to vex the most brilliant scientific and medical minds.

Neurodegenerative diseases, it seems, are already overwhelming us. In the midst of this urgent public health emergency and anticipating its future growth, most of us have been, and are still, counting on medical breakthroughs that will identify ways to prevent, more effectively treat, and ultimately cure Alzheimer's. Unfortunately, those breakthroughs have not yet happened, at least not in the ways we've been expecting. Based on the trajectory of the conventional U.S. medical model, a majority of us are likely still hoping and waiting for a pill that will cure all: all symptoms, all brain deterioration, all people with Alzheimer's. However, most of the pharmaceutical clinical trials, costing over $40 billion,[7] have failed to produce significant results. Between 1995 and 2021, six drugs, all of them expected only to treat symptoms rather than slow disease progression or mitigate the underlying biological process, were approved for Alzheimer's. Because of the expense of the trials with no medical or financial gains to show for them, a number of companies have drastically curtailed or altogether discontinued their Alzheimer's trials.[8] In 2021 and 2023, two new drugs received FDA approval in the U.S., one in the midst of a contentious controversy within the FDA itself over effectiveness, followed by dauntingly high costs ($56,000 per year), which Medicare refused to cover unless people were enrolled in a clinical trial specific to this drug.[9] By early 2024, it was reported that the U.S. pharmaceutical company providing this drug will stop clinical trials in May 2024 and will stop selling the drug in the U.S. on November 1, 2024. After the first eighteen months on the market, the revenue from sale of the drug "has been so small that the company no longer reports the details."[10] The second drug, produced by a Japanese company, produced research results showing mild effectiveness in removing amyloid plaques in the brain for a small number of people, but it had significant adverse side effects, causing a "wait and see" reaction from many professionals in the field. The low level of enthusiasm around this drug stems in part from current medical and scientific thinking that the amyloid plaques, historically considered to be the cause of Alzheimer's, could be just a symptom, an ongoing warning sign, not actually the cause of the disease. [11]

Some drug trials and applications with the FDA are still ongoing. In July 2024, another drug targeting amyloid plaques, produced by US pharmaceutical company Eli Lilly, received approval for use with mild and early Alzheimer's. Similar to the Japanese drug, both are administered by infusion, are expensive ($26,000 to $30,000 per year), may "modestly" slow the progression of Alzheimer's, and have "potentially dangerous side-effects, like brain swelling." Some physicians report being "thrilled" by this recent approval, now having another option to offer patients.[12]

However, according to neurologist, author, and Alzheimer's researcher Dale Bredesen, waiting for that magic pill—a "silver bullet" as he calls it—is old-fashioned thinking and ill-advised. He proposes that research teams need to be looking for "silver buckshot."[13] It's unfortunate that during this time of excessive gun violence in the U.S., Bredesen chooses the bullet/buckshot analogy to illustrate his point, but his analogy does align with our common way of approaching disease. When faced with an unwanted diagnosis, we often employ war language and intention. With singularly focused energy, we fight diseases; we battle them. We seek to defeat, to beat, to conquer every disease, and in this effort, we might actually trick ourselves into believing that death is an avoidable experience.

Bredesen's theory, shared by many other professionals in the field, is that Alzheimer's and other neurodegenerative diseases are not caused by any one thing, but are complex conditions arising from multiple concurrent conditions, including heart disease, diabetes, and obesity, for example. He identifies thirty-six factors that can help trigger what he calls "downsizing" in the brain. Therefore, a pill that is all things for all people with Alzheimer's is not likely to be discovered soon, or ever. Rather, treatment needs to vary from person to person.[14]

Alzheimer's caregiver, advocate, and activist Daisy Duarte, unfamiliar with Bredesen's buckshot theory, agrees with him none-the-less, reaching the same conclusion on her own. For the past twelve years, Daisy has been participating in clinical medication research designed to delay Alzheimer's onset, as well as speaking out about her personal experiences and learnings. As a person who has had fifteen members of her family die from early-onset Alzheimer's, who was primary caregiver for her mother, Sonia (one of the fifteen) and who has herself tested positive for the Alzheimer's gene, Daisy's voice is powerful. She is committed to doing everything she can to reduce her own risk for developing the disease and to inform and protect others. She is particularly concerned for her community. Hispanic and Latinx people living in the U.S. are 1.5 times more likely than white people to have dementia, and they tend to develop symptoms almost seven years earlier. Although they make up 18 percent of the U.S. population, they make up less than 1 percent of people participating in clinical trials at the National Institutes of Health.[15] Daisy is convinced that any pharmaceutical intervention proven to be effective for the Caucasian population may not be effective for the Latinx or Black populations, so she actively and passionately encourages Latinx people and individuals from other minority groups to volunteer for clinical studies.

Bredesen's wide-spreading buckshot protocol does include pharmaceutical interventions directed at reducing amyloid plaques for the small number of people they are so far shown to help. However, he more strongly promotes lifestyle changes, such as adding regular exercise, eating a brain/heart-healthy diet, nutrient supplementation, managing stress, sleeping well, avoiding traumatic brain injuries, and removing as many environmental toxins as possible—those found in food, household products, pesticides, building materials, etc.—as all are suspects for contributing to brain degeneration.[16] In his book *The End of Alzheimer's*, first published in 2017, Bredesen states his theories, his protocol, and his own encouraging research findings, noting, however, that his study included only a small number of subjects.

Bredesen's protocol was not my first introduction to the idea of lifestyle intervention for brain health. I first learned of this approach at an Alzheimer's conference in Massachusetts in 2009. So it's been a while now that scientists and physicians from around the world have known about, have been communicating about, and have been studying this connection.[17] This is good news. And bad news. The good news is that we can possibly do something, ourselves, to reduce our risk of developing dementia; Bredesen claims that we might even be able to reverse it.[18] In this effort, neurologist David Perlmutter calls us "the stewards of our own destiny."[19] But that's the bad news also. If we want to change the course of this disease, individually and collectively, we're going to have to change the traditional U.S. lifestyle, which is proving to be very hard on our bodies. Bredesen calls it the "fight of our lives" and encourages us to make changes now instead of waiting for symptoms to emerge.[20]

Acknowledging that the idea of making so much change could seem overwhelming, Heather Sandison, a naturopathic physician who specializes in treating people experiencing cognitive decline and founded the first senior living facility dedicated to Alzheimer's reversal, suggests that we be gentle with ourselves and begin with just one change. She recommends starting with a simple twelve-minute daily meditation called *Kirtan Kriya*, which has been shown by clinical research sponsored by the Alzheimer's Research & Prevention Foundation, to "improve cognition and activate parts of the brain that are central to memory."[21] Daniel Lieberman, professor of human evolutionary biology at Harvard University and author of *Exercised: The Science of Physical Activity, Rest and Health*, tells us that lifelong activity decreases vulnerability to disease and suggests that exercise is the most effective way of preventing Alzheimer's.[22] Kat Toups, functional medicine psychiatrist, says that meditation and exercise are the two best ways to change our brain for the better.[23] Knowing that genetics, alone, will not have the final say about Alzheimer's, or any disease onset, Daisy takes this kind of guidance seriously. She has significantly altered her self-described "party animal" lifestyle by changing jobs to reduce stress, eating a healthy diet (except potato chips—she can't give up potato chips!), meditating twice daily, and participating in various alternative treatment modalities. Daisy is admirably doing whatever she can to delay, and perhaps even avoid, the fate of her fifteen relatives.

"Human kind / Cannot bear very much reality," T.S. Eliot writes in his poem "Burnt Norton."[24] One reality about Alzheimer's that is particularly hard to bear is that the valiant pharmaceutical research efforts all over the world have been mostly unsuccessful.[25] Unchecked, Alzheimer's continues to devastate individuals, families, and societies. A second unbearable reality is that there isn't much doctors can do who are following the old fashioned prescriptive protocols and are treating the extremely complex medical condition of Alzheimer's with simple drug solutions.[26] And another reality: The most recommended treatment for those showing significant symptoms of cognitive decline is still the palliative care that Auguste D. received over a century ago, "providing basic comfort as patients wait to die."[27] This, traditionally, remains the common approach when the medical field declares, "There is nothing more we can do."

When Virginia Goldman was diagnosed with Alzheimer's in the early 1990s, her husband, Elliot, heard nothing optimistic from doctors, who at that time didn't even have the unhelpful drugs/false hope to offer. Living in a culture focused on conquering illness, he found himself standing uncomfortably at the intersection of his faith in medicine and the unbearable reality of Alzheimer's. Accustomed to the medical approach of making every effort to cure a disease, Goldman was not initially prepared for the submission that Alzheimer's demands. He ultimately recognized, however, the need to embrace the same type of care offered to Auguste D. and ensure Virginia's safety and comfort. In addition, he chose first and foremost to attend to her quality of life.[28] Adding quality of life to the palliative care model represents the evolution of standard care for the terminally ill over the past decades, with hospice organizations now leading the way.

While investigating nursing homes for Mom, I stumbled upon beautifully stated wisdom about a spiritual approach to terminal illnesses on the website of Luther Manor, a nursing home in Dubuque supported by a consortium of Lutheran churches in the county:

Cure may occur without healing; healing may occur without cure.

Cure looks at what sort of disease a person has; healing looks at what sort of person has the disease.

Cure seeks ultimately to conquer pain; healing seeks to transcend pain.

Cure is taunted by suffering; healing is taught by suffering.

These words prompted me to research the author of such thought-provoking comparisons, and I discovered that Lutheran pastoral theologian and chaplain Fred Reklau had recognized and documented many more contrasts between healing and cure.

Cure separates body from soul; healing embraces the soul.

Cure isolates; healing incorporates.

Cure combats illness; healing fosters wellness.

Cure fosters function; healing fosters purpose.

Cure alters what is; healing offers what might be.

Cure is an act; healing is a process.

Cure acts upon another; healing shares with a sister, a brother.

Cure manages; healing touches.

Cure avoids grief; healing assumes grief.

Cure encounters mystery as a challenge for understanding; healing encounters mystery as a ready channel for meaning.

Cure rejects death and views it as defeat; healing includes death among the blessed outcomes of care.[29]

These distinctions enlightened my thinking about what healing means in the context of Alzheimer's and all incurable diseases, reminding me that *cure* is a medical term and *healing* is a spiritual term. To heal means to "make whole." This is the life work of our souls and is not dependent on our physical well-being.

Reklau's interpretation of healing helped me to more fully appreciate the writing of Arthur Kleinman, psychiatrist, social anthropologist, Harvard University professor, friend to Elliot Goldman, and caregiver on the Alzheimer's journey with his wife, Joan. Acutely aware of the harsh realities of this disease, Kleinman believes the most effective treatment that physicians—or any healing professionals—can offer to people with Alzheimer's and their families is "some kind of caregiving and hope for the future."[30]

Dale Bredesen's protocol is all about hope for the future. He believes that the old-fashioned treatment for people with Alzheimer's leads only to despair and that the new-fashioned lifestyle treatment modalities he and many others are exploring and advocating offer us hope.[31] It's true that whenever we can do something to improve our own medical conditions, there is hope; but Bredesen's approach is still in the category of cure, still in its infancy, and still a long way off from making a significant dent in the numbers of people living with and dying from Alzheimer's. And so we all remain in the same place Elliot Goldman stood decades ago, where we need to care for people we can't yet cure, now millions and millions of them, for a long, long time. During my own efforts to embrace the reality of Alzheimer's, I realized and accepted the truth of Arthur Kleinman's words. Caregiving and hope *are* the cornerstones for healing—in the absence of cure, they are what's possible.

Caregiving

Elliot Goldman and Arthur Kleinman, both the primary caregivers for their wives, conclude that those in our society who truly have expert knowledge about Alzheimer's and the potential to bring about healing are the "spouses, children, friends, and the professional companions, aides, and nurses who do the actual caregiving—meaning everything from driving, walking with, reading to, feeding, bathing, and just being there for people whose brain is no longer capable of letting them be independent."[32] Through their writing, these now expert caregivers are our guiding lights in the wilderness. Goldman, writing about his personal experiences with Alzheimer's in the 1990s, was a trailblazer. By documenting and sharing the challenges and heartbreaks of his and Virginia's lives, Goldman charted new territory. He opened the door, giving others permission to reveal their truths about this disease and to share their thoughts, feelings, fears, frustrations, and confusion. His words of solidarity are a reminder that we are not alone.

Goldman understood the helplessness of people with Alzheimer's, describing it with exquisite accuracy. He alerted me about how important my role as caregiver would be: "The caregiver is the patient's mentor, her eyes, her voice, the experience she lives in."[33] Reading this for the first time, realizing the truth and the enormity of Goldman's statement, all I could do was take a really deep breath. Then I prayed for the courage to come close to every aspect of Alzheimer's, for the strength to stay with Mom until the end, and for the humility to ask for help.

When Alzheimer's caregivers arrive at the crossroads of cure and healing and find that only the road to healing is realistically open for passage at this time, many of us are, as Goldman was at first, unprepared, frustrated, and resistant. By describing Alzheimer's caregiving as a "defining moral practice," Kleinman gives us permission to release our dependence on medical science and the demand for a cure and to fully engage in the process of healing. Sharing an ancient Chinese perspective, Kleinman, who lived and worked for many years in China, writes, "We are not born fully human, but only become so as we cultivate ourselves and our relations with others." He reminds us that healing results from the practice of companioning people who are in great need. He considers companioning a "moral practice that makes caregivers, and at times even the care receivers, more present and thereby more fully human."[34] Modern Buddhist teacher, Tenzin Dasel, reminds us that we come into this world dependent on others. Broadening Kleinman's point beyond the caregiving relationship, Dasel says that we need each other to express our humanity. "This," he says, "is the human condition."[35]

Medical science seeks to cure diseases. Caregiving, from the relational foundation Reklau and Kleinman discuss, seeks healing for people afflicted with diseases. When we offer care in the context of relationship, this action leads to self-cultivation that, even as we experience our limits and failures, facilitates our own personal growth. Accordingly, Kleinman claims caregiving completes our humanity. He believes that Alzheimer's caregiving based in relationship and moral acts comes before—

and goes beyond—mind-driven modern medicine. He did not develop his compassionate way of seeing and acting in regard to Alzheimer's care in the classroom or the clinic. There he learned about cure. He developed his approach in relationship, the heartbeat of healing. In his new life, which consisted of daily care for Joan, Kleinman "learned to be a caregiver by doing it." He writes, "I had to do it. It was there to do."[36]

Michael Leach, publisher emeritus of Orbis Books, is the founding editor and regular contributor to an award-winning column in *The National Catholic Reporter* called "Soul Seeing":

> Soul Seeing columns are about looking at what is in front of our eyes and seeing what God has put in our eyes: love, mercy, goodness, beauty, grace, harmony, humility, compassion, gratitude, joy, peace, wisdom, salvation. Soul Seeing writers contemplate those moments when, without searching, they beheld something extraordinary in the ordinary, heard the "still, small voice of God" in a chapel or a forest or a subway train.[37]

Michael was also the primary caregiver for his wife, Vickie, who was diagnosed with early-onset Alzheimer's at age 57. His beloved died recently, after a journey lasting more than twenty years. One of Michael's "seeings," fifteen years into his caregiving life, was inspired by a documentary he and Vickie watched about Leonard Cohen, composer of the iconic song *Hallelujah*. At one point in the documentary, Cohen paraphrases the Hindu deity Krishna in the *Bhagavad Gita*. "You will never untangle the circumstances that brought you to this moment . . . . Embrace your destiny, your fate. Know what your duty is. Do it with love in your heart. And do it without hesitation."[38] Michael admits that for a time after Vickie's diagnosis, he was shaking his fist at God. But it wasn't long before he understood that his calling was to be with Vickie as she forgot and as she gracefully became more and more of the divine expression that was her true nature. "I'm good with it," he said. "The last few years have been the best of my life."[39] There is, indeed, peace, satisfaction, and even joy that comes from knowing you are embracing your destiny and doing your true duty.

Kleinman compares caregiving for someone with Alzheimer's to parenting, particularly mothering.[40] With this comparison, he ushers us onto the holy ground of duty. Caregivers will soon come to understand that this disease is calling us to transform our familial love and commitment into active caring. Like parents, our duty is to take responsibility for the well-being and fulfillment of someone else.

In our culture, we most often take our model of love from romance. Theologian Sam Keen argues that by stressing desire and excitement rather than "responsibility and care-giving as the central ingredients of love," we create "immense confusion about the relationship between love and care." When this happens, "we tend to think of care-giving as a burden that, unfortunately, comes with long-term commitments."

I have long believed that the deepest longing of every human soul is to love and be loved; that in loving and being loved we find meaning, purpose, and fulfillment in this life. Alzheimer's disease does not extinguish this longing. Influenced by ancient and modern spiritual teachings, I agree with Keen on this point: "Much of the meaning of our lives is created by tending, meeting, and taking responsibility for the well-being of others." Keen warns us, however, that it's easy, and quite common, to dismiss this idea. "After all," he writes, "news of most any day suggests that what makes the world go 'round is not love, but fear, greed, competition, cruelty, and the will to power."[41] As Erich Fromm told readers nearly seventy years ago in *The Art of Loving*, our culture has not encouraged us to explore the depths of loving, which includes care for the vulnerable among us. From the perspective of caring for the millions of vulnerable people with Alzheimer's, it's disheartening to realize that not much social progress has been made toward the blossoming of love. Fromm writes, "In spite of the deepseated craving for love, almost everything else is considered to be more important than love: success, prestige, money, power—almost all our energy is used for the learning of how to achieve these aims, and almost none to learn the art of loving."[42] From this perspective, our choices as caregivers—to move, to change our lives, to go to nursing homes every day and visit loved ones who don't seem to remember us, to value the lives of people with cognitive decline through fierce advocacy—are often met with confusion, skepticism, and even criticism by others.

However, the sacred importance of caregiving relationships has been a part of human consciousness since ancient times. According to Roman mythology, caregiving has the capacity to shape a being:

> Once when Care was crossing a river, she saw some clay. Thoughtfully, she took a piece of the clay and began to shape it.
>
> While she was meditating on what she had made, Jupiter, king of the Gods, came by. Care asked him to give her creation spirit, and this he gladly did. But when Care wanted her name to be bestowed upon it, Jupiter forbade this, and demanded that it be given his name instead.
>
> While Care and Jupiter were arguing, Earth joined the dispute. Since Earth furnished the clay from part of her own body, she expressed the desire for her own name to be conferred on the creature.

They decided to ask Saturn, the God of Time, to be their arbiter. Saturn made the following decision, which all believed to be a just one: "There is a dispute among you as to this creature's name. Let it be called homo-sapien for it is made out of humus—earth. Since you, Jupiter, have given its spirit, you shall receive that spirit at its death. Since you, Earth, have given its body, you shall receive its body. But most importantly, since Care first shaped this creature, she shall possess it as long as it lives."[43]

Devoted Alzheimer's caregivers are resurrecting this sacred understanding of care because we have experienced its relationship to elements of love beyond romance. Through our practice of caregiving, many Alzheimer's caregivers are realizing that the sacrifices demanded of us are making our lives richer with meaning, satisfaction, and expressions of true love than romance or sentimentality ever could.[44]

Caregiving took Arthur Kleinman to the depths of his being, where he met those sacrifices face to face and discovered what all caregivers come to know: This is *not* easy. He wrote, "Caregiving consumes time, energy, and financial resources. It sucks out strength and determination . . . . It can amplify anguish and desperation. It can divide the self. It can bring out family conflicts . . . . It is also far more complex, uncertain, and unbounded than professional medical and nursing models suggest."[45] Meeting all of these challenges, as caregivers must, unquestionably requires courage, commitment, creativity, learning, patience, and practice. Kleinman writes,

> The all-absorbing love I had for my wife and she for me, had more than sustained me and her through those uncertain years of building our professional lives, a family, and our own world. That fierce and joyful love

had animated those years, now gone forever, with a golden hue that expressed a shared sensibility of things being right and good and beautiful. During the terrible years of Joan's descent through neurodegeneration to blindness, dementia, paralysis, and a slow death, love had made it possible to endure the unendurable; it motivated my caregiving and her care-receiving.[46]

Love can make it all possible.

However healing and loving our caregiving efforts are, we're likely to encounter resistance and sometimes flat out rejection of them. Infants and toddlers, which people with Alzheimer's eventually come to resemble, are naturally receptive to the reciprocal practice of caregiving and care-receiving. Unfortunately, adults experiencing declining cognitive capacities, who need to practice receiving care and love, often don't realize that's what we are offering. They might perceive us to be controlling and bossy and be inclined to resist their new roles as care receivers for as long as possible. Their resistance is a by-product of a culture that places value on productivity, autonomy, and independence and interprets needing and receiving help as failure.

There will come a time in the progression of Alzheimer's disease when the afflicted ones' capacity to resist will decline. Should they live long enough to reach the end stages of the disease, this population will become completely helpless and dependent upon us for their survival.[47] They will essentially regress to infancy and will then be among the most vulnerable members of our society.

However, during the earlier stages of the disease, caregivers often engage in power struggles with people with Alzheimer's over life-changing, life-saving issues such as driving, attending adult day centers, bringing help into the home, or moving to care facilities. These complex struggles are often resolved only when something significant happens. For Mom, it was a car accident that took away her driver's license and finally the pronouncement by her doctor that she was not competent to drive.

There is no one right formula for ensuring that discussions or decisions about these issues will go smoothly. Whenever possible, however, and preferably before a tragedy happens, caregivers are encouraged to enlist the support of someone the person with Alzheimer's considers to be in a position of authority: a doctor, lawyer, family elder, boss, clergy, or someone else in a leadership role. It will be especially beneficial if these authority figures have sensitivity to and awareness about the dynamics of Alzheimer's.

My friend Diane is a parish priest in a neighboring town. A member of her parish, Miriam, was diagnosed with Alzheimer's. When the time came for Miriam to move to a memory care facility, her daughter Jessica, an overburdened, single working mom with three teenaged sons, couldn't cope with Miriam's resistance, and she sought Rev. Diane's help.

Before the move, Miriam's aging, sick dog had to be put to sleep, and her messy apartment had to be packed up and cleaned. The even bigger challenge was the need to convince Miriam that the move was necessary, good, and above all, happening. Jessica told Miriam that she had to move, but Miriam was not having it. Because of the role reversal of authority, it was hard for Jessica to convince her mother to take her seriously. When the priest (a clear authority figure for Miriam) arrived on the scene, however, and told Miriam that the move was happening, she accepted it, although she was devastated. Rev. Diane witnessed Miriam's sadness and offered her caregiving at its best—by sitting with her as she cried and comforting her with undivided presence.

Miriam didn't want change because she didn't realize that things could be better. As Rev. Diane explained what would be happening and how, Miriam became curious about many things, including why she couldn't ask Jessica any of her questions without emotions exploding. Rev. Diane replied, "Because this change is as hard for Jessica as it is for you." Indeed, moving people with Alzheimer's and dementia to assisted living or memory care centers against their will is very hard for their families.

For more than a week, Rev. Diane spent many hours each day with Miriam, explaining (and re-explaining) with kindness and compassion what was about to happen to her beloved dog, and the reasons for and details about the upcoming move. Miriam didn't want to leave her apartment, and she kept forgetting why she had to go. Rev. Diane calmly repeated the simple truth, "Because you have Alzheimer's, and you forget things sometimes. You need to be around people who can help you remember." Rev. Diane's calm presence each day kept the process moving forward—in baby steps—which helped Miriam get used to the idea of change.

One day, Rev. Diane engaged Miriam in a practical task. She arrived with an empty moving box for Miriam to fill with pictures to take to her new home. As they removed pictures from the walls, Miriam told stories of her life as she decided whether to take or leave each item. Rev. Diane helped Miriam identify the most important things to pack with a clear request: "Let's talk about things you'd like to take." Surprisingly, each list ended with "the coffeepot." Pictures and clothes and shoes and the coffeepot. The cat and the TV and the cactus and the coffeepot. When Rev. Diane mentioned to Miriam that she noticed the coffeepot was on every list, Miriam exclaimed emphatically, "I love my coffeepot!" They had a good laugh together over having a meaningful relationship with the coffeepot. Humor, patience, compassion, and simple truth were some of the ways that Rev. Diane was able to lessen Miriam's resistance.

After one of her afternoons with Miriam, Diane shared with me how excruciating it was to witness Miriam's torment and to feel so helpless. This is the plight of most Alzheimer's caregivers. Diane, however, was soothed by knowing that her investment of time and her kindness toward Miriam had made a difference. On the Sunday morning when Jessica was moving Miriam to the nursing home, she brought her mother to church before they left town. As Rev. Diane was greeting the parishioners after the Mass, Miriam came up to her, stopped, and looked right into Rev. Diane's eyes. Finally, Miriam said, "It's going to be OK," tacking on the question, "Isn't it?" Rev. Diane took her hands and replied with certainty, "Yes. It's going to be OK." They shared a long, warm hug. Then Miriam smiled at Rev. Diane and walked out of the church into the beginning of her new, OK life.

Hope

On my journey, I soon discovered a definition of hope that felt just right in the context of Alzheimer's caregiving. "Making a difference" is how Vaclav Havel defines hope: "Hope is not about believing that you can change things. Hope is believing that what you do makes a difference."[48] I soon realized that this kind of hope can show up in unexpected places. An article in *The Telegraph Herald*, our local newspaper, for example, brought me into a deeper understanding of Havel's hope.

In the spring of 2009, the Dubuque police chief, Kim Wadding, announced his upcoming retirement. During an interview with a reporter, he shared one of his most memorable moments from his thirty-year career in law enforcement: It was the face of a sixteen-year-old girl who was dying at the scene of a car crash. Wadding said, "I looked at her, and she was just so scared." It was obvious to him that the paramedics had tried everything to save her but could not. So he decided to give this girl as much peace as he could for as long as he could. He locked eyes with her and said, "Just look at me. We're going to get through this. This is going to be OK. Just look at me." He held her, and they looked at each other as he watched her just fade away. "It's a face you never forget," Wadding said. "And that's what keeps you going—those few seconds of comfort. I felt that she felt it."[49] At a Healing Moments workshop for Alzheimer's caregivers, I shared Chief Wadding's story. After the workshop, a staff member from the Alzheimer's Association came to me asking for clarity. "I don't understand how this is hopeful," he said. "She died!"

That's right. She died.

But in her final moments, Kim Wadding made a difference in her life. And clearly, this girl made a difference in his life.

Many years ago, a friend introduced me to the writing of David Steindl-Rast, a Benedictine monk who is also a Zen Buddhist. Steindl-Rast, like many theologians, had searched his heart and mind and experience in a quest to define God. He ultimately defined God as "surprise," saying no other definitions can ultimately be sustained.[50] This story about Chief Wadding's memorable moment was so surprising to me—I guess I had expected a different kind of moment from a police officer— and so I looked prayerfully and deeply into this story, looking for God. What I found was encouragement on the caregiving journey. Like this girl's injuries, Alzheimer's is terminal. Unlike this girl, however, who had only moments left to live, people with Alzheimer's can live with the disease for decades. Our challenge is to help those afflicted with Alzheimer's get through the time they have, moment by moment, with a good quality of life. We can make a healing difference in their lives. And as we help them, what then happens for us? As we live into the answer, we might be surprised to find that they make a healing difference in our lives too.

When I visited Iowa the summer after my sibling moved away, my intention was to assess various possibilities for being with Mom. One was the possibility of moving to Dubuque from Boston to be with her full-time. Well-meaning friends and colleagues challenged this idea. They expressed disbelief and concern that I would consider leaving my established life and career opportunities in Boston and move halfway across the country to care for someone who barely spoke and, most of the time, probably wouldn't even know who I was. My initial response to their argument was, "Well, I know who she is. And who she is needs me, now more than ever before."

However, as I spent more time that summer with Mom and her neighbors in the nursing home, I began to question the premise that people with Alzheimer's don't know their loved ones. I saw the nursing home residents light up like fireflies when their sons, daughters, spouses, friends, and cherished caregivers came for visits. Faces that were often blank burst into smiles as soon as they noticed their loved ones approaching.

Etty was Mom's neighbor on the Alzheimer's wing of the nursing home. Her husband was away for the winter, and although they had spoken on the phone, she hadn't seen him for six months. On the first day he returned, he respectfully greeted her, asking if he could hug her. Etty cautiously hesitated but then agreed. He took her out for lunch, and when they returned, he kissed her goodbye and left her at the nurses' station. With a dreamy gleam in her eye, like a teenager in love, she shouted out to everyone, "I'm going to marry that man!"

She didn't remember that he was already her husband, but something in her knew they belonged together.

Perhaps her spirit recognized his spirit. That's what I felt was happening between Mom and me during those weeks I was with her assessing a possible relocation. One afternoon, she was absorbed in looking at and touching the new clothes I had laid out on her bed earlier in the day. When I walked into the room, she looked up from the clothes. Quickly, she recognized me. I knew this from the wide smile that spread across her face. As she clutched her new flowered blouse to her heart, Mom's shining blue eyes looked at me—really looked at me. Then she said slowly but distinctly, "You. You. It's you!" Her face and eyes expressed awe. Hearing this, seeing this, I felt as if I was, at that moment, a visiting deity—or at least the most important person in my mother's world. It was a moment of pure recognition and belonging, a deeply human *ubuntu* connection, even if she wasn't exactly clear about the relationship between us.

After those seven weeks with Mom, I returned to Boston in turmoil. My life in Boston was fulfilling and happy and I couldn't imagine myself thriving in my small Iowa hometown. I sought counsel from respected friends, colleagues, and counselors, who mostly discouraged the move. Only my spiritual director recognized the longing of my soul to be with Mom, and she encouraged me to follow this call. The turmoil intensified.

One hot September day on a sunny beach north of Boston, I crouched at the shoreline and watched tiny sand crabs skittering in and out of the water. As my mind focused on the crabs, a calmness came over me and a question posed to me long ago during a session of the Life/Work Directions vocational program rose into my consciousness: "What would you do with your life if you found out that you had only six months to live?" A clear answer came quickly. I would finish my semester of school, keeping the commitments I had for teaching classes and leading workshops, and then I would go to Iowa. Then I asked myself another question: "If you knew that your mother would die in six months, what would you do?" Instant clarity: I would move to Iowa tomorrow.

Without doubt or delay, I began to make arrangements for the move to Dubuque. I completed my teaching and workshop commitments in Boston, spent six weeks during December and January in Iowa with Mom, and officially relocated in February, 2008. When friends and colleagues asked me why I was doing this, I explained that, when I arrived in Iowa in July, my mother couldn't get up from a chair without assistance. She couldn't walk, feed herself, or catch a ball. When I left in September, she could do all of those things and more.

I told a friend how I "cued" Mom to get out of a chair without assistance by telling her the steps in the process: "Put your hands on the arms of the chair. Now push up with your arms. Now push up with your legs."

He remarked, "Oh, so she has to relearn how to do things."

"That's not exactly it," I replied. "Mom's not relearning. Although she has the physical strength and ability to stand up, she doesn't remember how to initiate this action. I'm noticing her remaining abilities and then helping her to use them."

The sad truth was that Mom would not regain the capacity to stand up from a chair on her own. For a while, however, she could do this with minimal cueing, such as slight pressure on her elbow and the verbal suggestion, "Let's stand up now."

People with Alzheimer's have remaining abilities that are unrecognized, unused, and too often lost forever from inertia and atrophy. Mom needed me there to help her maintain her abilities for as long as possible. Unfortunately, it's often more practical and efficient for nursing home staff to lift a person from is a chair than it is for them to offer cues, wait for the cue to register in a decaying brain, and then patiently allow the person to actually follow the cue and perform what has been asked. This quicker fix is detrimental to people with Alzheimer's, because for them the old adage is especially true: If you don't use it, you lose it.

As my plans evolved to be with Mom during the home stretch of her life, I explained to inquiring colleagues and friends that, during the weeks I spent with her, I was making a significant difference to her well-being and quality of life. This mattered to me. I couldn't stop the course of Alzheimer's disease or change the fact that my mother would die, but I saw that, in the midst of these harsh realities of life, healing was possible— healing was happening. I felt that I was living Vaclav Havel's definition of hope; I believed that my presence in Mom's life was making a difference in important and meaningful ways.

As we search to understand what hope might mean for individuals and societies caring for people with Alzheimer's disease, we need to consider various contexts for hoping.

Over one hundred years after Dr. Alzheimer discovered the mysterious plaques and tangles in Auguste D.'s brain, we are probably still holding onto the hope that science and medicine will identify ways to prevent, treat, and cure this disease. This kind of hope, based on logic, reason, and trust in traditional methods, could offer some consolation to a fearful population.

Finding hope becomes more challenging, however, within the context of caring for the millions of Americans who currently have Alzheimer's and the millions more who will have it by 2060. This reality is daunting, especially as we consider the impact Alzheimer's disease and related dementias have on tens of millions of family caregivers. These "informal" caregivers, who contribute millions of unpaid hours of care, often suffer significant financial loss and are susceptible to illness, depressions, anxiety, and often, early death.[51]

In an effort to find someone or something that will change unbearable realities, most of us still tend to look outwardly for hope. True hope for Alzheimer's, however, requires us to first accept the realities that humankind cannot bear and embrace suffering as a natural part of the human condition. On this topic, saints and poets, both ancient and modern, have insights to share. Julian of Norwich, a fourteenth-century Christian mystic, shares her perspective: "During our lifetime here we have in us a marvelous mixture of both wellbeing and woe."[52] Four hundred years later, poet William Blake expressed a similar life view:

Man was made for joy and woe.
And when this we rightly know,
Through the world we safely go. [53]

From the springboard of these truths, hope inspires us to accept that life includes pain, loss, decline, grief, and death. This inevitability of the human condition becomes personally and socially significant in ways that have ethical consequences. Only by accepting the realities of Alzheimer's, which brings us face to face with what theologian Teilhard de Chardin calls "a universal power of diminishment and extinction,"[54] do we have the option to transform it into an experience that is, in essence, life-giving.

In the face of this universal power of diminishment, we caregivers realize that hope is not "out there." The possibility for hope exists within every one of us. Through the practice of conscious and compassionate caregiving, we can make a difference. We can alleviate the suffering of people with Alzheimer's.

Knowing my mom's life story, I realized that she had not been protected, nurtured, loved for who she was, or encouraged to be all she could be. How then could she have passed this kind of love and nurturing on to me when I was a child? My spiritual intention in moving to Iowa was to love Mom in this lifetime so her soul would learn and remember love and be able to love more fully in her next lifetime. Through this intention, which I thought was all about me caring for Mom, I made the most glorious and surprising discovery. Naively, or arrogantly perhaps, I was convinced that I would be healing Mom's soul. Over time, however, I most humbly discovered that she was also healing me. Mom was making a difference for me! *She* was being hope—for me. From the beginning of Mom's journey through Alzheimer's, she surprised and inspired me. She beckoned to me from across the threshold of Alzheimer's, inviting me into her world in Iowa, where I built a wonderful new life for myself. Most importantly, Mom offered me countless opportunities to be present in the moment, to practice giving and receiving unconditional love, and to recognize the presence of God in every beautiful and terrible corner of life.

Caregivers and their loved ones with Alzheimer's have opportunities every day to manifest hope for each other. It happens in between us—with a smile, a touch, a gentle voice, and a loving look in each other's eyes. It happens through witness and empathy, responsibility and solidarity, recognition and belonging. We can't yet change the prevalence or the course of Alzheimer's disease in significant ways, but every one of us—caregivers and care-receivers alike—can make a difference in someone's life. We can *be* hope.

5 The Value and Beauty of Every Person

While I was sitting with Mom and holding her hand during the Rhythm Time activity at her nursing home, our eyes met and she smiled. With gusto and joy, we were shaking maracas with our free hands and singing along to old familiar songs such as "How Much Is That Doggie in the Window?" and "Take Me Out to the Ball Game."

My eyes, drawn away from Mom for a brief moment, gazed across the expansive room and noticed what seemed to be a sea of people in wheelchairs, each alone. Most of them were diagnosed with Alzheimer's or dementia. I wondered why more family members weren't there, enjoying this experience with their loved ones. Being with Mom and participating in this activity together was actually a lot of fun for me, and Mom clearly loved and appreciated my company. I saw this in her eyes and smile as I helped her participate more fully than she could on her own.

My wandering thoughts led me to recall a recent article in the local newspaper that was advertising the annual Alzheimer's Association Memory Walk. A well-meaning but clearly uninformed reporter used metaphors that I considered distasteful and offensive to describe people with Alzheimer's disease. Through his narrow vision, the reporter saw "empty shells" and "octogenarian Beach Boys, able to mount the stage yet unable to present anything new."[55] With one stroke of his pen, this reporter had managed to demean people living with Alzheimer's as well as the Beach Boys! Obviously, he had never been to Friday morning Rhythm Time! There was always something new happening among these beautiful old souls. On this day, Etty was dancing her version of what looked like the twist; Mary and Tom, a resident couple, were holding hands and looking at each other with moony eyes as we all sang "For It Was Mary"; Isabel was singing in German; Susan offered to pay for everyone's lunch with the Monopoly money in her red purse; Mom and I were attempting a wheelchair polka; hands were clapping, feet were tapping, faces were bright with interest and joy.

Because misinformed media coverage could influence people to formulate opinions and stay away from family members and nursing home residents with Alzheimer's, I wrote a letter to the newspaper editor. I shared my perspective, letting the population of Dubuque know that, through my eyes, my mother and her neighbors were not empty shells. The newspaper printed my letter, and I was pleased to plant seeds for another perspective to bloom and grow.

A combination of misinformation and fear about Alzheimer's causes many in our culture to conclude that people with Alzheimer's are useless. From an economic perspective, especially, they are seen as a burden for families and societies.[56] Many families and friends of people with Alzheimer's are juggling priorities, and if a person is considered "gone," then deciding to spend limited time and attention elsewhere becomes an easier choice. How I wish everyone could witness what I saw looking back at me from within that sea of wheelchairs: beauty within vulnerability, in-the-moment happiness, gratitude for any kindness, earnest efforts to engage in life at every opportunity, and, especially for Mom and me, celebration for one more blessed day together.

How I wish everyone could feel the warmth I felt when, at times, I experienced the nursing home as being like a college dorm, where residents are friends on a shared journey to a similar destiny, looking out for each other and enjoying each other's company. After dinner one Saturday night, Mom and I were in her room watching *The Lawrence Welk Show*. Mom relaxed in her wheelchair while I stood behind her brushing her hair. Music, companionship, and peacefulness filled her room. These energies may have drifted out into the hallway and beckoned to Mom's neighbor, Etty. Like a college girl from down the hall, Etty walked uninvited into Mom's room and smiled. She spoke words that didn't add up to a sentence, but I replied anyway with a warm welcome. After she sat down on Mom's bed, Etty and I exchanged a few more words; Mom looked at Etty with interest. Then Etty sprawled out on the bed, arms tucked up behind her head, feet crossed, making herself quite at home. I was delighted, and turned the TV so she could also see. We all watched together for a while in the loveliness of silent presence. Soon, Etty was humming along with the TV band and vocalists.

Then an aide came in and tried to shoo Etty away, telling her this wasn't her room, telling me it wasn't sanitary for her to be lying on Mom's bed. I insisted that Etty could stay with us, right where she was on Mom's bed. We were having such an enjoyable visit. Before Alzheimer's, Mom was a very sociable person, and I was sure she shared my delight about her friend initiating this visit.

Empty shells? Unable to offer anything new? Not through my eyes. What I saw was pure gold, shining brightly.

The essays "Memory: The Community Looks Backward" and "Hope: The Community Looks Forward" in *God Never Forgets: Faith, Hope, and Alzheimer's Disease*[57] were my first introduction to Stephen Sapp, then professor and chairperson of the Department of Religious Studies at the University of Miami. These engaging essays inspired me to personally contact Stephen, who graciously agreed to a phone interview. This was the beginning of a treasured mentorship and collegial friendship.

During our first conversation, Stephen shared with me his unique outlook about Alzheimer's disease formulated over twenty-five years of study, combining ethics, theology, science, and personal experience. He surprised me, though, when he started talking about how much he enjoyed eating sweet corn. It was an abrupt turn of topic, so I thought. But still, it made me chuckle. Stephen lived in Florida. Really—what could he possibly know about corn? A person hasn't truly tasted excellent sweet corn until they eat an ear picked fresh from an Iowa field! But he told me how much he loves eating steamy, buttery sweet corn—on the cob, of course. After he's devoured the tasty kernels, he said that he throws the cob away, believing, as most of us do, that it's now useless.

As it turned out, Stephen wasn't actually talking to me about corn. He was talking about whether, and how, our culture values elders and people with disabilities, particularly those with Alzheimer's or other forms of cognitive decline. With sadness in his heart, Stephen believes that most in our society assume that people with Alzheimer's have nothing more to give; no potential left for serving the world. Based on all the misconceptions about this disease and the observations we make with what ancient Hebrew prophets describe as "eyes to see but do not see,"[58] it's understandable how we mistakenly conclude that the potential of people with Alzheimer's is all used up. As a society, we tend to devalue beings and things when their potential is not blatantly evident; as a result of this devaluing practice, we are tempted to discard, shut away, or ignore this population of people with Alzheimer's without even being curious about them.

Then Stephen was back to talking about corn. His metaphor moved on to include revelation and discovery. This grain was first developed from teosinte, a wild grass, over seven thousand years ago by Indigenous people living in present-day Mexico. Since then, corn has accompanied people migrating throughout the world and has been cultivated into numerous varieties. Throughout the centuries, the potential for corn kernels (seeds) has multiplied exponentially, and thousands of uses have been discovered and utilized, including farm animal feed, pet food, antibiotics, baby food, condensed milk, sweetener for fruit juices, food starch, peanut butter, flour, alcohol, and even textile products. Until recently, when it was discovered that the cellulose biomass of corn stalks, husks, and cobs could be converted into ethanol fuel, these now valuable resources were seen as useless and discarded. It took humans almost seven thousand years of coexistence with corn to discover that stalks, husks, and cobs still have something to offer, even after they have completed their primary role of aiding in the production of corn kernels. More and more about the ever-increasing, ever-valuable potential of corn continues to be revealed.

As I considered this slow process of revelation and discovery, I realized that the inherent potential was there all along—waiting. Waiting to be discovered by the human mind. The corn didn't have the capacity to reveal its own value, so in order to notice the hidden potential, people actually had to look for it. People were looking for it. Most recently, we were desperately looking, particularly for alternate and renewable forms of fuel.

It's not the corn's fault that it has taken so long for more of its inherent value to be discovered. It's not exactly humanity's fault either. It took evolutionary time for science and technology to develop the capacity for recognizing and harvesting the fullness of the corn's potential. But most importantly, the realization had to dawn on the human mind that we need *all* of what corn has to offer. This kind of realization is often an inspiration for exploration and, ultimately, discovery.

So it is with recognizing the value of individuals with Alzheimer's. Our whole world needs to notice and respond to their still-hidden potential, and it's up to us—those who know and love them—to begin our own explorations, to discover their value and beauty, to reveal it, and to give them the opportunity to express it.

As I continued to explore Stephen's corn metaphor, it expanded even further to include cultivation. Although corn contributes monumental value to the world, it does not exist naturally in the wild. It can only survive if it's planted, cultivated, and protected by humans. Similarly, as their abilities decline, people with Alzheimer's can survive and contribute the value that has been divinely implanted within them, only *if* their lives are cultivated and protected. Cultivating their potential and protecting their hearts, bodies, minds, and souls is our divine purpose—as individuals and as a society.

Sue Bender, author of *Everyday Sacred*, offered me another creative, if unlikely, metaphor to ponder: a white enamel kitchen pot. Bender shared the experience of her friend Gale Antokal, who taught a graduate art class called "The 100 Drawings Project." The assignment for this class is to take a single ordinary object and draw it one hundred times. After teaching this class for years, Antokal finally decided to join her students in the drawing project. She chose a white enamel pot from her kitchen as her object. In Bender's analysis, this intriguing project for art students requires them "to find new techniques, materials, and ways to work—to take risks and exceed limits."

Bender observed Antokal as she worked on this project "for hours, day after day," seeing and drawing her pot, becoming familiar with it through constant studying, and ultimately becoming emotionally attached to it—even taking it on family vacations! My favorite artistic depiction was of the pot reflecting the "many tiny colored lights at night by the water's edge at Piazza San Marco" in Venice, Italy. In the process of observing the pot as a model for artistic expression, Antokal had, without intention, imbued "this most ordinary object . . . with meaning."

Bender reports that she wondered often and long about Antokal's pot, ultimately concluding, "If there are one hundred ways to see an ordinary white pot, imagine all the possibilities for viewing with fresh eyes an 'average' child, an 'average' marriage . . . . If you can take a white enamel household pot and begin seeing it brand new each time, *you can do it with anything.*"[59] Just imagine the possibilities for viewing, with fresh eyes, people with Alzheimer's.

A couple years into my caregiving journey, already familiar with the writing of James Ellor, a gerontologist from Baylor University and author of the essay "Celebrating the Human Spirit," in *God Never Forgets: Faith, Hope, and Alzheimer's Disease,* I had the honor of meeting him in person at an Aging in America conference in Chicago. In his writing and in his heart, Jim confirmed and supported my growing belief that people with Alzheimer's still have potential and purpose. He writes, "I, for one, believe that the millions of [Alzheimer's] sufferers, who can no longer read, no longer speak, still have a thing or two they can teach us, particularly about the love of God."[60]

The idea that people with cognitive loss, who can't read or speak, have a thing or two to teach us sets up a contradiction for most of us. But contradictions are often the greatest teachers of all. For example, religious scholar John Dominic Crossan points out that in the Christian New Testament, the parables of Jesus consistently invite those *with ears to hear* "to experience the world differently, so differently in fact, that expectations about the way things normally go might be completely reversed."[61] Reversals in thinking have enormous potential to enlighten us in profound ways if we can become open to having our worldview shattered and to the challenge of reimaging how we then might live. Consider this possibility: Rather than being useless, people with Alzheimer's and dementia could be our most important teachers in the school of life and love. However, if our attention is hopelessly fixed on the obvious losses of Alzheimer's, this might seem impossible. As we attempt to change our perspective, keep in mind Bender's encouraging thought: "Maybe the most sacred things are the hardest to see, because they are so obvious."

Essential things are often obvious, *and* still they can be easy to miss. Once recognized, however, then of course, we notice what's obvious, and wonder how we could have missed them! Consider the story of the Sufi dervish Mullah Nasrudin:

> Every day for four years, Nasrudin smuggled valuable treasure across the border of his homeland, Persia, into Turkey. Because the guards saw him prospering, they knew Nasrudin was somehow hiding precious cargo, and they inspected every corner of his belongings, including the saddle of his donkey. They could find nothing. Many years later, after Nasrudin had moved away, he encountered one of the border guards, who asked him, "Please tell me now, what were you smuggling?" With a broad smile and proud laugh, Nasrudin replied, "Comrade, I was smuggling donkeys!"[62]

The open secret about the value of people with Alzheimer's is hidden to many, especially when we are besieged by the endless details of everyday life. But for those determined to find the secret, it will become hard to miss. Therefore, when Alzheimer's caregiving is added to our everyday lives, it's important to slow down and simplify in order to focus. And to open ourselves to insights coming from unexpected places. Antoine de Saint-Exupéry's classic children's book *The Little Prince*, for example, offers simple, timeless guidance for recognizing the sacred in people with Alzheimer's: "It is only with the Heart that one can see rightly; what is essential is invisible to the eye."[63] When we look at someone with Alzheimer's with ordinary eyes instead of our hearts, many of us may see someone whose purpose and potential are over, someone who would be better off dead, or someone who seems already dead.

On national television, the influential televangelist Pat Robertson claimed that Alzheimer's is "a kind of death."[64] Dr. Robert Stern, Boston University professor and Alzheimer's researcher, sees people with Alzheimer's differently, and firmly refuted Robertson's comment: "A person with Alzheimer's is always alive, always filled with feelings, always able to connect at some level. To think or say otherwise is absurd, naïve, inhuman."[65]

If we look really closely at people with Alzheimer's through the lens of our hearts, we see even further and deeper than do the inquiring eyes of the scientist who studies the corn, the imaginative eyes of the artist who sees meaning in ordinary objects, or the grief-stricken, loving eyes of family members and friends. If we look through the eyes of one seeking connection with the creator and sustainer of life, we might be surprised by the potential and beauty these individuals with Alzheimer's still possess. From the ancient world of fourth-century Rome, Augustine of Hippo, considered by many to be one of the greatest Christian thinkers of all time, tells humanity that "our whole business in this life is to restore to health the eye of the heart whereby God may be seen."[66] Shining out from within every person, including people with cognitive decline, is the spark of divinity.

Through my unique perspective and experiences, I have noticed that people with Alzheimer's have the potential to inspire us and teach us; love and heal us; amuse and befriend us; calm and comfort us; touch us physically, emotionally, intellectually, and spiritually; energize and enlighten us; empower us; forgive us; nurture us; open our hearts; bring out the best in us; and bring meaning and purpose into our lives. We may be surprised to realize that people with Alzheimer's still have the capacity to show us how to be humble, trusting, courageous, and receptive, to be authentically ourselves in this present moment, and to be guileless and innocent. We may be surprised to discover that, if we look beneath memory loss and declining cognitive and motor abilities, people with Alzheimer's can reveal to us the true value of life—theirs and ours. From within their inherent and indestructible ability to give and receive love, beauty and value radiate—and bring joy.

There are definitely secrets hidden on this Alzheimer's journey. One thing we often miss is this enduring desire and capacity for love. Caregiver Sol Rogers found the key while his beloved wife, Rita, who had Alzheimer's, was living in a nursing home. Out of a desire to help other Alzheimer's family caregivers, Sol sent his story to the helpline office at the Massachusetts/New Hampshire chapter of the Alzheimer's Association, asking them to let others know his good news:

> I have a wife in a nursing home with an advanced stage of Alzheimer's. She can't get out of bed, can hardly move her arms, and can't talk at all. To get out of bed

she has to have a large lift that requires 2 people to get her in a wheelchair. I visit her every day and had become very depressed, couldn't sleep very well, and my body was shaking. I thought I was getting a nervous breakdown and would end up in a hospital.

Then an idea came to me (probably from God). I told the aide to have my wife in bed the following day when I came to visit. She got the OK from her bosses for me to get into bed with her. I took off my shoes, asked workers to get her as far over on the bed as they could so there would be room for me and got in. I cuddled close hugging her and kissing her and telling her how much I loved her. In the meantime, I asked her if she loved me, but no answer. Then I said to tell me yes or no. Then she said "yes," the first word she had spoken in a couple of months. I was ecstatic. I was never so happy in my life.

Now when I come to see her everyday, they have her in bed. I get in with her for about an hour. Then they get her up in a wheelchair. I am now a happy man. I am less depressed and sleep much better. I guess love does conquer all.

I would like to get this message out to the thousands of husbands and wives who would benefit from my experience. I hope you can help in this matter.[67]

During a conversation I had with Sol, he added a p.s. to this story: "After she said this 'yes,' Rita was talking again, and laughing at my jokes for about four months. Once I asked her if she thought I was handsome. She said, 'No. Cute.'" He laughed and hugged her!

Another capacity of people living with Alzheimer's that often goes unnoticed is their ability to continue to influence us, *if* we pay attention. Before experiencing symptoms of cognitive decline, Liz was the dedicated, competent, and formidable director of Waypoint Services, a non-profit organization that provided food, shelter, and low-cost day care to victims of sexual assault and domestic violence. Her love and compassion for this vulnerable population of women and children showed in everything she did professionally. Throughout Liz's journey with dementia, which was first diagnosed as Alzheimer's but, based on her symptoms, was more likely frontotemporal dementia (FTD), she retained her assertive personality, her concern for vulnerable women, and her ability to lead, influence, and teach in ways that changed lives. The key to unlocking this open secret was the willingness of Sondy, her wife, and Jacobi, the director of the care center where Liz lived for two and a half years, to follow Liz's lead and to humbly learn from her. Because of this environment that fostered open hearts and minds, Liz's "fierce" and "strong" leadership was revealed and flourished.[68]

Moving into a care center was a difficult transition for Liz, and on day one, her assertive personality surfaced. Liz was not happy being away from home, and her subsequent behavior was likely fueled by FTD symptomology. She got physical with the staff and hit another resident. She was pretty quickly transferred to a local hospital for psychiatric evaluation and medication assessment to manage her behavior, which is common practice when people with dementia are displaying acting out behaviors that are considered violent.

During the effort to stabilize her with medication that would both help and be tolerated, Liz was in and out of the psych unit at the hospital over the next year. Knowing that the psych unit was not designed for supportive memory care, each hospital transfer put Sondy into a state of despair. Liz's third hospital stay happened early in the Covid-19 pandemic, and due to the lock-down restrictions, Sondy was not allowed to enter the hospital. She imagined the fear and confusion Liz must be feeling and knew that Liz would not be able to speak up about medication effects and side effects. Feeling powerless and panicky, herself, because she didn't have any input or control over what was happening inside the hospital, Sondy conjured up Liz's leadership for this situation by asking herself the question: What would Liz do? Well, it turned out Liz would email the CEO of the hospital and insist that she be allowed to be with her wife to support and soothe her and to assist in the medication management decisions. The imagined nudge from Liz to be assertive and her internalized voice offering specific guidance worked. Sondy sent an email to the CEO, stated her case, and was allowed to be with Liz. This helped to calm and heal them both.

On Liz's first tumultuous day at the care center, director Jacobi was faced with a decision to make: Could their care center safely and compassionately manage a resident with advanced dementia and such complex behaviors—or were they in over their heads? As Jacobi wrestled with the practicalities of staffing, stress, and quality of care, a different kind of question entered her mind: If we don't, who will? Well, they did. This choice led to a satisfying care center life for Liz, and for Sondy as her visitor and supporter. It also led to positive changes in the care center protocols for memory care since Leader Liz was always looking for ways to make the staff more efficient and compassionate, always coming up with ideas she did not hesitate to share for as long as she was able to do so; and, it led to life-changing learning for Jacobi.

After Liz's death, Sondy was concerned that Jacobi and the staff would remember Liz for all the wrong reasons. When hearing this, Jacobi quickly relieved Sondy of that notion. She said, "I am always going to remember Liz—as the person who reminded me to sit down and shut up, because I ALWAYS have something more to learn; as the person that taught me that sometimes you must push back and challenge those more powerful than you to evoke change, even it if scares the hell out of you to do it; [as] the person who taught me to fight for what I believe in, stand up for others when they no longer can, and to be stubborn enough to prove everyone wrong . . . . But most of all, I will remember Liz as the person who solidified my belief that 'if I don't, who will?'"[69]

As a spiritual director, I take seriously my intention to recognize and respond to the movement of the Spirit of Life in all aspects of creation. One evening, a particularly surprising and challenging experience brought to life for me Jim Ellor's belief that people with Alzheimer's can guide us into deeper relationships with God.

It was the holiday season. As I walked down the long corridor, admiring the festive holiday decorations, I noticed Ruth. She appeared restless and agitated. As I passed by her chair on my way to the craft room, Ruth leaned forward and reached out to me with her delicate hand.

Almost whispering, she said, "Can you come here? I have to ask you something."

Moving close to her and taking her outstretched hand in my own, I bent down and looked into her eyes. "OK," I said.

With grave sincerity, she asked, "Is Santa real?"

From the urgency of her expression and the firmness of her grip, I knew the answer to this question was really important to Ruth, so I didn't respond immediately. I looked closely into her eyes, and there I saw the answer.

"Yes," I said, returning her firm grip. "Yes, Santa is real."

She relaxed her grip ever so slightly and replied, "I thought so. But they are trying to tell me there isn't one."

"Who's telling you this?" I asked.

"Well, I don't want to say," she replied. "I don't want to get anyone in trouble."

"Oh no. You mustn't tell then," I said, reinforcing her choice to protect the doubters.

Still clearly upset by the quandary, Ruth leaned closer to me and asked, "But what should I do now?"

Time stopped. I took her hands in mine and looked again into her eyes. I felt a moment of true connection happening between us, and replied, "You just keep believing. You just keep believing."

"Yes," she said, taking a slow breath of relief. "Yes. I'll do that."

"Just keep believing," I repeated this over and over like a mantra, more to myself now than to Ruth.

"Thank you," Ruth said, her sweet smile revealing a row of missing front teeth. "I feel so much better." She let go of my hand and sat back in her chair with a sigh of relief, peaceful at last.

Ruth is not the real name of the one-hundred-year-old woman who asked me if Santa is real. I didn't know her name when we spoke. Although she also had Alzheimer's disease and lived in the nursing home on the same floor as Mom, I had never before met her or even seen her.

Receiving a question about Santa's existence from this stranger had caught me by surprise, and at first, I wasn't sure how to respond. Mom was no longer talking, so my skills for verbally meeting people with Alzheimer's in their world were a bit rusty. But I did remember the importance of being present in this moment and the healing implications of meeting people with Alzheimer's in their current reality, which for Ruth might have been Christmas, 1915. I did my best in a confusing and stressful moment for her, and she felt better.

After I left Ruth and walked on toward the craft room to work on a project with Mom, I noticed that I felt better, too—light, peaceful, joyful—in the Christmas "spirit." As I later reflected on our conversation, I realized it was both an endearing and profound experience for me. I felt inspired at a deep level. From the intensity of her question, Ruth could have been asking me if there is a God. Given the course of Alzheimer's disease, every afflicted person—and their families and friends—might have spiritual doubts.

This encounter with Ruth reminded me of David Steindl-Rast's definition of God as surprise. Everything about this conversation was a surprise for me: a one-hundred-year-old woman asking about Santa, finding the healing answer in her eyes, and the power of my own words to bring comfort to someone in confusion and distress. I was also surprised by my suggestion to keep believing. It was an expression of my own faith: In the face of doubt, fear, and resistance, keep on believing in the possibility of goodness.

After Mom went to bed that night, I looked for Ruth to say good night but couldn't find her anywhere. For a fleeting moment, I wondered if Ruth was real, if the profound experience had actually happened. Of course, she was real; of course, it happened. A few months later, I officially met Ruth and enjoyed her company for almost three more years. But on that night, my hope for Ruth was that she slept peacefully, still believing that life can and does bring good gifts even in the midst of loss. I certainly slept well in this belief.[70]

When Mom began her journey through Alzheimer's, I was too terrified to even open a book about it. As her companion through the years, however, I have been given countless opportunities to confront my helplessness and fear. Somehow, I have managed to continuously welcome and embrace these opportunities. Within this embrace, I have come to see people with Alzheimer's through the eyes of one who seeks meaning and value and beauty in every person and every experience of life. Subsequently, Mom and my new friends with Alzheimer's have guided me into closer relationships with them, with myself, and with God. I have seen their beauty and their value and have fallen hopefully in love with them. Through my love for them, I have discovered satisfaction in life beyond my imagination, beyond my hope.

To consider people ravaged by a relentless disease such as Alzheimer's to be of value individually and socially, reversals in thinking and imagining are essential. In a culture such as ours, where youth and external beauty are practically worshipped, these reversals are especially challenging.

At a dementia conference in Massachusetts, I met Olivia Hoblitzelle. She shared heart-opening vignettes of companioning her husband, Hob, through Alzheimer's. His greatest fear related to his disease was "of being a nuisance." A devout and practicing Buddhist, Hob discussed his fear with his guru, Jim, whose reply reminds us that care receiving is another opportunity to consider life's challenges as lessons in becoming more fully human. "If you feel like you're being a nuisance, Hob, then you're going to have to learn to live with those feelings, too: letting people care for you, learning to receive. Consider all this a spiritual discipline!"[71] Hob is not alone in this concern. Almost every older and disabled person I've encountered has vehemently said, "I don't want to become a burden." Mom and her neighbors remind me that we may not have a choice about diminishing to the point of dependence, but what if caregiving for people with Alzheimer's and dementia doesn't have to be a burden?

As I gazed out over the sea of wheelchair orphans at Rhythm Time, my thoughts drifted to Victor Hugo's insightful words from *Les Misérables*: "The beautiful is as useful as the useful . . . . Perhaps more useful." My attention returned to Mom and "The Beer Barrel Polka," performed with dedication by a woman who has played the accordion for more than fifty years. Mom's eyes followed me as I swayed and hopped in rhythm, careful to stay within her line of vision. She smiled and tried to tap her feet. I saw this tapping attempt, and my heart swelled with love and pride. I smiled back. Mom and her neighbors in that room all had the potential to beam forth the beauty and light of the divine force of the universe, and those who are paying attention will notice and celebrate the barely perceptible foot tapping.

6   Redefining Self

When Auguste D. first met Dr. Alzheimer, she described the anguish of her condition by saying, "I have lost myself."[72] Her medical records don't elaborate on what Auguste meant by this declaration, but most likely it was her memory loss and cognitive decline that brought the first identified Alzheimer's victim to the point of wondering about life's most important existential questions: Who am I? What is my "self"?

French philosopher René Descartes pondered these same questions in the seventeenth century, reaching this conclusion: "I think, therefore I am." His conclusion expresses the common definition of *self* as it was understood by dominant European philosophy and theology during Auguste's lifetime, including in Germany where she lived. Although this definition remains dominant in twenty-first-century American culture, modern theologian Richard Rohr asserts that Descartes' statement "was probably the lowest point of Western philosophy."[73] Neuroscientist Antonio Damasio evaluates the logic and persisting impact of Descartes' statement in his book *Descartes' Error: Emotion, Reason, and the Human Brain*. Through his important research, Damasio has brought to our attention the valuable roles our bodies and emotions play within the processes of brain activity and reason.[74]

In the context of societies where the self was, and is, considered fundamentally rational, disembodied, and solitary, it's understandable, and heartbreaking, that people with Alzheimer's disease experience their memory loss and other cognitive diminishments as a loss of self. However, if alternative understandings of self were accepted and valued, would people with Alzheimer's or other diseases of dementia continue to experience their decline of cognitive memory and abilities as an existential loss of self?[75]

During the 1970s, feminist theologians and writers brought forth their understanding of the human self as *relational*. Damasio presented his similar understanding in research first published in 1994. These insightful explorations of self, refuting Descartes' narrow definition, include our bodies, our feelings, our relationships, and our communities.[76] As we apply this more holistic understanding of self to people with Alzheimer's, we—and they—will be able to recognize the ever-enduring self. Within Mom, and within the hundreds of residents with Alzheimer's and dementia living with her at the nursing home, I met the self that remains throughout the long course of Alzheimer's.

The Embodied Self

As I considered the necessity of approaching Alzheimer's from the perspective of holistic healing, I became consciously aware that one of the body's remaining capacities was its ability to heal itself. On a quiet Saturday morning, from the deserted hallway of the nursing home, I heard a resident named Iris weakly calling for help. I peeked into the hallway from the door of Mom's room and saw Iris lying on the floor. I rushed to her side and saw that her shoe was untied. She must have tripped over her dangling shoelaces and fallen. Her face was already showing bruising, and she was crying in pain. After reassuring her that I would bring help, I sprinted to the nurses' station. Because Iris couldn't articulate the source of a specific injury or describe her pain, a couple days passed before she was taken to the hospital and it was discovered that her arm had been broken in the fall.

Seeing Iris day after day, I witnessed her embodied memory for healing. The black-and-blue bruises on her face changed colors every day, to purple and red, then green and yellow, and finally they disappeared. At the same time, the broken bones in her arm, protected by a cast, were knitting themselves back together. In the exact amount of time it would have taken for my broken bone to heal itself—six weeks—Iris's broken arm was repaired. Her healing process was, for me, a shining demonstration that Iris and I were alike. In many ways, our bodies were similarly functioning and remembering. Throughout my daily observation of Iris's healing, what most intrigued me was the coexistence of healing and decay. Her teeth were continually falling out; she was losing weight and losing words; she was walking less. But by healing her wounds and various subsequent infections, Iris's body continued to reveal her aliveness.

People with Alzheimer's will react to physical pain throughout the course of the disease. One night, during my first trip to Iowa when Mom was experiencing moderate-stage symptoms, she was washing dishes and something happened. I didn't know what, but she started saying over and over in a plaintive tone, "Little finger, little finger, little finger." She clutched her finger. I asked what happened, but she said only, "Little finger." I examined her finger; there was no blood. So I held her finger for a minute, applying pressure. Then, not knowing what else to do, I kissed it. This was a moment of confusion for us both. Mom couldn't tell me what had happened; I didn't know if her finger was broken or burned or pinched or bruised. I felt helpless and wanted to cry. Should I take her to the emergency room? While I was trying to decide, the pain must have subsided—healed by the kiss. Mom relaxed and returned to the dishes.

In the end stages of the disease, when Mom couldn't say what hurt, she expressed her pain by grimacing, wincing, shaking, and when the pain seemed to be at its worst, her eyes rolled back into her head. At these times, she was unresponsive, her body limp. This was frightening to me, but Mom was taking care of herself. She knew exactly what to do to get through the pain, and she knew how to communicate her distress to those around her who were knowledgeable and observant so she could get the help she needed.

In addition to reacting to painful sensations, people with Alzheimer's respond appropriately to touch that is gentle and loving, or brusque and rough. Various forms of gentle healing touch may have wide implications for improving the quality of life for people with Alzheimer's. When Mom was in the hospice program, one of the benefits was a biweekly massage. The massage therapist told me that one of his male clients surprised his daughter by liking the massage. The daughter was shocked that her father allowed the massage therapist to touch him at all; that he liked it was beyond her comprehension. People with Alzheimer's who have previously resisted being touched might change their preferences, so it's important not to make assumptions that could deprive the embodied self of healing.

Mom also appeared to love her massages, which were gentle, unlike the deep tissue massage many younger people use for releasing muscle tension. During her massages, Mom either kept her eyes wide open, watching every motion but resisting none, or closed them, wearing a blissful, peaceful expression on her face. Because she was in and out of the hospice program, she didn't receive massages regularly. In between professional massages, I continued offering her gentle, healing touch by massaging her face, neck, shoulders, hands, and feet.

Families and friends often wonder what to do when visiting people with Alzheimer's, especially in the late stages as verbal communication wanes and other shared activities, such as playing cards or games, are no longer possible. During these stages, I chose to initiate activities with Mom that I enjoyed, such as listening to music, watching a particular program on television, or just looking out her window at the beautiful countryside surrounding the nursing home. I would stand behind her and gently massage her shoulders. This became a shared activity that greatly enhanced our connection and our well-being.

An opportunity for Mom to receive more healing touch found me at the grocery store. Linda was stocking shelves when I asked her a question about where to find a product. We started talking, and she mentioned that she was training to become a reflexology practitioner. For her internship requirement, she was looking for clients to practice on for free. Remembering that one of my spiritual direction teachers talked about her ministry of reflexology to nursing home residents, I volunteered Mom. Over the next several months, Mom received weekly reflexology treatments, which involved gentle massage of and light pressure to specific points on her hands and feet. After the first appointment, I arranged for the sessions to happen when I wasn't there, so Mom would have more company to make her days interesting. Linda brought music and oil and her loving presence into Mom's life.

According to Dr. Robert Stern, "There is all kinds of research out there that the body and mind respond to touch in very positive ways. Whether it will actually have an impact on the progress of [Alzheimer's] is very unlikely, but providing someone with a connection ... can only be positive for both."[77] I'm sure Mom enjoyed the healing touch of reflexology, and perhaps it helped to strengthen and heal her body in certain ways. She couldn't say how her body was being affected as a result of the treatment, but clearly, a special relationship developed between Linda and Mom. After Linda completed her training program, she had to charge for her services, which we couldn't afford, but she continued to be a friendly presence in Mom's life. She sent cards. She visited and brought flowers. Mom smiled in her presence. The experience of reflexology had bonded them. Physical touch can reach beyond words, beyond reason, into the heart of who we really are and what truly nourishes us: relationship.

Damasio writes that our sensing body states are "inherently ordained to be painful or pleasurable." Without the reactivity of the body, "there would be no suffering or bliss, no longing or mercy, no tragedy or glory in the human condition."[78] It was my deliberate intention to assist Mom in experiencing bliss and mercy and glory for as long as her self was living in her body.

The Emotional Self

Neuroscience researchers in Iowa have scientifically proven that emotional memory is retained by cognitively impaired people whose brains have damage to the hippocampus, as is the case with Alzheimer's.[79] Having emotions and emotional memory shows, beyond doubt, that people with Alzheimer's have not lost their selves. The research supporting this claim indicates that people with cognitive loss can still experience an emotional stimulus in the moment. Although they cognitively forget the stimulus quickly, the emotional reaction generated by the stimulus, for better or for worse, will be retained for long periods of time.

People with Alzheimer's can experience and express a range of emotions throughout the course of the disease, including joy, gratitude, anger, and fear. According to Paul Raia, people with Alzheimer's are very emotional, and their emotions are usually appropriately expressed given their interpretation of their experiences, although this appropriateness may not always be evident to or appreciated by observers.[80]

Sadness. One morning as I crossed the parking lot of the nursing home, I saw Etty's husband and their dog get into their car and drive away. When I got upstairs, Etty was standing in the middle of the hallway, weeping. She always recognized me as a familiar person, and when she saw me on this day, she walked toward me. I opened my arms, and she melted into my embrace. I held her as she cried. She seemed comforted, and when she stopped crying, she led me to her room to show me her stuffed dog. Nursing home staff, unaware of Etty's recent family visit and departure, wouldn't have been aware of the rational cause and effect of her tears.

Joy. Once a month, a country singer came to Mom's floor of the nursing home and entertained the residents. At the first concert we attended together, Mom's smile and the sparkle in her eyes indicated obvious joy. To further demonstrate her appreciation and happiness, she attempted to clap. She raised her hands, moved her arms (by herself, without any cueing from me), and then clapped her hands together—once. She couldn't seem to remember how to unclap. And so, her hands remained clapped as she continued to enjoy the music. She tapped her toe as her whole face smiled, and her eyes gazed with admiration at the singer. After the concert, I helped her stand (hands still clapped together), and before I could direct her toward her room, she walked away from me, making a beeline toward the singer. I followed her and told him about her clapping effort. He took her hands into his, looked into her eyes, and said, "Thank you so much." Her smile told me that this event and this contact with the singer had made her day.

Gratitude. Isabel asked a nursing home staff member who was stocking the bathrooms if she could please have another roll of toilet paper. "Sure," the aide said, and she went off to get an extra roll. Then Isabel asked for another roll. This would make three in her bathroom, but the aide said, "Sure." After receiving the third roll, she asked if it would be possible to get a box of tissues. "Sure," the aide said again. When the aide placed the box of tissues in Isabel's hands, she smiled brightly and said, "Thank you so much. I think this is the nicest thing anyone has ever done for me." "How easy it was," the aide told me, "to make her so happy." Because many people with Alzheimer's can no longer verbally express their appreciation, this was also a particularly special, day-making moment for the aide.

Anger. In the dining room, most residents were accustomed to sitting in regular places. Maxine sat at a table with another woman resident and her husband, who was there to assist her with meals. One day there was an empty chair at their table. When I started to pull the chair away so I could sit by Mom, Maxine erupted into anger. "You can't take that! That's my sister's chair! She's coming today!" I had accidently violated unspoken dining room rules: Don't agitate Maxine. Don't try to help her eat; don't touch the chairs; and don't sit at her table. Not wanting to agitate her, but needing the chair, I asked, "Well, do you think it would be OK for me to borrow this chair until your sister arrives? I want to sit by my Mom." "Of course," Maxine replied, showing a big toothy smile sorely in need of dental intervention. "Thank you," I said. "Let me know when your sister gets here, and I'll return the chair." "OK," Maxine replied. Then she added, "Do enjoy your lunch with your mother, dear." Anger transformed into cooperation. Maxine was able to respond in a friendly way to a clear request that made sense to her. Maxine's sister never arrived that day— or any day. She had passed away a decade earlier.

Fear. When feeling threatened or afraid, people with Alzheimer's will express fear, and if they can, they will protect themselves. Marta, a high-school friend whose eighty-seven-year-old mother Gwen had Alzheimer's and was in a nursing home in Oregon, described an incident she witnessed. While trying to give Gwen her medication, the nursing home aide startled her. Because the room was crowded, the aide shoved a spoonful of applesauce laced with ground-up pills at Gwen's mouth from behind her. Marta reported seeing a flash of panic in Gwen's eyes. In that instant, she was startled and frightened by the sudden approach of the spoon. With an instantaneous self-protective reaction, Gwen swatted at the air, hitting the aide's arm. The aide had not followed the prescribed protocol of getting Gwen's attention, making eye contact, and explaining that she had a spoonful of applesauce and medicine for her. Perhaps this aide was unaware that people with Alzheimer's often have compromised peripheral vision and that they eventually forget what spoons are and what they're for. What Gwen most likely saw and felt, therefore, was a foreign object being shoved into her face from out of nowhere. She was frightened and logically reacted by trying to protect herself.

Damasio's research confirms that human feelings "are not a luxury," and certainly not useless: "They serve as internal guides, and they help us communicate to others signals that can also guide them."[81] Gwen's immediate response was guided by the "emotional action program we call fear." This program, which was not taken away by Alzheimer's, "can get most human beings out of danger, in short order, with little or no help from reason."[82]

The Cognitive Self

When people with Alzheimer's can no longer speak, we could easily conclude that they can no longer hear or understand what's being said to them and around them. On the contrary, long after people with Alzheimer's have lost the ability to speak, they retain receptive speech: the ability to hear, comprehend, and respond to verbal language. Although many presume that people with Alzheimer's are "absent of will," researchers refute this presumption by revealing that they, "surprisingly, still communicate through gestures and some spoken language in the face of 'quite severe deterioration.'"[83] Michelle Bourgeois, professor of Communication Sciences and Disorders at Ohio State University, explains, "Persons with Alzheimer's will attempt to get us to understand with whatever remaining skills they have, so we need to stay with them, even when they challenge our limits of creativity, imagination, and patience."[84]

One rainy day at the nursing home, Mom and I walked together up and down the long hallways. The day-shift nurse was sitting at the desk as we passed by, and we stopped to chat with her. Being naturally curious about people, I asked how long she had been working there. It had been over twenty years. She said that when people learned she had worked in a nursing home for so long, they often asked her how she could work with the elderly. "Wasn't it depressing?" Mom must have heard "the elderly . . . depressing" because she clearly took something personally and was offended. She clenched her teeth, presented an angry look, and pounded her fist on the counter. The nurse and I looked at each other, stunned. The nurse took gentle hold of Mom's clenched fist and reassured her that she loved taking care of her. Then the nurse said to me, "Well, this has been an important lesson. I'll be more careful about what I say."

One night I arrived at the nursing home after dinner. The dining room aide had moved several chairs out into the hallway so she could clean the dining room floor. Six women, including Mom, and one baby doll were seated in these chairs in a line against the wall. I asked the aide if I could play ball with them and she found a multicolored beach ball for us to use. During the game with these six women—Etty, Lena, Iris, Ilene, Regina, and my mom—I learned something important about the capacity of people with Alzheimer's to understand and respond. I started by throwing the ball to Etty. She caught it and threw it back. I threw the ball to Lena, the woman sitting next to Etty, and then all the way down the line. After every woman had a chance to catch the ball and throw it, or bat it, back to me (at this point Mom could only catch; she had forgotten how to throw), I started again with Etty. This predictability got boring for me quickly, so I decided to mix it up. I threw the ball to each woman in random order, not just once but multiple times. I wanted to see if they were paying attention to the game. They weren't always, and either missed the catch entirely or were startled when the ball hit their hands. Then I began calling out each woman's name before I threw the ball to her, still in random order. As each woman heard her name, she immediately turned her attention to me. We made eye contact before I tossed the ball, and the catch success factor was almost 100 percent. So, then I tried another experiment. Before throwing the ball, I called out "Mom," and not one of them, including my own mother, looked at me. This reminded me of one of Dale Carnegie's principles: "Remember that a person's name is, to that person, the sweetest and most important sound in any language."[85] After that experience, I began using Mom's given name, Jeanne, when I talked with her. I wasn't sure if she knew she was my mother, but I was very sure she knew that she was Jeanne. I wanted her to be comfortable around me, and calling her Mom might have confused her about our relationship. I continued this practice until the last couple weeks of her life, when I started to call her Jeanne-Mom.

People with dementia can understand and respond to requests and do things further into the disease process than we might think.[86] However, bringing out their abilities to respond requires patience. When the weather cooperated, Mom and I went for walks outside almost every day. Since she lived on the third floor, an elevator ride was required. I remember the first magical time we walked to the elevator and I said to Mom, "Push the button down." At the time, I didn't know how much language she understood or how much she could do. As we stood at the elevator door, I saw her looking at the buttons— for a long time, it seemed to me. Then I noticed her arm slowly rising, her finger slowly pointing and finally pressing the arrow facing down. It took time, I assumed, for her brain to register the instruction and then to pass that instruction on to her body; then it took more time for her body to respond. Based on delayed responses, we could easily assume that the capacities of people with Alzheimer's are "gone," and push the elevator button ourselves. Mistaken assumptions and impatience could prevent caregivers from knowing that people with Alzheimer's can still do things and still want to do things.

My efforts to recognize and bring forth Mom's remaining cognitive capacities enhanced our ability to continue relating and enabled us both to feel joy over her accomplishments. I could see joy in her eyes and her smile, and it warmed my heart every time. Once inside the elevator, Mom could also respond to my instruction to push the button with the number of the floor we wanted. "Push one," I'd say. Beaming with pride, Mom would push the lighted round number 1 button. With tears in my eyes, I beamed right along with her.

The Relational Self

Alzheimer's does not take away the desire or the ability to form and appreciate relationships. Although Ilene and Alice lived on different wings in the nursing home, they met during lunch in the dining room for the residents with Alzheimer's. Through some kind of communication, they came to recognize each other as compatible companions. They walked hand in hand down the hallways after lunch, having a conversation in sentences unintelligible to others but seemingly satisfying to them. One day as I passed them and said, "Hello," Alice reached out to me. She took me by the arm and shared very clear words of wisdom. "You just take it as it comes, and you give thanks to God for another day." Alice and I became good friends.

Most residents in the nursing home continued to manifest the innate human desire to connect with others and to be useful and helpful. They were actively engaged in helping to clean the dining room after meals. Mom washed the tables; John wanted to sweep; Regina was always gathering up the dishes. Mom and her neighbor Etty enjoyed pushing others in their wheelchairs. Once when an aide and I were helping Mom to stand up from her wheelchair, Lena saw us from across the hall. She came right over and offered to help Mom. We carefully guided, assisted, and supervised Lena in helping Mom to stand, and Lena seemed happy and satisfied to be of help.

Fulfilling their desire to remain useful and productive helps to maintain the self-esteem of people with Alzheimer's. Keeping them actively involved in tasks at which they can succeed (such as folding laundry, setting the table, assisting with cooking, dusting, filling bird feeders, and watering flowers) helps them to sustain a good quality of life for a longer time.

After Miriam, the woman with Alzheimer's we first met on page 74, moved to the care center, her life was more than OK. In fact, she flourished. She voluntarily took on the role of "assistant" caregiver. Her interactions with the other residents involved helping them get acclimated when they first moved in, helping them stand and walk, and introducing people to each other. Rev. Diane concluded that, in Miriam's mind, she became the person she wanted to be when she retired, "the helper." "So often in our conversations," Rev. Diane said, "Miriam talked about going back to work at Walmart because she loved her job there as 'greeter.' She was convinced that her mind would work better if she could do this. Interesting. It seems that she was right!"

Violet, who was ninety-four and in the middle stages of Alzheimer's, demonstrated during her most lucid moments— often to the dismay of the staff—that Alzheimer's did not necessarily destroy a person's capacity to affect and influence people and situations. For me, one of Violet's most endearing qualities was that she did not hesitate to express her opinions. She was the most reliable food critic, almost daily stating her thoughts about the quality of the food she was served. If Violet said, "This is the worst chili I've ever tasted," I usually asked the kitchen to send Mom a grilled cheese sandwich and tomato soup, her favorite meal. Since Mom couldn't tell me whether or not she liked something, I watched closely for her reactions and listened to Violet's reviews.

One spring, the nursing home administration decided to replace the air conditioning system. Unfortunately, the timing coincided with an unexpected and severe heat wave in the Midwest. It was over ninety degrees outside and extremely humid. The third floor of the nursing home was almost unbearable. One particularly steamy night, as everyone capable of expressing their discomfort was doing so (mainly staff and family members), Violet took up the cause of helping her neighbors. In the dining room, she loudly stated the obvious and barked an order: "It is too hot in here! Somebody, get a fan." All the aides ignored her. She kept demanding a fan. Considering her request to be disruptive, one aide tried to shuffle her out of the room. "I'm not going anywhere!" Violet assertively resisted. "I'm staying right here until you get some fans to cool off these poor people!" Which they finally did. This incident brought to mind the parable from the New Testament about a neighbor who comes knocking at midnight to borrow bread for an unexpected guest. The request is granted, not from generosity or because of neighborliness, but because it was the only way to get the annoying knocking to stop![87] Ask and you shall receive is the moral of the story. But Violet demonstrated that in order to be effective in our asking, persistence might be necessary. Ask and ask and ask . . . and then you shall receive. This was such an inspiring and empowering model for speaking up on the caregiving journey on behalf of the powerless.

The propensity of people with Alzheimer's to hold, feed, and care for baby dolls demonstrates their remaining instinct for nurturing. At first glance, giving dolls to elderly people and others with cognitive decline might appear demeaning. But dolls, teddy bears, and other soft, cuddly creatures bring them comfort and company. The night I was playing ball with the group of six women and one baby doll, I witnessed the nurturing instinct in action. The doll was sitting on a chair next to Etty. A rogue toss of the ball bounced off the doll's head and knocked her onto the floor. Etty reacted to this injury to the doll with horror, glaring at me like I was a murderer. She picked up the doll and cradled her. She carried the baby doll to her room, put the doll into her own bed, covered her up, and sat with her until it was bedtime. A retired teacher, Etty didn't have children of her own. She was, however, the most protective of the dolls and the most visibly reactive if any seemed injured.

Both men and women were attracted to the dolls. John had been a single parent to his seven children after his wife died giving birth to their youngest son. John loved caring for the baby dolls. His gentleness with them was remarkable. All of the residents regularly held the dolls; some would hold them, coo at them, and rock them for hours. They enjoyed talking dolls, crying dolls, soft dolls, and especially the ones that resembled real babies. Often the residents were more interested in engaging with the dolls than they were in eating. At meals, some of the residents attempted to share their food with dolls and teddy bears. It was messy but very sweet. A few times, young aides brought their real babies to visit the residents—this was a highlight in everyone's day. As were puppies who visited.

The instinctual energies of the libido are also still alive in people with Alzheimer's. This became especially evident at Mom's nursing home when Rick came to work as an aide on her floor. Tall, dark, handsome, and very kind, Rick became an instant favorite among the many female residents. With dazzled eyes and giggly, groupie-like smiles, they followed Rick up and down the hallways like a brood of ducklings lined up behind their mother.

Remaining energies of the libido can propose challenges as well. One resident, who evidently forgot he was a priest, flirted with and attempted to touch the young female aides. In response to such situations, many nursing homes offer the option of same-gender aide care. This was helpful to the aides in Mom's nursing home because some of the male residents were flirtatious, even flirting with me. Some flirted in ways that were charming, others in ways that were gross. I didn't react negatively to either approach because I saw the flirting as a glorious reminder of humanity shining through Alzheimer's. However, when I knew this was a potential factor in a male resident's behavior, I didn't get close enough to risk being touched or grabbed.

Sometimes the residents flirted with each other. At lunch one day, Mom and I sat at a table with Bert and Regina. Bert thought Regina was his wife, and he repeatedly touched her hand and asked her to go to his room. Regina was shocked and offended. Blushing, she firmly responded, "No! I'm married." Her response was clear, but she was overtly flustered. After this episode, the staff seated them at separate tables.

Care facility stories of residents with Alzheimer's meeting and forming romantic or special relationships with other residents are common—even if they are married to someone else. In the movie *Away from Her*, a wife with Alzheimer's explains to her husband her attraction and connection to another male resident. "He doesn't confuse me," she says. This is another reminder that we can maintain and nurture our relationships with people with Alzheimer's if, throughout the disease process, we can remember to meet them in their worlds.

Violet's ninety-five-year-old boyfriend took the bus from downtown every day to visit her. One day at lunch, she told me they were engaged. "How wonderful!" I exclaimed. "And when is the wedding?" I asked. "It was supposed to be in the spring," Violet replied. "But I might have to postpone that if I haven't lost enough weight to get into my wedding dress."

The Spiritual Self

Dr. Allen Power has worked as a physician and advocate for people with dementia for decades. Drawing on evidence from his own experience, he concludes, "Even people with advanced dementia can experience well-being and growth."[88]

In addition to wanting to enhance Mom's well-being, a big part of my inspiration for choosing to be with her during the last part of her journey through Alzheimer's was my belief that the instinct for growth is in every one of us—from birth until death. This includes, of course, people with Alzheimer's. We all have the momentum for physical growth; if we live long enough, we will grow into decline of body and mind. But we will also retain the potential to grow emotionally, spiritually, and more deeply into our humanity. These were the areas of growth where I felt I could be of service to Mom. A wise teacher once said that our purpose for being born is to help each other get through it all to the other side of life. "We're all just walking each other home," said spiritual teacher Ram Dass.[89] I came to Iowa to support Mom's growth process and to help her get to the other side—home. I understood that making this choice would involve sacrifices, which I readily accepted. I was quickly surprised and humbled, however, to discover that, from a spiritual perspective, there was more to it. By helping Mom, I received much more than I gave, enhancing my spiritual and emotional growth, on many levels, and deepening my connection to all of humanity.

Teresa of Avila, a Catholic saint, wrote about spiritual growth and self before Rene Descartes was even born. She was aware of the limitations of the human mind, and her definition of self is considerably more expansive than his. "It seems to me," she writes, "that the soul is a different thing from the faculties and that they are not all one and the same." She continues, "Each of us possesses a soul, but we do not prize our souls as creatures made in God's image and so we do not understand the great secrets which they contain."[90]

As Alzheimer's disease progresses, it claims memory and cognition. It claims speech and movement. It does not, however, claim the self, the soul, which, according to Western theologians and Eastern spiritual teachers going back into antiquity, is endowed with an immortal essence. The Hindu scripture *The Bhagavad-Gita*, composed in the first century AD, describes the self in the Second Teaching:

> Our bodies are known to end,
> but the embodied self is enduring,
> indestructible, and immeasurable;
> therefore, Arjuna, fight the battle![91]

On the surface, *The Bhagavada-Gita* chronicles the resistance of warrior Arjuna to fighting in a just war. It is a heartfelt, authentic conversation between Arjuna and his teacher, Krishna. As the story evolves, we realize that war is a metaphor for the challenges in life we all would rather avoid. Challenges like Alzheimer's and caregiving. The instruction to Arjuna to "fight the battle" is also an instruction to us to do our duty—to be the best caregivers we can be—because the self of our loved ones is alive and well and will be as long as breath animates their bodies. Those who define *soul* as "relational potential" have recognized this enduring self "even in the persons most severely affected by dementia."[92] If only we could perceive and know the souls of people with Alzheimer's, what treasures we might discover!

> When ignorance is destroyed
> by knowledge of the self,
> then, like the sun, knowledge
> illumines ultimate reality.[93]

In 1992 (more than thirty years ago!), psychologist Steven Sabat and Rom Harre, philosopher of psychology, argued that the "so-called loss of self is contingent on the failure of those around a person with dementia to respond positively to fragile clues of selfhood" that are not lost even in the end stages of the disease.[94] Noticing these fragile clues was a spiritual practice for me, and it brought me so much joy.

Perhaps anticipating a forthcoming, Descartes-like conclusion about the self as defined by mental faculties, Teresa reached a conclusion in direct contrast to this idea. She says, "The important thing is not to think much, but to love much. Do then, whatever most stirs you to love."[95] Indeed. Theologian Sam Keen echoes her thoughts in his book *To Love and Be Loved*: "In the depths of our being, in body, mind, and spirit, we know we are created to love and be loved. Fulfilling this imperative, responding to this vocation, is the central meaning of our life."[96]

Teresa's words are equally applicable and meaningful for caregivers and people with Alzheimer's. According to Australian researcher Stephan Millett, if Alzheimer's caregivers "are helped to understand the inner life of a person with dementia, to look at them from the inside out, so to speak, they will be more likely to act for the sake of the individual with dementia and exercise sympathetic care."[97] Empathic caregivers are more likely to love than think; and effective, loving caregiving has the potential to advance both well-being and growth for care receivers and caregivers.

Because inevitable and relentless physical decline reminds us that death is ever near, we don't naturally consider the aging bodies and beings among us as valuable. We usually don't open ourselves up to embrace what Olivia Hoblitzelle, inspired by Teilhard de Chardin, calls the "grace of diminishment,"[98] and we rarely consider aging or illness to be a universal power that will ultimately transform into life-giving factors. In the fifteenth century, Dutch theologian and Catholic priest Desiderius Erasmus wrote, "Bidden or Unbidden, God is present."[99] Similarly, whether or not we accept and embrace the life-giving possibilities coexisting within the diminishments of Alzheimer's, they are still present.

In people with Alzheimer's, I have witnessed—over and over—an enduring resilient capability and an ever-growing openness to giving and receiving love. In body as well as spirit, people with Alzheimer's who have lost cognitive abilities still know that they are created to give and receive love, and they will instinctively seek to fulfill their vocation by forming and deepening relationships when given the opportunity.

Hannah, one of Mom's neighbors at the nursing home, was ninety-two. In the winter, she became ill and stopped eating. Everyone thought she would die. Although she was weak and thin, she surprised us by surviving. She began to eat again—even feeding herself. She once again smiled, walked, talked, and engaged with others. One evening as I walked into the dining room to assist Mom with her dinner, Hannah saw me and smiled. She extended her delicate, now bony hand to me. Her hair had been styled in the beauty shop, and her fingernails glowed like sun-drenched, hot-pink peonies. I smiled with pure joy seeing her in this remarkable condition. I took her hand and held it. Our eyes met. Neither of us spoke, but the intimacy of the connection between our hands and our eyes brought tears to Hannah's eyes; then to mine.

"You're beautiful," she whispered in her slight, gracious southern drawl. My joy and my smile widened. I hugged her. She hugged me back, holding me close in a long embrace. When I looked into her eyes again, she drawled in a stronger voice, "I love you."

The stresses of my day drained out of me, and I felt transformed by the power of this surprising interaction. I took a long, deep breath and replied, "I love you, too, Hannah," feeling it to the depth of my being.[100]

In our society, we debate over which part of a human is most valuable: body, heart, mind, or spirit. Which deserves the most respect? The most care? The most attention? As I ponder this, it seems absurd to even ask the question. Until death, the parts are inseparable. According to Stephan Millett's research, "people with dementia continue to perceive and feel and to create a life-world"[101] in spite of diminishing cognition. Years ago, one of my most important mentors, ethicist and author Stephen Post, was presenting at a conference in India. During his keynote address, he spoke about the personhood of people with dementia, saying, "Deeply forgetful people should never be feared or devalued, bullied or derided." He added that certain capacities, such as kindness, mirth, and creativity, could be revealed once their minds are freed from cultural constraints.[102] In response to these comments, a Hindu philosopher stood in the crowd and emphatically stated, "Correct, we must uphold equal regard and respect because the moral worth of a person is based on consciousness alone, not on memory or rationality. Namaste: we must honor the sacred consciousness of all people."[103]

People with Alzheimer's are conscious. Although some seem unresponsive, they are not in a coma—a state of deep unconsciousness. They are not brain dead. Stephen Post reminds us that "someone who is deeply forgetful is as conscious of beautiful fall colors or exhilarating music as anyone else. *Equality of consciousness is more fundamental to moral considerations than equality of intellect and memory.*"[104]

The souls of people with Alzheimer's—the immortal essence, the reflection of God, the relational potential, the "self"—remain strong and shining throughout their lifespan. Until their last breaths, people with Alzheimer's and dementia *are*.

Since love and relationship, even more than cognition, define who we are and enliven our beings, I offer this alternative, inclusive, everlasting definition of selfhood: *I long to give and receive love—therefore, I am.*

7 Into Our Hands

Communication attempts by people with Alzheimer's, especially as the disease progresses, can be confusing for caregivers, but sometimes people with Alzheimer's have trouble understanding our words and actions as well. Perhaps we talk too fast. Perhaps we're not facing them and making eye contact as we talk. Perhaps we don't know that they can't differentiate between consonants and that "Let's get in the car" sounds like an invitation to get in the "star." Perhaps we move too quickly or approach them in ways that feel threatening. Perhaps our body language or tone of voice doesn't match our words. Cognitively impaired people, being highly sensitive and intuitive, will notice such discrepancies, reminding us that they may be more aware of our feelings than we are. Although they may not be capable of processing the implications of our feelings, words, and behaviors, they will notice and react to them.[105]

In confusing interactions, people with Alzheimer's could be like scared improvisers who, seeking safety, try to block our offers. When Gwen was startled by the aide shoving a spoonful of pills into her face, for example, she tried to block an action she perceived as threatening by swatting at the spoon.

Unfortunately, Gwen's intact emotional action program, cuing her to respond appropriately to fear, got her into, rather than out of, danger. Her self-protective swat apparently frightened the aide and the entire nursing staff. Subsequently, they took big steps to prevent this action from happening in the future.

Their success in this endeavor still haunts my dreams. According to Marta, Gwen's daughter, the aide reported Gwen's flailing swat to the charge nurse as "acting-out behavior." This category includes behaviors that are considered potentially dangerous to the person, other residents, or staff. Apparently, the aide considered a swat to her spoon-holding hand by a frail, eighty-seven-year-old woman as potentially dangerous. What happened next was standard procedure. Gwen was referred for psychiatric evaluation on the recommendation of the nursing home. The psychiatrist was told that Gwen was "acting out" by hitting people and refusing her medication. That was clearly an overstatement, or a misinterpretation, of the actual event. Gwen was admitted to the psychiatric hospital and prescribed antipsychotic medication and a sedative. Because she couldn't report side effects, she was overmedicated; perhaps wrongly medicated given the controversies at the time over prescribing anti-psychotic drugs for people with dementia. When Gwen returned to the nursing home, she was confined to a wheelchair. She slept most of the day slouched and slumped over the side of the chair. During the night, she was awake, agitated, and disoriented. Trying to get up on her own, she repeatedly fell out of her bed or chair, resulting in bruises and cuts on her legs. She slept through many of her meals. Because she was diabetic, missing meals altered her blood sugar in medically alarming ways. Additionally, she retained fluids, and her limbs became swollen. Although she was very groggy, Gwen was taken to every meal. In semi-lucid moments, she tried to eat and drink, and she ended up gulping her fluids. Previous to her hospitalization, Gwen did not need any help with her meals, so no one was helping her now, or even watching her. Another family member at the nursing home told Marta that Gwen was choking on her food and spitting up her gulped fluids. Soon she aspirated both food and fluid, and developed aspiration pneumonia. Three weeks after the incident with the medication aide, Gwen was dead.

In this chain of events, Gwen was not the only scared improviser. The nursing home staff, administrators, and the doctors who medicated Gwen all responded to perceived aggression in ways that contributed to the tragic outcome. "In reality," improviser Keith Johnstone tells us, "everyone more or less chooses what kind of events will happen to them by their conscious patterns of blocking or yielding. [An improvisation student of Johnstone's] objected to this view by saying, 'But you don't choose your life. Sometimes you are at the mercy of people who push you around.' [Johnstone replied], 'Do you avoid such people?' 'Oh!' [the student] said, 'I see what you mean.'"[106] People with Alzheimer's, however, *are* at the mercy of the benevolent/evil, informed/ignorant world. They usually don't have the option to avoid caregivers who push them around. Nor do most of them have the ability to say what they need, object to mistreatment, or require or request that caregivers become educated about Alzheimer's disease so they can be communicated with clearly and cared for properly. And when they do retain these abilities, they aren't always taken seriously.

Marta shared the day-to-day details of Gwen's condition with me, and over those three tragic weeks, asked many times, "What would you do?" Unfortunately, my responses didn't have much impact. Marta's stepfather, who was in his late eighties and somewhat confused, himself, was Gwen's "responsible party" at the nursing home. He was, therefore, the only one empowered to make medical decisions on her behalf. Like most family members of nursing home residents, he consistently approved the recommendations of the nursing home. Although Gwen had other children, Marta was her mother's most consistent companion. She encouraged her siblings to try to influence their stepfather, but they didn't want to upset him by challenging his decisions.

During Gwen's last weeks, Marta visited every day, becoming frantic because she was powerless to help her mother. She was angry about what had happened with the medication aide and distraught by the outcome of her mother's attempt at self-protection. Marta didn't want her mother medicated in the first place, but because she wasn't the official decision maker, she had no say about her mother's treatment. Because of the gulping, choking, and swallowing problems at meals, Marta moved mountains to finally convince her stepfather to attain a speech therapy evaluation for Gwen. This resulted in dietary changes to softer foods and thickened liquids, which, if implemented sooner, could have prevented the pneumonia that caused Gwen's death.

While keeping vigil at Gwen's deathbed, one of Marta's brothers admitted that he thought her dying was for the best. He then said that living with dementia was no kind of life. This attitude, shared by many in our society, is probably the reason why these sudden deaths of previously healthy individuals with dementia remain uninvestigated, and why the staff of so many care centers still remain uneducated about the specific needs of this population.

Each family touched by Alzheimer's will have experiences of conflict or cooperation that are as unique as the manifestation of the disease process. Caregiving responsibilities often bring out family conflicts that have been dormant for years, and invariably will separate those who can and can't handle it.[107]

Conflict within my own family complicated my desire to care for and accompany Mom. My sibling and I had parted ways almost thirty years earlier over disparate recollections of my abusive childhood experiences. However, I had been told that Alzheimer's sometimes has the ability to bring families together, so I was open to this possibility. Our vastly different ideas about Mom's needs and what constituted appropriate care for a person with Alzheimer's, unfortunately, widened the gap. My sibling, who was living with Mom during the onset of the disease, believed that preserving Mom's sense of independence was the top priority. Preserving autonomy is an important approach in the early stage, but when the progression of the disease puts a cognitively impaired person in danger, appropriate interventions become essential.

During my weeks with Mom in 2004, when she was in the moderate stage of her disease, I perceived her to be in danger. We went for a walk one afternoon, and when we reached a busy intersection, I paused to look both ways for oncoming traffic. Mom, however, pulled me by the hand into the street, and, without looking, started to cross.

"Wait," I said. "There are cars coming."

"That's no problem," Mom answered. "Cars have to stop for me."

I recognized other potential hazards to Mom's well-being. If her meals weren't prepared for her and her eating wasn't monitored, she probably didn't eat anything all day except candy from the bowl kept on the dining room table. Allowing her to have unrestricted access to alcohol, to use the stove unsupervised, and to wash dishes without having someone check the water temperature, all seemed like activities fraught with opportunities for injury. When I heard stories about Mom walking the dog, getting lost during below-zero days of winter, and wetting her pants, I really worried.

I insisted on taking Mom to physicians for an evaluation so her condition and her needs could be better understood as we determined a course of care. Through my later reading and study, I learned from gerontologist and theologian James Ellor that "the first place for advocacy" for a person with Alzheimer's is "ensuring that the impaired person has proper diagnosis of the disease."[108] I felt validated and relieved that I had followed my instincts and was able to at least do this to care for and protect Mom.

From my first encounters with Mom after the onset of Alzheimer's, I felt able and willing to handle her care. However, my sibling had acquired medical and financial power of attorney for Mom, and I was, like Marta, cast into the role of powerless bystander. For several years I was unable to care for my mother in any meaningful way. It was agony.

After my sibling moved, the path became clear for me to relocate to Iowa and become Mom's on-site companion and advocate. Although I was now living two blocks away from Mom, my sibling, who lived far away and visited rarely, didn't want to relinquish her control over Mom's care. It made logical sense to me that, as the person who was in the nursing home every day spending time with Mom and interacting with the staff, I should be the decision maker. After much soul searching, many sessions of legal counsel, great financial expense, and several court hearings, I was named Mom's legal guardian. Family conflict persisted, however. Although I grew weary of legal wranglings, I knew at a deep level that this struggle was part of caring for Mom. Knowing what had happened to Gwen and accompanying Marta through her frustration, despair, powerlessness, and loss, I knew that my legal expenses, the emotional turmoil, and the conflict with my sibling were worthwhile, and unquestionably my duty in service of Mom's care.

My new role as guardian, however, brought me face-to-face with decision-making that could prolong or shorten Mom's life. The awesomeness of this responsibility caught me by surprise. In several situations, I anguished over what to do. Mary Anne, another caregiver who had been through similar experiences and feelings, coached me by saying that, no matter what I decided, I would probably feel some despair and guilt. Hearing this was oddly comforting. I prayed that Mom's time for death would be inevitable and obvious regardless of what I decided. Thankfully, it was so.

A basic necessity of care for a person with Alzheimer's is a committed and involved companion tenderly giving love and attention, and an informed advocate fiercely monitoring medical, in-home, and nursing home care. Two years after the death of his mother May, my friend and colleague Steve spoke with a tinge of grief about his own "reserved, nonconfrontational" personality. He was tender, but he backed away from being fierce.

For his whole adult life, Steve has been an impassioned social justice advocate for the vulnerable. Consequently, he was surprised and disappointed by his inability to fiercely advocate for his mother on a personal level. In one instance, assisted by his wife, who is a nurse, he did successfully fight to prevent the nursing home and doctors from prescribing psychotropic medications to manage May's "behaviors." Steve was very clear that his mother was not the behavioral problem; the aides caring for her were. He was able to protect his mother in the way Marta could not protect Gwen. Ultimately, however, he could not protect her completely. One of the aides "let it slip" to Steve that May was given too much of a particular drug and that her kidneys were compromised and failing as a result. This would eventually lead to her death. Feeling defeated, he surrendered the fight and chose to be completely, compassionately present at his dying mother's bedside. He still carries within his mind, however, the imprinted images of incompetence and neglect that harmed his mother, and wonders if he should have pursued legal action against the hospital and the nursing home. Within his heart, he carries regret for his lack of fierce intervention on his mother's behalf, believing that he could have made different, better decisions for her.

Loretta, on the other hand, was an intentional, relentless, and fierce advocate for her mother, Doris, wanting her to be always treated with dignity. Eighteen years before Doris was diagnosed with dementia, mis-steps in Loretta's own medical care would influence how she cared for her mother. She had learned, the very hard way, not to make compromises in health care decisions. When she was in her twenties, Loretta experienced serious gynecological issues. She saw her doctor often, who repeatedly concluded that nothing was wrong; this was normal menstrual discomfort. Finally, because every month Loretta passed out at work from the pain and her co-workers had to call 911, her boss intervened, saying, "We love you, Loretta, but we can't keep calling an ambulance every month." Her boss suggested that she see his wife's gynecologist, and although the doctor was not taking new patients, he heard Loretta's story and agreed to see her. It turned out that Loretta had a very severe case of endometriosis (a condition resulting from the appearance of endometrial tissue outside of the uterus and causing pelvic pain). It took thirteen years, forty-seven hospitalizations, and twenty-one surgeries to resolve her condition. During this time, Loretta's new gynecologist ran into her previous gynecologist at a medical convention. He updated her on Loretta's condition and progress and asked why she had not evaluated Loretta for endometriosis. The other gynecologist replied, "Oh? I didn't think Black people got that." Anyone with a uterus, regardless of race or culture, is at risk for this condition.

After having this kind of dismissive, overtly racist medical experience, Loretta was prepared to act in a no-nonsense, assertive way when Doris encountered comparable race-related attitudes in her quest for dementia care, and she did act. She fired Doris' neurologist on their first visit. The doctor was aggressively insisting that Doris take the drug Aricept for what he described as mild dementia. She was resisting the idea, saying that she already took two pills. At this point, Loretta spoke up and said, "She doesn't have to take medication if she doesn't want to." Hearing this, the doctor snapped and blurted out, "That's what's wrong with you people. You don't want help; you just want to complain." Assuming "you people" was in reference to their race, Loretta's fierceness emerged, but ever so graciously. She stood up; she did not argue or curse; she gathered up their purses and coats; she took her mother by the hand; and they walked out of that doctor's office. She was not going to let her mother be in a situation where her needs and preferences were not taken seriously, where she was not treated with respect and dignity, and where race was obviously an issue for the doctor. They changed neurologists immediately.

Even though nursing home administrators, nurses, and aides, as well as physicians, may resist our input, family members and guardians must speak up on behalf of people with Alzheimer's because they cannot advocate for themselves. Although many of us do try to be proactive advocates, often the troubling situations don't seem to change in the short term. Some brave family members report infractions to state agencies, but generally, they can only effect change in the most egregious cases. More timid family members will complain to friends but never to the nursing home administrators for fear of staff retaliation against their loved ones. I was shocked to consider this possibility of retaliation, but apparently it happens in spite of a Resident Bill of Rights in most facilities promising that complaints can be voiced without fear of negative consequences for residents.

There were known incidents of abuse in Iowa care facilities during the years I was Mom's companion at the nursing home. One male aide had molested female residents with dementia all across the state. He was fired from several nursing homes but then quickly hired at others where he committed the same abuse. He was eventually caught and prosecuted. No one wants to think about these possibilities. We take our loved ones with Alzheimer's to state-inspected care facilities, expecting them to be safe and cared for. Although this expectation is reasonable, it is not always satisfied in the ways we want or in the ways our loved ones need. Even if things don't seem to change after we voice concerns and complaints, this doesn't mean that family members should give up and become silent. Our loved ones with Alzheimer's need us to speak for them. A staff member from the Alzheimer's Association advised me to advocate assertively for Mom. She said I would know my advocacy on Mom's behalf was effective if, when Mom passed away, the nursing home administrators were happy to see me go. I'm quite sure they were!

Steve, Marta, Loretta, and all the caregivers who do our best, need to be kindly reminded that we have shared our tender hearts with our loved ones. Although Steve and Marta could not prevent tragic outcomes, they were attentive, compassionate, empathic caregivers for their mothers; they felt their mothers' suffering and sought to relieve it. Their care "healed" their moms. Hopefully, this awareness will help—in time—to heal them as well.

My story of family conflict, Steve's story of regret, Marta's story of helplessness, and Loretta's story of medical neglect and racism are not unique. Numerous family members of people with Alzheimer's have shared similar haunting stories with me.

Unfortunately, the neglect, abuse, and financial exploitation of people with Alzheimer's is much more common than any of us would like to think.

The abuse and exploitation of New York socialite and philanthropist Brooke Astor by her son Anthony Marshall made headlines across the country. In 2009, the ABC news program *20/20* heightened my awareness about the exquisite vulnerability of people with Alzheimer's. Philip Marshall, Brooke Astor's grandson, recognized the neglect and abuse that his grandmother was enduring under his father's care. Encouraged by Brooke's friends to "do something," Philip reluctantly filed a petition to challenge his father's control and to become his grandmother's guardian and conservator.

Aware of the reality that every family conflict of this nature begins and ends in heartache, Philip Marshall and I shared the same internal turmoil: We wanted to care for our loved ones with Alzheimer's, but we didn't want to drag delicate family issues into the court system and thus into the public view. At the beginning of the Marshall family conflict, Philip naively hoped it could all happen quietly. He had no idea the heartache at the end would include nationwide news coverage and his father being sent to prison for financial exploitation of a dependent adult.[109]

Because many caseworkers from the Department of Human Services still hold the attitude that elder abuse concerns are a family matter that can and should be resolved within the family,[110] most of these cases never reach a prosecutor's office. The millions of dollars involved in the Astor conservator petition, however, caught the attention of the Manhattan District Attorney's office, and I was exceedingly grateful for the media attention to this story. Philip's courage gave me strength to continue my efforts to obtain the legal right to decide what was best for Mom.

As I tried to understand the process by which abuse could develop as Alzheimer's renders people living with the disease more and more vulnerable, I was once again enlightened by James Ellor:

[For family members] whose relationship with the senior have been difficult or abusive there is a sense of unresolvable anger ... the lack of resolution can turn into vengeance when the angry family member becomes legally responsible for the person with Alzheimer's. It may also turn into neglect, a result of the deep conflict of emotions between a feeling of filial responsibility and anger that enveloped the relationship.[111]

From the reports about the relationship between Anthony Marshall and his mother, abuse in childhood and unresolved anger certainly could have been at the root of his neglect, abuse, and exploitation of his mother.

Accurate statistics regarding the prevalence of elder abuse in the U.S. are not readily available because it is "a largely hidden, private matter," and agencies gathering the data—law enforcement and social services—are not often involved. In addition, "research and funding lag behind efforts in the comparable and related disciplines of child abuse and intimate partner violence." However, over the past two decades, The National Center on Elder Abuse (NCEA) has made strides in naming the problem, identifying areas of need, and organizing its efforts to expand research and interventions. The NCEA defines a "vulnerable adult as a person who is either being mistreated or in danger of mistreatment and who, due to age and/or disability, is unable to protect himself or herself."[112] According to Stephen Post, people with Alzheimer's are a particularly vulnerable population of elders "in need of special protections from those without dementia, who are capable of a myriad of abuses of power."[113] In a 1991 article about elder abuse, E. T. Lucas describes the chilling reality that continues thirty years later: "People with dementia ... are socially outcast, unwanted, marginalized, and oppressed. A remarkable amount of elder abuse and neglect falls upon people with dementia, not just because caregivers are exhausted or ignorant, but because people with dementia are defenseless and easily victimized."[114] Quoting studies from 2016 and 2020, the National Center on Elder Abuse indicates that

> Nearly one in two older adults with cognitive impairment experiences abuse. In addition to being dependent upon others for assistance, elders with dementia are more likely to experience deficits in memory, communication, and judgment that make it harder for them to identify, prevent, and report mistreatment. Many may also be reluctant to report abuse by caregivers and others upon whom they rely. Older people with dementia are often at an increased risk of mistreatment because of pre-existing medical and mental health weaknesses.[115]

When Mom moved to the nursing home, a zippered change purse disguised as a small stuffed frog survived the garage sale of her life and moved with her. This frog's belly held a religious medal Mom put there years before and some coins I added for card-playing wagers and treats from the ice-cream truck. One day, on our way to get ice cream, I opened the zipper of the frog purse (which had been kept on Mom's bookcase with other stuffed animals) and found that all of her money was gone. Presumably, one of the staff members must have taken the money. This is a clear example of people with dementia being defenseless and easily victimized. Even if Mom had seen someone taking her money, she couldn't have protested at the time or verbally identified the thief.

Sadly, too many people with Alzheimer's are victims of physical, emotional, sexual, and financial abuse; however, "harm" to this vulnerable population can also result from "the absence of love and care," according to Stephen Post.[116] Without question, taking pocket change from someone who can't speak represents the absence of care as well as the absence of respect and regard. If Mom was awake at the time of the theft and witnessed someone violating her in this way, it surely caused harm to her heart and her spirit. The experience may have left her feeling fearful. This type of theft happens so often in nursing homes that residents are warned to keep valuables in the safe. It happened to my friend Mary after she and her husband moved to an assisted living facility. Mary had put $400 cash into a metal box kept in the closet on a shelf. A few days later it was gone. She reported it to the management, but they didn't take her seriously. She has dementia, after all. Surely, she misplaced it. The perpetrators of these small and large violations are rarely identified.

It's notable that Mom's religious medal was left behind in the zippered belly of the frog. Since it was the same size as a coin, the thief, unconcerned about being caught, must have looked at each item, choosing only to take the money.

National research conducted by the Illinois Department on Aging in 2011, the most recent national data I could find, suggests that "elder abuse is seriously underreported because most people aren't informed, don't want to get involved, or don't know how to report an abusive situation." The report describes some of the challenges involved with protecting vulnerable elders from abuse:

- Only one out of thirty cases of elder abuse is reported. A woman interviewed in the film *Silent Crisis* reported being robbed of her life savings by her trusted, very wealthy daughter. The elder woman initially resisted telling anyone because she was ashamed and didn't want people to know that her own child had done this to her.

- Thirty-eight percent of reported abuse cases concern elders who are living with their alleged abuser. This represents a difficult challenge for social service caseworkers for gathering information and developing and monitoring a care plan.[117]

I met Felicia at a dementia care conference in New England. Her father was living in the southeast with Felicia's brother. A local social worker at a senior center noticed some problems and filed a complaint of neglect with the Department of Health and Human Services (DHS), and caseworkers initiated an investigation into her father's care. Throughout this investigation, relatives continually contacted Felicia with alarming reports about her father's care and condition. Felicia tried to intervene, but her brother told her to stay out of it. Although she didn't completely comply, Felicia kept her distance because she was afraid of her brother's volatile temper.

When Felicia heard her father had lost an alarming amount of weight, she ordered Meals on Wheels for him. After a few meals, her brother cancelled the service, explaining that their father didn't like the food and it was a waste. Felicia asked her father if he liked the food delivered by Meals on Wheels, and he said, "It's better than nothing." Indeed, it is. When Felicia heard that her father wasn't taking his Alzheimer's medication, she attempted to have visiting nurses come. They weren't allowed in the house. This was also what happened when her father's physician ordered a needs assessment.

After listening to the reports from her relatives, Felicia asked them to repeat their concerns to the DHS caseworkers. Not one of them agreed to do this. Like a chorus in a song, each person responded to Felicia's request to talk to DHS with the same words: "I don't want to get involved." Their reasons varied. One elderly relative told Felicia that she was afraid there would be negative consequences to her for speaking to "authorities." Felicia understood and accepted their decisions, but receiving their well-meaning reports of her father's unmet needs only made things worse for her. Having this information increased her worry, and since she couldn't intervene in a meaningful way, it also increased her feelings of helplessness and despair. Her father continued to suffer since DHS took no action.

Unfortunately, staff members in nursing homes who witness their colleagues mistreating or neglecting residents most often say nothing. One aide in a nursing home saw another aide hit a defenseless woman in the bath. By the time the grapevine informed the administration about this incident several months later, the abusive aide had moved out of town and the woman had died. The aide who had kept quiet was immediately fired. He didn't speak up at the time, fearing retribution from the abusive aide. He learned, however, that there are consequences for not speaking up as well.

Steve and I, and others who advocated for our loved ones with Alzheimer's living in nursing homes, were shocked by some nursing home and medical professionals' neglect, abuse, and objectification of this population.[118] Steve experienced it as "inhumanity." I experienced it as appalling and fought to make changes and healing choices, at least for my mother.

During Steve's investigation of nursing home placements for May, as well as the years he spent as his mother's companion and advocate, he became aware of classism in the world of Alzheimer's care. In some parts of the country, elders with financial resources are able to live in newer, cleaner, better-equipped facilities with private rooms and more highly trained, more caring staff. When I was investigating care facilities in Massachusetts, many of those that accepted Medicaid residents tried to convince me that housing four residents with Alzheimer's in one room was good for them. "They tend to isolate, so we don't let them spend much time in their rooms. And when they are in their rooms, they aren't lonely." This was definitely a good financial plan for the for-profit nursing homes, but newer recommendations for caring for people with dementia would not support their rationale.[119] In other parts of the country—Iowa, for example—some nonprofit facilities provide each resident with Alzheimer's a private room and bath. The administrators cite "dignity" as their rationale, and there is no differentiation due to Medicaid status.

In most areas of the country, elders without any financial resources or without any concerned family members will be taken care of—perhaps in lesser-quality facilities, perhaps in fabulous ones—by state and federal monies through Medicaid and Medicare. It is critical that we continue to support our vulnerable elders through these programs.

Contemplating the prevalence of and various explanations for elder abuse, particularly the issue of unresolvable anger, I recognized the deep significance that leaving home had for my own healing and, ultimately, for Mom's healing. Some people, aware of the intense vulnerability that is characteristic of Alzheimer's, perceive them as people who can be easily manipulated, abused, and exploited. Others respond with a desire to protect them. Between these polar opposite responses is a vast range of intentions toward vulnerable populations, including complicated, sometimes unconscious, motivations for caring. Acknowledging and exploring our own confusing feelings can present opportunities for caregivers to experience meaningful personal growth and to expand our relationships with our loved ones.

When my life journey intersected with Mom's Alzheimer's diagnosis and I touched the true meaning of vulnerability, something surprising and completely unbidden occurred. Witnessing Mom transform from an empowered, competent, independent woman to a confused, vulnerable, dependent, diminishing elder caused my heart to instantly widen. My heart ached to protect her and to care for her.

Had the intersection with Alzheimer's happened during an earlier phase of my life's journey, however, my heart would not have guided me to Iowa, into painful family dynamics in order to care for Mom. When I left my abusive childhood home thirty-three years earlier, I wandered in a wilderness of despair that involved denying my pain with substance abuse and other addictive behaviors. In my late twenties, overcome by unhappiness, I started therapy and made a deliberate effort to embrace my feelings and resolve my anger at my mother for not protecting me. It was a long, difficult, painful process.

I have a distinct memory of a conversation with my doctor about my relationship with Mom that happened about fifteen years before she was diagnosed with Alzheimer's. I was wondering about the wisdom of staying in contact with her, given that most of our conversations and visits resulted in long-lasting despair for me. My main question focused around Mom's assets, even though she was not a wealthy person. Would she still leave me something in her will if I broke off contact?

My doctor responded with practicality: "If your mother lives long enough, she will probably require some kind of nursing home care, and most likely, all of her assets will be used for her long-term care needs. So don't let money be your guide in this. Stay connected with your mother *if* you want to, *if* doing so is helpful to your healing." At that juncture, I chose to maintain contact with Mom from a distance that felt safe to me. Although I was angry at her and hurt by her constant rejection of me, my desire to love her was not extinguished. And I never stopped wanting her to love me.

My doctor's practical prediction did come true. By the time Mom died, all of her financial assets were gone.

After Mom visited me in Maine in 2003, I revised my own will to include a trust for her care, should she need financial support. My heart had opened to her and widened enough that I wanted to provide for her physical safety. Being in her presence, however, and caring for her myself—these options didn't enter my heart or my mind.

A year later, when I spent time alone with Mom in Iowa and intimately touched her world, I more fully witnessed and experienced her vulnerability. When she recognized my kindness and asked me to stay and take care of her, my willingness emerged and did not retreat. After another three years, I willingly made the necessary sacrifices and overcame sometimes daunting obstacles to move to Iowa and care for her.

My desire to do this, and even more my willingness, amazed me. Many who knew me and who knew the details about my childhood and my historically troubled relationship with my mother were stunned and disturbed by my decision. By acknowledging and resolving my anger, I became open to caring for Mom and thereby transcended the past, rooting myself in the compassion I felt for her in the present.[120] Many people in Iowa who witnessed my commitment to Mom's care remarked to me, "She must have been such a wonderful mother, that you would care for her so dearly." I smiled, leaving them with their own conclusion. I have learned that the reasons for caring—or not caring—for a family member with Alzheimer's are as unique as every family's history and every individual's healing journey.

I met Coleen at Mom's nursing home. Her mother Ilene lived across the hall from Mom. As Ilene began to show signs of "something wrong," she resisted Coleen's wanting-to-be-helpful presence in her life. Ilene was angry and directed her anger at her daughter. She accused Coleen of causing the problems she was having and manipulated other family members into doubting and criticizing Coleen. In her fear and confusion over the changes she was experiencing, Ilene lashed out at the person closest to her, perhaps believing that pushing Coleen away would resolve her own difficulties. Although Coleen stepped back and asked her brothers and sisters-in-law to watch over her mom during this time, she was not pushed away. She was always there in the background—aware, waiting, and ready. One day, Ilene's resistance was over. She called Coleen and asked her to come. Coleen left work and went immediately to her mother's side. Ilene said sadly, "I think something is wrong." Coleen replied, "I do too, Mom. I do too. But whatever it is, I'll be here. And we'll get through this." For over fourteen years as her mom's dependable companion and advocate, Coleen kept the "vow" she made to her mother that day.

"The truest test of any society," according to French philosopher Simone de Beauvoir, "is how it treats the aged, those who are an unwanted reminder of our frailty and mortality."[121] Alzheimer's disease, like nothing else we have yet experienced, has a profound way of shining a light on the truth of who we are— as individuals, as communities, and as a society. Alzheimer's can bring out both the best and the worst of human nature. My friend and ministerial colleague Carl Scovel pointed out that one important reason a society cares for its vulnerable people is that we all witness this caring; and then we trust that we, too, will be cared for when we are in need.

There comes a developmental point in Alzheimer's when those afflicted will have no choice but to trust others—to trust *us*—for their support and care. Clinical social worker Marty Richards explains that they trust us not out of desire, and not because we have earned their trust, but because of pure necessity.[122] At every moment, whether we are actively caring for someone with Alzheimer's, or waiting in awareness and readiness to give care, it's imperative to recognize that these exquisitely vulnerable people with Alzheimer's trust *us*. Into our hands and hearts, they *must* commend their fragile beings. People who are afflicted with Alzheimer's have not chosen their situations of frailty, dependence, and declining capacities. We, however, can choose. We can choose our attitudes and our reactions to their ever-changing, ever-increasing needs.

In the multicultural, multiracial, economically diverse country that is the United States, we have more yet to do to demonstrate to our society that we can be trusted with the care of this vulnerable and diverse population of people living with Alzheimer's. Recent research is showing us that "older Black and Latinx individuals are more likely than older white individuals to have ADRD (Alzheimer's disease and related dementia)," and that the increased risk factors for minority populations are related more to social, lifestyle, environmental, and economic reasons than to genetics.[123] "Racial and ethnic disparities in old age are likely to reflect a cumulative effect of disadvantage across the life span."[124] Since the seeds for the complex brain changes associated with Alzheimer's can germinate "a decade or more before memory and thinking problems appear,"[125] it would benefit individuals as well as all of society—for generations to come—if early health interventions were available for all. Perhaps the crushing tsunami could be averted.

Minority groups are also more at risk for a dementia diagnosis to be delayed, completely missed, or for the condition to be misdiagnosed.[126] Caregiver Daisy's mom, Sonia, was first assumed to be "crazy" by her neighbor who found her outside and barefoot in the snow on her way to work. The doctors diagnosed Sonia with depression; then mad cow disease; and later with Jakob's disease. A mad cow disease specialist in Australia referred Daisy to a specialist in New York, who referred her to a specialist in St. Louis near where she lived. After an evaluation in St. Louis, Sonia was diagnosed with early-onset Alzheimer's. She was fifty-five.[127] An inaccurate diagnosis like this can delay "access to timely and effective early interventions and recommendations, resulting in worse outcomes for the [person with Alzheimer's], caregiver and family."[128]

The vulnerability of people with Alzheimer's is a sacred invitation to individuals and to society to be trustworthy. To respond appropriately to this invitation, caregivers and others with authority and power need to learn about, accept, and embrace the realities of living with Alzheimer's. We all need to observe how the realities of this disease are manifesting in each afflicted person, in each afflicted family, and in each afflicted culture and racial group. This is, indeed, a challenge. It may, however, be the most fulfilling and rewarding challenge we will ever face.

Into our hands these dear ones with Alzheimer's disease have entrusted the care and cultivation of their fragile beings. May our tender hearts make us compassionate and trustworthy caregivers. May our fierce hearts empower us and make us effective advocates.

III

Spirit-Inspired Caring

"Where does the wind come from Nicodemus?"
"Rabbi, I do not know."
"Nor can you tell where it will go."

"Put yourself into the path of the wind, Nicodemus.
You will be borne along
by something greater than yourself.
You are proud of your position,
content in your security,
but you will perish in such stagnant air.

"Put yourself into the path of the wind, Nicodemus.
Bright leaves will dance before you.
You will find yourself in places you never dreamed of going;
you will be forced into situations
you have dreaded
and find them like a coming home.

"You will have a power you never had before, Nicodemus.
You will be a new man.
Put yourself into the path of the wind."

—Myra Scovel

When I moved to Iowa to be with Mom, I understood that making some sacrifices was a part of the decision. I left an established life, including wonderful long-sought, long-prepared-for professional opportunities. I still feel sad, sometimes, when I consider what I left behind. Additionally, there have been and continue to be some undesirable consequences for me. Yet I have no regrets. My decision to move was the right decision for Mom. And it was the right decision for me; of this I feel certain.

During my decision-making process, and my relocation and transition, I carried the poem *The Wind of the Spirit* close to my heart. This poem first became a guiding light for me in 2003 while I was seeking wisdom about shifting the focus of my ministry to spiritual direction.

I later discovered, quite by accident, that the poet, Myra Scovel, was the mother of my colleague, Rev. Carl Scovel. Ultimately, the truth of this poem guided my decision to care for my mother when Alzheimer's struck; it also chronicled the outcome of my "yes." As Myra's poem predicted, by putting myself into "the path of the wind," I found myself living in Dubuque, Iowa—a hometown I never dreamed of returning to; I was drawn into a situation I previously had dreaded—caring for a dependent, vulnerable mother who hadn't protected or cared for me when I was dependent and vulnerable; and this never-dreamed-of, dreaded circumstance, surprisingly, became a "coming home."

When I began this journey, it was inconceivable that a nursing home filled with people in various stages of Alzheimer's would become a holy land or that words like *suffering, Alzheimer's, gratitude, meaning,* and *joy* would be spoken in the same sentence, flowing sincerely from my healing heart.

Into the path of the wind . . .

8   Points of Surrender

Years ago, I attended a monthly Centering Prayer group. It was our practice to first pray in meditation for twenty minutes and then read together and discuss a spiritual text. One night the leader brought a reading that offered a theological explanation for the terms *letting go* and *surrender* within the context of spiritual living. After the reading, everyone reacted with, "Huh?" It seemed too complicated, too esoteric, bewildering. At this point, a young man in the group, an attorney, offered imagery that clarified my understanding of the difference between these terms and their spiritual meanings. "Letting go," he said, "is like being in a boat that's tied to the dock. We untie the rope." "Surrender," he said, "is being in the boat, without an oar, drifting in the waves, with trust in God."

After Mom moved to the nursing home and while I still lived in Boston, I was in regular contact with her by phone. She didn't talk much by this time, but the nurses told me she listened attentively and hearing my voice brought an ear-to-ear smile across her face. One day, she found the words to clearly blurt into the phone, "I miss my house!" I sighed, took a breath, and replied, "I know you do, Mom. I know you do." It was heartbreaking to know how much Mom missed and wanted to return to her home of sixty years.

One of Mom's friends had called earlier and told me of a visit with her. When the friend tried to leave, Mom clung to her, sobbing, begging to be taken home. It seemed to me that Mom was experiencing what theologian Marcus Borg calls "life in exile." She was separated "from all that was familiar and dear," and now, on the margins of society, she felt the depth of her powerlessness. Borg writes that "the feeling of being separated from home and longing for home runs deeply within us ... and life in exile is marked by deep sadness and an aching loneliness."[1] The solution to exile is, of course, "a journey of return ... a homecoming." For Mom, there was to be no going home to her house. My coming home, however, brought Mom into connection with a familiar and dear person, and helped us both journey "home" to a "place where God was present."[2]

For many people with Alzheimer's, assisted living facilities, memory care units, or nursing homes eventually become a necessity. My mom was vehemently opposed to this idea, which she communicated to me clearly through her volatile reaction when I proposed that we visit an adult day center and by her reference to nursing home living as being "garaged." This reality, however, is an important point of surrender that many people with Alzheimer's and their families often must face. Although we may have promised our loved ones that we will not move them to nursing homes "no matter what," although we may fear our loved ones may die shortly after moving to a care facility, and although other family members may condemn us for making this choice, Alzheimer's often presents circumstances we can't foresee and can't manage in our homes. In the presence of these circumstances, "no matter what" is overpowered by Alzheimer's.

As Sam Keen explored the sacred relationship between love and care in American society, he noticed that we have "transferred as much as possible our responsibility for care to the 'caring professionals,'" whom he refers to as "care-sellers."[3] Keen's observation regarding the transfer of care from homes to facilities is accurate. But in many cases, necessity, rather than the desire to transfer responsibility, is the motivation. The reality of his chilling reference to care-sellers, however, makes the necessary letting go and surrender to this choice feel even more difficult for families. When caregivers come to this point of surrender, it's important to be empathetic to our loved ones' resistance, to understand their feelings of separation and exile, to seek guidance and support in facilitating this lifestyle change, and to practice forgiving ourselves for not being more than we are and not doing more than we can.

An eighty-something woman I knew put herself in jeopardy because she didn't realize the enormous emotional stress and physical strain she would encounter while trying to care for her husband with Alzheimer's at home. I met Georgia at mom's nursing home, and she told me of her reluctance to move Roger into a care facility. She surrendered only after Roger fell on top of her. He weighed 250 pounds, and she was a fragile 105 pounds. The fall broke her arm, which was a lucky outcome because she could have been killed.

Adult children who want their parents to live with them might work outside the home and therefore be unable to provide the kind of care, attention, socialization, and supervision needed by people with Alzheimer's, especially as the disease progresses. In these circumstances, home care and adult day programs can offer support for those who can afford them, and the surrender to nursing home care could be delayed.

The ability to afford twenty-four-hour in-home care still might not be a match for the power of Alzheimer's. Two of my friends attempted to keep their moms living independently in their own homes. Both found it to be a highly stressful challenge: hiring and keeping track of personnel, making sure all shifts were covered, making sure the care was appropriate, figuring out what to do if an aide couldn't make it because of illness or weather. One of these friends, who lived in New England, heard a story about a woman with Alzheimer's who, on a day her home health aide hadn't come, wandered outside, slipped on the ice, and froze to death. Within a week, he moved his own mother into an assisted living facility.

The aging "industry"—including adult day programs, assisted living facilities, memory care units, and nursing homes—is growing rapidly to meet the needs of our aging population, particularly those of people with Alzheimer's who have the most demanding and daunting of needs. The facilities are unquestionably a personal and social necessity.

For various reasons, some family members do what my mom feared and so horrifically referred to as "garaging." They drop their loved ones off at care facilities and wash their hands of any further responsibility. Some of them, exhausted by their previous caregiving endeavors, feel relieved that others can take over. Unfortunately, many family members never return. Ever. This absence of family engagement with the residents and staff of nursing homes is another heartbreaking reality of Alzheimer's disease. At this point, people with Alzheimer's must surrender and adjust, since their power to change anything about this reality has vanished.

When people learned that I moved from Boston to be with Mom, some thought I had made a martyr-like choice. Others were unimpressed with my commitment to care for her, citing the freedom I had in my life to do so. Apparently, I wasn't shifting my priorities in ways that seemed meaningful to them. It's true that I wasn't a member of the "sandwich generation."

I didn't have children who needed my attention at the same time I was caring for Mom; I didn't have a spouse or job that prevented me from moving. My life, however, was complicated in other practical ways: health considerations, the need to relocate across the country, disrupted living situations, doctoral studies, financial pressures, family conflicts creating legal turmoil, and demanding work.

Caregivers who shared their experiences with me also had complicated practicalities in the context of their busy lives. Mary Anne and Coleen were striving to meet the needs of their mothers with Alzheimer's, their young children, and their spouses, all while working full-time. Coleen even returned to college and got her bachelor's degree in business during this time. Carl and Steve were caring for their moms and their families in addition to the demanding work of parish ministry, which required them to meet the pastoral needs of hundreds of parishioners.

Although our complications were different, we had one thing in common: None of us considered caregiving for our mothers as optional. It became something we *would* do. Along with Arthur Kleinman and Michael Leach, it was something we had to do; it was our moral duty. We all organized our lives around this priority; we set up schedules and stuck to them. When a person's needs or a specific activity can't be optional, we human beings always seem to figure out a way to make time and find energy for it. This figuring out process ultimately requires us to surrender to the reality that this need can't be changed and so we must be willing to rearrange our priorities.

Changing priorities is something parents do all the time— often automatically, usually willingly, and sometimes joyfully. Later in life, however, we don't expect to have to make radical changes in our priorities or our patterns to care for our spouses, parents, siblings, or other relatives. Alzheimer's disease is shaking up old patterns, though, and inviting us to change our individual and social priorities and respond to the changing realities of need.

Many spousal caregivers feel anger and anguish over Alzheimer's appearing just after they reach retirement. Their plans to move to a warm climate, to travel the world, to visit children and grandchildren, to relax, have likely been cancelled, or at best, altered. Caregivers have to adapt. But trying to convince them to be happy about it would show our lack of understanding about how this disease impacts more than the person who has it, as well as our lack of understanding about how emotions are healed and transformed. Emotions need to be welcomed and embraced, not pushed away. In this case, the loss of a previously imagined future causes disappointment and heartbreak and needs to be met with compassion.

Daisy's priorities changed in a heartbeat. It happened the moment she saw her sister standing on her front walk with her mom in tow. When Daisy and her siblings learned that their mom, Sonia, had serious health concerns, including cognitive decline, and could no longer live independently, Daisy's brother, a police officer in Chicago who lived close to Sonia, agreed to have her move in with his family. He thought his wife could help with the caregiving needs. That lasted a month. Sonia then moved to Missouri to live with Daisy's sister. That lasted a week. And there they were, at Daisy's house, the least likely child to be prepared for this duty. She was in her early thirties, not married, didn't have kids or any experience that might have qualified her to care for a dependent person, owned her own business (a sports bar), was a partier, and had many wounds from being slapped down by society because of her lesbian identity. But OK, this was happening. Sonia moved in, and Daisy had an "instant child."

At first, Daisy took Sonia to work with her every day at the bar, always giving her something to do. Sonia loved to sweep. As her mom's needs became greater, Daisy sold the bar and went to work managing her sister's restaurant, where her schedule could be flexible. Caregiving needs became even greater, and it was obvious more would need to change. Sonia begged not to be put in "a home." Daisy promised. Daisy, who is Latina, said it is part of her culture for families to keep their loved ones at home. "It's frowned upon to put them in a home. They took care of us when we were little, and now we need to take care of them when they are old." Finally, Daisy stopped working to become a full-time caregiver, and they lived, frugally, on Sonia's teachers' pension. The challenges continued to grow, however, and caregiving became really difficult, physically and emotionally. One day, Daisy's sixteen-year-old nephew, Martin, noticed she needed help, and he offered to move in with them to help out with Grandma. Promising his mother that he would stay in high school and attend every day, he moved in. They became a dream-team (Sonia's Angels) offering care, along with Daisy's friend, Andi. And then, a kind of miracle happened, Daisy was able to foster, and then adopt, a young boy, Jaden, who added so much joy, playfulness, and love to the caregiving team.

Daisy could have felt like a victim as she faced all that was required to continually adapt, shift, and change her life in order to meet her mom's ever-demanding needs, but she didn't. In fact, as the caregiving years went on, she felt more and more empowered, more and more at peace. After her mom died, Daisy declared the past eleven years of caregiving to be the best of her life.

In order to integrate Alzheimer's caregiving into an already over-busy life, it could help to think of it as a spiritual practice or discipline. To factor any spiritual practice into our lives, this is how to begin: We develop a practice to which we can willingly and realistically commit; then we make the practice a priority by choosing to do it no matter what. In order to do this, something else will most likely have to be given up. Mary Anne, Coleen, Carl, Steve, Daisy, and I committed to caregiving in this way, and caregiving became a regular part of our daily life routines.

Choosing to make our not-easy caregiving roles a priority requires a profound shift in our attitudes and in our actions. At first it may seem impossible, but with practice, it becomes doable. As with any spiritual practice, we all struggle at the beginning because it's truly an effort to integrate a new priority and routine into our lives. Developing a regular schedule works best. For example, visit Monday through Friday at lunchtime; Sundays for lunch; Saturday mornings while doing errands; on the way home from work on weekdays; Monday, Wednesday, and Friday for dinner; or Tuesday for dinner and a walk. The important first step in succeeding with any spiritual practice is choosing a schedule that can be maintained.

When I first arrived in Iowa, Dominican Sister Mary Owen, my friend and spiritual direction colleague, helped to guide me through my process of shifting and surrendering. Mary Owen was a nurse and had spent a large part of her ministry in nursing homes. Coaching me, she said, "In order to really appreciate what elders in decline have to teach us, we need to go close enough and stay long enough to see their beauty and value." Once we can see, once the spiritual practice of caregiving becomes part of our lives, caregivers may be surprised by unexpected moments of gladness and a deep sense of satisfaction.

Some family members and friends of people with Alzheimer's will have the best intentions to visit their loved ones regularly. Unfortunately, our best intentions are often met with emotional complications, which are perhaps the greatest deterrent to active caregiving. One resident in Mom's nursing home told me that her only daughter didn't come to visit because she "couldn't stand" seeing people in wheelchairs. Many other family members told me they don't visit because it's just "too hard" for them to see their loved ones in a diminished capacity. It's not because they don't care. It's because it stirs up uncomfortable thoughts and feelings—emotional complications—that most of us don't know how to endure. It's truly terrifying to see the possibilities that life might have in store for us. Everyone, including every resident, knows that nursing homes are usually the last stop before death. No one wants to think about that. I understand. But I also know that emotional complications, once addressed, can be overcome.

One evening, as I walked the two blocks from my new Dubuque home to the nursing home where Mom lived, I was surprised to notice a bounce in my step. My heart felt light and open and joyful. I hadn't felt like this earlier in the day. "Why now?" I wondered. By the time I arrived at the door to the nursing home, my joy was bursting out all over.

Recognizing that joyful anticipation is not the universal response to visiting relatives, friends, and loved ones in nursing homes, I had to reflect a bit to understand why I felt this way. I realized that spending time with Mom and others with Alzheimer's was a pleasure and a relief because they are people without pretense. Their spontaneous authenticity refreshed me. They always seemed happy to see me, and without having any perceptible expectations of me, they graciously and gratefully received whatever attention and kindness I was able to offer on any given day. I realized that, having come close enough and staying long enough, I now recognized value and beauty in their presence.

Lightness, openness, and joy were not always my responses to nursing homes or to people with Alzheimer's. When Aunt Milly had Alzheimer's, she lived in a care facility for fifteen years until she died in 1991. During one hometown visit when I was in my twenties, Mom convinced me to accompany her on her weekly visit with Milly. My dearest aunt did not recognize me. Her bulging eyes were blank and her hands clutched a baby doll. She was leaning over her wheelchair, drooling. The unintelligible, garbled noises she made finally drove me from the nursing home to the car, where I waited for Mom—feeling traumatized. As we rode home in silence, I was surprised that Mom didn't criticize my reactivity or my abrupt departure. We never talked about it, but I had the impression that she understood. She never asked me to go again.

I wasn't drawn back into nursing homes until 2004, when it became evident that Mom's disease was progressing and she would eventually need constant skilled care. Over the next two years, I visited a number of nursing homes with Alzheimer's units both in Massachusetts, where I lived at the time, and in Iowa, where Mom lived. My tour of one beautiful state-of-the-art facility specializing in Alzheimer's care for people in various stages of the disease took place during the activities time, which involved ball playing. More than twenty residents sat in a circle in chairs and wheelchairs. Some were leaning and drooling and garbling words. Some clutched dolls or teddy bears. A staff member stood in the center of the circle, throwing a large soft ball to the residents, who then did their best to bat it, or catch and throw it back to the staff member.

It's humbling to admit that my initial internal responses to the nursing home environment were not much different than they had been when I tried to visit Aunt Milly twenty-five years earlier, although my external composure was more restrained. I didn't bolt out of the facility in a traumatized state.

After witnessing the ball-playing scene, however, I did make a hasty, albeit slightly more gracious, exit.

After I assisted Mom with her dinner, we would usually go for a walk together. During nice weather, we walked outside, but on cold or rainy or dark winter evenings, we walked the long corridors of the nursing home, four hallways on each of three floors. As we passed by the rooms, I often glanced in, mostly looking for decorating ideas for Mom's room. Sometimes I would see residents in their rooms. Occasionally, seeing them would awaken me to the idea that someday I could be living in one of these rooms. This possibility frightened me, and I would go home on those nights and weep—for Mom, for the other residents, and for my future exiled, lonely, and frightened self.

In the midst of these recurring times of lament, I prayed for the strength to embrace my own emotions. Sometimes, from within the turbulence of my fear, I would hear echoes of encouragement from my friend and caregiving companion, Mary Anne. She had heard the myriad of reasons people offered for not visiting nursing home residents, many from her own siblings. In response, her eternal hopefulness and her clarity of need shone through. She hopes that, when caregivers' hearts are fearful, we will be able to overcome our resistance and be there for our loved ones with Alzheimer's—because they need us. During the times when my practical and emotional complications made the world of Alzheimer's feel impossible for me to touch and I felt so alone on this journey, I turned to a poem by Sufi mystic Hafiz for comfort and strength:

> Don't surrender your loneliness
> So quickly.
> Let it cut more deep.

Let it ferment and season you
As few human
Or even divine ingredients can.

Something missing in my heart tonight
Has made my eyes so soft,
My voice
So tender,

My need of God
Absolutely
Clear.[4]

Each time I encountered roadblocks called loneliness and fear, I asked for inner and outer help to get beyond them. Each time I was tempted to turn away, I intentionally worked to shift my attention to Mom and her needs. Although it was productive to recognize and acknowledge my feelings of loneliness, fear, helplessness, and despair, it wasn't especially comfortable. However, after consciously meeting and accepting as valid every one of these challenging emotions, I was always able to return to the nursing home the next day, always filled with joy on my mission to care for Mom. One of my teachers, Janet Ramsey, would describe my process and my ability to "bounce back" as "spiritual resiliency." She believes our ability to be resilient can increase with practice, and that possessing this ability becomes more important as we age and our losses accumulate.[5]

On the evening that my feelings of lightness, openness, and joy caught my attention, I was on my way to lead the ball game for the residents on Mom's floor. No longer running away in fright, I had become the person tossing the ball to drooling, leaning, word-garbling, doll-clutching, smiling, grateful people in various stages of Alzheimer's. I was the joy-filled person in the center of the circle, calling out their names and connecting with each person through eye contact, gentle touch, smiles, and laughter. These people were no longer nursing home residents to me. They had become individuals with names and personalities, with likes and dislikes, with abilities and disabilities, with joys and sorrows, and with families—some who visited and brought joy to the residents and some who didn't visit until death was imminent. Many of the residents had become friends and were part of my daily life. They were friends with life histories (whether or not they could tell me about their histories, their histories existed and informed their interactions). They were friends who possessed the potential to love me and to teach me about living—and dying. There is a Buddhist proverb, "When the student is ready, the teacher appears." These blessed, darling, vulnerable, wise people with Alzheimer's, many of whom had been cast aside like unwanted orphans, had become my important companions and teachers.

Psychiatrist James Gordon explains that we often don't feel the "need to be aware when all is going well" and "life is on kind of an automatic pilot."[6] Without our approval, a diagnosis of Alzheimer's disrupts our patterns and turns our habitual momentum inside out, giving us an opportunity, a mandate perhaps, to shift away from automatic pilot and to wake up. During my journey with Mom through Alzheimer's, I came to understand that waking up is one kind of challenge. Staying awake is another. Because I trust that there are life-giving secrets within every aspect of life, I knew I needed to stay awake—to all aspects of Alzheimer's, including my uncomfortable feelings—in order to find the hidden secrets.

Family members of nursing home residents with Alzheimer's, from all across the country over two decades of conversations, have explained to me that they don't visit more often—or at all—because seeing the conditions of neglect and the substandard care their loved ones were receiving caused them to feel distressed and helpless. They reported finding their loved ones in undignified situations, painful positions, hungry and thirsty, sitting in soiled clothing, and suffering from medication side effects that the nursing staff didn't notice. My caregiver friend and Alzheimer's activist/advocate, Lynda, shared the anguish she experienced over witnessing "horribly and inexcusably negligent behaviors" by professional caregivers in the memory units where her husband, Richard, lived during his last years. They simply did not understand Alzheimer's or how to care for those with the disease. This is inexcusable. Lynda said that she would maintain a happy demeanor with Richard but often had to leave his bedside and retreat to her car, where she would weep over what was happening to him. However, she didn't let this, or anything, defeat her resolve to be there for Richard; she kept going back, day after day, to make sure her husband's experience of life as a person living with Alzheimer's was as good as it could possibly be. She came to recognize the power of just being with him, and referred to this as "ministry of presence."

After making similar observations of subpar care in regard to Mom, I discussed my concerns with nursing home staff. Sometimes I felt heard, sometimes not. Occasionally things improved. After all of these conversations, however, I usually felt helpless to make any meaningful changes in Mom's life. It's not just in the nursing home setting that Alzheimer's caregivers will feel helplessness; it's a recurrent experience all throughout our journeys with our loved ones.

As if life with Alzheimer's and family caregiving weren't challenging enough, then came the Covid-19 pandemic! I adapted my workshops for Zoom and was honored to continue my work with caregivers. At the end of every workshop, I always left time for questions and discussion. During this time, all of the questions from family caregivers with loved ones in care centers revealed their frustration about not being able to see their loved ones. Almost panicky, the caregivers were asking what more they could do to care for them. I offered some practical suggestions for what "to do," since that was specifically what they asked for. But they had already thought of and done everything I suggested: calling daily, video chats, sending cards and gifts, sending photos, window visits. You name it, they were doing it. But what else? They wanted to know! With desperation, they kept asking, "What else???" I quickly realized that these caregivers were suffering terribly in this situation of not being able "to do" anything to relieve their loved ones' loneliness—or even more pressing it seemed, their own loneliness. Listening to them, I would imagine my own despair if I had moved to Iowa and a month later was not allowed to see my mom! My imagined suffering was intense. Devastating. Those who were at home with a loved one with Alzheimer's with no place to go, no outside stimulation, and no relief from the togetherness revealed their experience of a different but similar kind of suffering. It was all about helplessness. Suggestions of what "to do" were not what any of these caregivers needed. What they needed was to recognize their own suffering and to find guidance and comfort for coping with a situation over which they had no control. What they needed was to surrender.

Viktor Frankl was a man who influenced me greatly in my life, especially when I was younger and embarking on the healing process for the abuses from my past. His guidance resurfaced, however, during the Alzheimer's journey. A Jewish-Austrian doctor who lived from 1905 to 1997, Frankl was a neurologist, psychiatrist, author, and survivor of four different Nazi concentration camps. In his book *Man's Search for Meaning*, Frankl writes, "When we are no longer able to change a situation—just think of an incurable illness . . . we are challenged to change ourselves." Although we can't change this "unalterable fate," we can, perhaps, change our attitude.[7] I encouraged caregivers to begin paying attention to their own feelings and trying to meet some of their own needs using mindfulness meditation practices. I presented the idea that noticing ourselves and listening to ourselves can lead to good self-care and good caregiving. This suggestion represented a shift in focus for most, but it was actually one of the saving graces during my own time as a caregiver. I came into the caregiver role with my own chronic illness, one I had surrendered to decades earlier, and I had to pay careful attention to meeting my own needs as well as Mom's, including my emotional and spiritual needs.

The Alzheimer's journey, in or out of pandemic restrictions, is no time to be trying to exhibit our independence; it's a time to surrender and to ask for help. Caregivers are urged to reach out to therapists, support groups, spiritual directors, Alzheimer's coaches, 24-hour help lines from Alzheimer's agencies, family members, care center staff, friends, and clergy for support.

As I weighed the pros and cons about moving to be with Mom, my friend, a nurse in a veterans' nursing facility, offered me a warning. She said that because of limited staff and time, residents who have family members looking out for them receive more attention and ultimately better care. The overworked, sometimes undertrained, and often under-valued certified nursing aides have been known to forget or neglect their required responsibilities while caring for our loved ones. This can happen in even the best care facilities, especially at this time when staffing numbers continue to decline due to Medicare and Medicaid cuts, decreases in health care workers resulting from Covid-19 restrictions, the aftermath of the pandemic burn-out experience, and the general growth trend of the population (more older adults and fewer younger people to meet the escalating need).[8] It's estimated that between 2020 and 2030, 1.2 million more new direct care Alzheimer's and dementia workers will be needed than in any other single occupation in the U.S.[9]

One of my greatest challenges in caring for Mom was trying to ensure that the nursing home delivered the care they had recommended and promised, what they called a "care plan." I interpreted the care plan as a sacred covenant to care for my vulnerable mother. In the beginning, I fretted over the details of this plan. I lost sleep worrying that Mom's head wouldn't be elevated to the proper angle when a substitute aide put her to bed and that she would choke during the night. Even though I knew that there was no way to beat death, I did not want my mother to die from this kind of oversight. I also knew that I couldn't possibly monitor the nursing home care twenty-four hours a day.

In the midst of this worry, the thinking of theologian Abraham Joshua Heschel brought me awareness and comfort. According to Heschel, there are two ways of knowing reality: reason and wonder. Through reason, he explains, we try to make the world conform to our existing concepts of how things should be. In my mind, the nursing home should be implementing— to perfection—every aspect of Mom's care plan. After all, they developed the plan! This reasonable expectation, however, had the potential to create great misery. Because I saw this misery manifested in other nursing home families who relentlessly demanded perfection from the staff, I carefully attended to Heschel's thoughts about wonder. Through wonder we seek to adjust to our world, to pursue authentic awareness of that which is.[10] Wonder requires letting go—and staying still until the truth can reveal itself.

My worry about Mom's care eventually evolved into a grace-filled surrender. I accepted that many things in the nursing home, everything about Alzheimer's disease, and the time and circumstances of my mother's death were beyond my control. I was face-to-face with what theologian Richard Rohr refers to as the "spirituality of imperfection." I knew the limits of my power and acknowledged all that I couldn't change, fix, or make into what I wanted it to be. When we become aware of and surrender to our own powerlessness, according to Rohr, we have to transform. "Great healing," he said, "is always about transforming."[11]

Ultimately, my daily view of the monumental task of caring for the flood of elders, particularly those with dementia, flowing into Mom's nursing home led me to feel admiration for the facility's mission. I matured into a greater understanding of their strengths and limitations, as well as an acceptance of their imperfections, identifying what could and could not be changed.

My surrender to the limits of nursing home care, however, did not in any way lead me to conclude that Mom, or any person with Alzheimer's, is undeserving of better, more informed, more compassionate, and more enlightened care than many are currently receiving. About this, I retained my resolve and manifested the courage to speak. One issue that I raised repeatedly was finally investigated, and a facility-wide problem with the computer charting process was discovered. So by relentlessly raising this issue, I brought about reform within the nursing home and perhaps improvement in the lives of other residents as well as in Mom's.

The Alzheimer's Association and others, including authors Joanne Koenig Coste and Marty Richards, have introduced the word *carepartners* into the practice of Alzheimer's care. Their common intention, by coining this term, is to emphasize the reciprocity of love and care that flows between people with Alzheimer's and their families, friends, and communities. To believe that our relationships with people with Alzheimer's are about more than their neediness and our giving them care requires a shift in attitude about and understanding of Alzheimer's. The purpose of introducing the word *carepartners* into our vocabulary is to empower people with Alzheimer's and inform families and friends that people with Alzheimer's remain an integral and contributing part of our relationships. Considering each other as partners in caring speaks to the covenantal relationship of givers and receivers. When this shift in attitude happens, caregivers may feel less burdened, and people with Alzheimer's may feel more valued.[12]

When I was visiting Mom during the summer of 2004, she facilitated an experience of reciprocity of care that enlightened me about the carepartner relationship. Shortly after my arrival, I noticed scratchiness in my throat, the usual beginning of an allergic reaction. Later that day, I had a sore throat and mentioned it to Mom when I suggested that we have tea together. The next morning, when I was making breakfast, I saw a bottle of aspirin at my place at the table. Still trying to get a handle on what kind of medication Mom was taking, I asked her, "What's the aspirin for?" She replied, "It's for you. You said you had a sore throat." I was surprised and impressed that she remembered, and so very touched that, through the ravages of Alzheimer's, my Mom still wanted to take care of me. "Oh, yes, Mom, I do. Thank you so much," I said as I hugged her. Without taking the aspirin, or any other medical intervention, my sore throat went away quickly, and the anticipated allergic reaction didn't happen. Perhaps Mom's exemplary effort at carepartnering had stimulated my immune system enough to heal me.

After Mom moved to the nursing home, I expanded my understanding of carepartnering to include the staff. The nursing home provided Mom with her basic needs: shelter and food, baths and toileting, appropriate furniture and linens, laundry services, and assistance with the tasks of daily living. I provided her with clothing, companionship, more assistance with the activities of daily living, attention, fun, and love. The nursing home scheduled activities and outings; I accompanied Mom to the activities and on the outings, helping her to participate in and enjoy them. As the structure of the nursing home evolved to include more state-of-the-art care for dementia residents, I was able to select the nursing aides I wanted to work with Mom. I chose aides who were mature, devoted to elder care, and seemed to have naturally developed a friendship with her. They were especially kind to her and attentive to the details of her care plan. They helped her maintain her capabilities, such as walking, and encouraged her to continue to grow. These aides and I communicated well, and they kept me informed about Mom's accomplishments and any changes in her habits and behavior. We were Mom's eyes, recognizing what she needed; and we were Mom's voice, keeping each other informed of her ever-changing abilities and needs. I came to truly feel that the nursing home and I were in a cooperative carepartnership for Mom, each of us providing what the other could not.

In spite of her increasing limitations, Mom continued to demonstrate her desire to care for me. In the evenings, an aide would help her stand up from her wheelchair. Once she was standing, we hugged. I put my arms around her and she put her arms around me. She held me so tightly that it could only be described as holding me like she would never let me go. Sometimes we swayed to music, but mostly we just stood and hugged, and I would scratch her back. I know Mom loved this time for hugging, because she always had a broad smile and an ecstatic look on her face. She also made a purring sound. At this stage of her illness, her fingers were constricted and her hands almost constantly curled into a fist. Often while I was scratching her back, I could feel her fingers uncurling and ever so slightly moving back and forth. She was trying to scratch my back while I scratched hers. Mom could barely move any part of her body voluntarily, and yet she was making a clear effort to be my carepartner. She was trying to give me the same kind of physical pleasure and comfort I was giving her. Her efforts moved me deeply.

Mom's desire to be an active carepartner reached beyond me to the staff who cared for her with love and devotion. Alexis, her primary aide on the afternoon-evening shift, had a unique gift for interacting with people with dementia. Maybe it was the tone of her voice or the encouragement on her face, but something about Alexis brought out impressive responsiveness. Mom and Alexis became close.

One night, however, Mom caused Alexis a moment of worry. Toward the end of her life, when her hands were curled, Mom's grip became viselike. To get her to let go of something, we often had to pry open her fingers, gently of course. On this night, Alexis was crouched on the floor in front of Mom's recliner, putting on her shoes. Slowly, Mom reached out her arm and put her hand on top of Alexis's head. Alexis was afraid that Mom was going to grab her hair and not let go. Then she would be stuck there, probably in hair-pulling pain, until someone happened by to rescue her. But Mom didn't grab Alexis's hair. She very gently stroked the top of her head, just as I had stroked and massaged Mom's head. Mom was making an effort to give Alexis the same kind of comfort and pleasure she had received from me.

Once caregivers can shift their attitudes away from the presumed solitariness of their role and open their hearts to include the possibility of carepartnering, there is ample opportunity for everyone in the partnership to experience healing.

A colleague recently mentioned how much she hates the word *surrender*. This is understandable. In our culture, *surrender* is most often used in the context of warfare and carries a connotation of defeat, loss, or failure. In the context of the spiritual journey, however, surrender is an acknowledgment, and ultimately, an acceptance of reality. Some might be more comfortable with the Buddhist notion of *detachment*. Others might prefer the less emotionally charged phrase *letting go*, an active phrase that gives us agency and control. But *surrender*—defined by Webster's as "to give oneself up, as into the power of another"—seems to best describe both the requirement and the gift for caregivers on the spiritual journey through Alzheimer's. As their brains deteriorate, people with Alzheimer's will naturally, gracefully evolve into surrender. Similarly, this disease is asking caregivers not for combat but for cooperation. The power of Alzheimer's is still so great that, for now, only surrender will bring us spiritual victory and peace of mind and heart.

9   The Dance of
   Yes and No

In between yes and no, there's a dance that happens in all of our lives. It's a dance of discernment and choice as old as recorded history. In the book of Deuteronomy in the Hebrew scriptures, God speaks to Moses about this dance: "I have set before you life and death, blessings and curses. Choose life . . ."[13] The guidance in this passage is clear, but identifying the choice that says yes to life and blessings might not be so clear. If we choose to say yes to someone or something, it usually means we're simultaneously saying no to someone or something else. As we attempt to recognize and choose our caregiving attitudes, priorities, and practices, our dancing in between yes and no will be in full swing.

A Testament of Devotion, by Quaker missionary and revered theologian Thomas Kelly is a classic in the spiritual direction formation process, and it was the first book I read for my training program. This book lit a passion within me for the spiritual quest that has never extinguished. Other readers felt the same, including Kelly's fellow Quaker Richard Foster. In his introduction to the 1992 publication of the book, Foster brought into focus for me the intricacies of the dance of yes and no.

Foster began reading Kelly's book while waiting at bustling Dulles International Airport for his flight to Los Angeles. He describes himself as exhausted from "a hectic schedule of 'muchness' and 'manyness,'" and from this place, he felt as if Kelly's words were speaking to him. "We feel honestly the pull of many obligations and try to fulfill them all. And we are unhappy, uneasy, strained, oppressed, and fearful we shall be shallow." Soon, though, came the words that resonated with Foster's soul and facilitated a personal transformation, which began right there in the airport. "We have hints that there is a way of life vastly richer and deeper than all this hurried experience.... We have seen and know some people who seem to have found this deep Center of living, where the fretful calls of life are integrated, where no as well as yes can be said with confidence."

Kelly's certainty that people can find a divine center of living that supports their ability to confidently say no as well as yes shook up Foster because that ability was foreign to him. He could easily say yes, because doing so usually supported his "egoistic view" of himself as spiritual and self-sacrificing. He worried, however, what others would think of him if he said no. Right then and there, in the midst of airport chaos, Foster paused and prayed for "the ability to say no when it was right and good."

Very soon, Foster was invited into the dance. Shortly after returning home from his travels, a denominational executive presented him with an enticing professional opportunity. Oh, how he wanted to do this, but then he heard the date. It was scheduled on the same night he had already said yes to spending time with his family. Foster chose to say no to the denominational executive and yes to his family commitment.

He describes the result of this choice as "electrifying." "I had yielded to the Center .... That simple no coming out of divine promptings set me free from the tyranny of others. Even more, it set me free from my own inner clamoring for attention and recognition and applause."

With humility, Foster then confesses his embarrassment that such a small and seemingly insignificant incident facilitated this important inner transformation. "But there it is, a trivial event, yet it changed everything for me .... At least I know that often the genuinely significant issues are decided in the small corners of life."[14]

Jewish theologian Martin Buber reminds us often to hallow (make holy) our everyday experiences. He explains that the transformation from life-draining responses, such as an automatic yes to all requests, to life-giving, "holy" choices, does not happen inside us alone. Buber is convinced that our transformations can only be manifested *in relation* to another.[15]

In the Christian New Testament, we find an example of how "Yes," spoken in relation has the potential to manifest transformation. Matthew 15:21-28 tells the story of a Canaanite woman who comes out of the crowd, shouting at Jesus, "Have mercy on me .... My daughter is tormented by a demon." Disturbed by the woman's persistence, the disciples urge Jesus to send her away. Jesus explains to the woman that he has been "sent only to the lost sheep of Israel." The woman then presents herself to Jesus from the deep center of living, revealing her bravery, her humility, and her dignity. She kneels before him, saying, "Lord help me." Jesus, however, remains unmoved and continues to say no. Finally, in response to her plaintive cries for help, he further explains his position, "It is not fair to take the children's food and throw it to the dogs."

The woman then speaks words, which, through meditation on this passage, I recognized as the improvisational theater practice of *Yes, and.* "Yes, Lord, yet..." she begins. It's her yes, her acceptance of Jesus's explanation, that facilitates a transformation in him and results in the healing of the woman's daughter. Unlike the Pharisees, who are always arguing with Jesus, challenging him and pushing him into defending his argument and maintaining his power position of teacher or prophet in order for his point to be received, the woman simply accepts and agrees with Jesus's position. She says, "Yes, Lord." She shows her respect and understanding; then she offers her perspective: "...Yet even the dogs eat the crumbs that fall from their masters' table." The courage and humility of her earlier actions and pleas have not opened Jesus' heart, but her yes opens first his mind, because she has acknowledged what he said as valid, and then his heart. From this place of openness, he chooses to step into what Buber calls "direct relation"[16] with her. He chooses to override his bias toward healing only the Israelites. From his divine center, Jesus says no to his previous limited understanding of his mission, and he says yes to the radical choice to heal a Canaanite. "Woman, great is your faith! Let it be done for you as you wish." And her daughter is healed instantly.[17]

The "Yes, and" practice of improvisational theater requires that we first learn to validate and accept the offer extended to us by saying yes. The practice then invites us to *advance the offer* by saying "and...." We then have the opportunity to add our own inspired truth (or inspired, imaginative therapeutic fiblettes, if necessary in the situation of dementia caregiving). Choosing this life-affirming response often encourages a connection to flourish. The opposite step in the dance is to *block the offer* by saying no, denying the other, and/or arguing and creating a struggle for power and control.

Inspired by Foster, the Canaanite woman, and Jesus, I carried their examples of saying yes and no from the divine center into the nursing home and into every interaction I had with Mom and her neighbors. In the place that Mom referred to as a garage, with people in the midst of cognitive decline, I looked for opportunities to hallow the everyday experiences of life with Alzheimer's disease. Repeatedly, I was offered life or death, blessings or curses. I consciously tried to choose life and blessings.

Because of my school schedule, Mom had been living in the nursing home for four months before I was able to travel to Iowa during my winter break to see her. Those first days I spent with her turned out to be about much more than visiting. Those days, and all the years that followed, became an immersion experience in Alzheimer's reality and care, providing limitless practice in the life-changing dance of yes and no.

Throughout Mom's first months at the nursing home, the distressing departure episodes—which included her clinging, begging to be taken home, angry outbursts, and crying— were constant. Every time someone visited Mom and left her, there was an emotional scene. My desire to help her avoid this upsetting experience became my first lesson in saying no when it was right and good. I was surprised to discover that, in order to say yes to what Mom needed, I had to say no to myself, to my beliefs and habits about what constituted a proper good-bye.

When it was time for a visitor to leave, my habit was to walk with them to the door, to express gratitude for their time and presence, and to say goodbye with a kiss, hug, or touch. I learned this habit from my gracious mother. However, this very habit of acknowledging that our time together was over, expressing gratitude and sharing a physical connection now caused emotional turmoil for Mom. She didn't want her visitors to leave without her; she didn't want the connection to be broken by goodbye; she didn't want to feel abandoned. Accepting where Mom was in the disease process and accepting her ever-changing needs were the places where I needed to express my yes.

I began a new approach to leave-taking. As the time approached, I told Mom that soon I would have to go away for a while. I told her where I was going (to have lunch and a rest), and when I would be back (5:30, in time to have dinner with her). When it was the actual time for me to leave, however, I made sure Mom was occupied in other ways. The first time I tried this was after lunch. We waited together in Mom's room for the aide to come and help her to the bathroom. When the aide arrived, Mom and I walked across her room. She looked happy walking with me as we held hands. When we reached the aide, I gave Mom's hand to her. As soon as they made eye contact, Mom was fully engaged with the aide. They walked away from me and into the bathroom together. Mom never looked back. There was no distress for her in this process of my leave-taking. The aide told me there was no emotional upset. Instead, Mom napped away the afternoon in a happy glow from our time together. Her happiness was still glowing when I returned at 5:30.

On other days, I waited until Mom had dozed off in her chair or I arranged to stay until she was walking with someone else to meals or an activity or on her way to have a bath. From my first visit with Mom in the nursing home until the day she died, it was always hard for me to leave her. But by being aware of timing, Mom's schedule, and her attentiveness to other people, things, and activities, I could make sure that the separation was not stressful for her. Although it was a less than satisfying goodbye for me, and at times required me to stay a bit longer than I had planned, the choice was right and good for Mom.

My experiences with Mom during the early and middle stages of Alzheimer's, reading *Learning to Speak Alzheimer's*, my conversations with the psychiatrist and the improv teacher, and the possibilities for healing and transformation I discovered in my spiritual reading had solidified for me the critical importance of *acceptance* in the presence of Alzheimer's disease. Reinforcing my learning, a friend shared a fascinating research study on stress-related disorders among dementia caregivers. This study determined that acceptance is one of the most effective coping techniques for reducing caregiver stress.[18] This knowledge motivated me to fully accept the ever-changing landscape and the challenges of Alzheimer's. It wasn't easy, but integrating improvisation with my spiritual practices helped me to accept what was and then notice what was possible. Acceptance became a way of saying yes to Mom as well as to my own well-being.

After I moved to Iowa and gained more in-depth knowledge and experience from interactions with people with Alzheimer's and their caregivers, my understanding of saying yes in the context of Alzheimer's care became more refined. I discovered that the idea of saying yes doesn't actually translate into literally saying yes, which could have catastrophic consequences. One woman I met at a dementia care conference told me that her husband wanted to sit in his lawn chair in the middle of a lake. In improv class, that desire could initiate an entertaining scene. In real life, though, it's dangerous. In order to avoid conflict in that situation, some creative, compassionate improvising would be necessary. Since it's highly possible that he didn't realize the lake was made of water and couldn't be walked on, or sat on, one initial intervention could be to tell him he will sink and to show him the water is not solid by splashing. However, logic cannot be counted on as an effective intervention. Keeping him safe is the priority. But being curious about his need and what he was trying to accomplish by taking the lawn chair into the lake, saying "yes, I understand," and then offering alternatives, would likely lead to the most healing solution.

Saying yes in the context of Alzheimer's is not about agreeing with or showing approval for an offer extended to us by a person with Alzheimer's. It's about adopting an attitude of acceptance and affirmation. Figuring out what was happening for Mom—what she was feeling and what she needed—was, at times, like the most complicated Sudoku puzzle, often bringing me face-to-face with that dreaded feeling of failure. But accepting her, affirming her, and guarding her self-esteem were my goals, and so I puzzled on.

Reality orientation, which many caregivers still try to implement with people with dementia, is the direct opposite of acceptance and affirmation. Reality orientation is about changing people and correcting people. Being constantly corrected is annoying and demeaning for anyone. I don't like it, and I'm sure people with Alzheimer's don't like it either. Unfortunately, I heard endless corrections happening in the nursing home on a daily basis. "No. This isn't your milk." "No, you can't go in there. It's not your room." "No. I don't work on Friday. I work on Monday. How many times do I have to remind you?" "Oh, no. This is not your husband. Stay away from him. You're bothering him." "You can't take that. It's not yours." These negations and corrections were issued relentlessly, presumably with good intentions. Perhaps those offering the corrections thought they would make some kind of lasting difference as they might with children, who will remember and learn from the stated boundaries.

As I sat with Mom in the resident lounge, assisted her with her meals in the dining room, and walked with her through the nursing home corridors, my ears were constantly barraged by these corrections. Listening to them wore me out and made me feel vicariously annoyed. One day, thinking there had to be another way to interact, I recalled a scene I had witnessed while walking along the beach in Maine. A man was standing at the shoreline while refreshingly cold waves washed over his feet and ankles. Using his arms to beckon to his daughter who was playing in deeper water, he called to her, "Honey, come in closer to shore." This sweet invitation brought me to a halt and a moment of awareness. If I had been the parent, concerned for my child's safety, I probably would have done what my parents did—issue a firm order that sounded like this: Don't go out so far!

"Honey, come in closer to shore" versus "Don't go out so far." The energy of the first statement carries a concerned but loving invitation. The second is a correction, carrying with it the clear message that the child has done something wrong.

On two separate days, I witnessed scenes in Mom's nursing home representing these polar opposite messages. And I observed the powerful effect these differing messages had on the feelings and mood of someone with Alzheimer's.

In the nursing home, all of the residents had plastic nameplates that slid into metal brackets attached to the wall next to the doors of their rooms. One day, Regina, one of the residents, appeared in the doorway of the dining area with the biggest smile on her face. In her hands was a large stack of nameplates, which she had collected from all the rooms on the floor.

"Oh my, Regina, you've collected the nameplates!" remarked Kathy, the regular companion aide assigned to the dining room. As Kathy, who was a natural yes-sayer, received the nameplates from Regina's hands, her eyes were round with surprise. "I do believe you got them all," she said with a glint of amusement in her voice. "Good job. Thank you."

Regina's smile remained, and she seemed so pleased with herself. She stayed close by Kathy throughout lunch. Later that afternoon, Kathy walked around the floor with Regina hand in hand. As they replaced all the nameplates, Regina tried to read the names and was visibly proud of her ability to help reinstall the nameplates.

The next day, Regina again appeared in the doorway of the dining area. Again, she had a big smile and her hands full of nameplates. On this day, a substitute aide was working.

"*Oh no*, Regina!" the aide screeched. "These are not yours. You can't do that."

Snatching the nameplates from Regina's hands, shaking her head, and looking very angry, the aide muttered, "Bad. This is very bad."

Regina's smile instantly disappeared and she slouched in despair. She turned around, walked out of the dining area, and went to her room. She spent the rest of the day alone, in bed, refusing meals. Observing these two scenes, I felt Regina's joy and pride on the first day and her sadness and shame on the second day. One aide was affirming. She said yes and accepted Regina's offer. The other aide was correcting. She said no and blocked Regina's offer. The correction and the subsequent depression, however, didn't deter Regina from collecting the nameplates in the future.

Correcting people with Alzheimer's and/or denying their realities is likely to result in them becoming ashamed or angry. Those who feel ashamed will become depressed and they will withdraw; those who become angry could strike out verbally if they're still able to talk; those who are able to voluntarily move their bodies sometimes strike out with physical force. Christian theologian and ethicist Stephen Pattison explains that whenever an experience causing someone to feel ashamed is "bypassed or ignored, rage and aggression [are] likely to occur."[19] Ashamed and angry people with Alzheimer's can't explain or process their feelings or reactions, but their feelings will arise nonetheless. They will react and act accordingly. If the nursing home staff aren't specifically trained to say yes through validating, investigating, and interpreting these behaviors, residents are often responded to with psychotropic medication to control their "acting out behaviors" rather than with understanding and empathy.

Inspired by the first rule of improvisation, my main intention in my dances of yes and no with Mom and her neighbors was to make them "look good." Instead of reminding them of errors (from my perspective), judging them harshly, negating their reality, or attempting to reorient them into my world, I committed myself to interacting with them in ways that accepted them, affirmed them, made them feel important, and enhanced their sense of worth and dignity. The scenes with Regina brought to life my reading and research. As my professor, Earl Thompson, pointed out, "Every interaction we have with others is fraught with the possibility of creating shame or healing pride."[20] Regina's reactions over the name-plate incidents heightened my awareness of my own words and actions. I became more conscious of my impact on all those around me, especially vulnerable people with Alzheimer's, who are highly sensitive to emotions and emotional energy. An entire floor of residents could feel upset in various ways from witnessing corrections, negations, and emotional outbursts.

Martin Buber's thinking further informed me about the spiritual implications of the improvisation practice "Yes, and . . ." in the context of Alzheimer's caregiving. When we affirm people with Alzheimer's by saying yes to their realities, we step into direct relation with them; we recognize and acknowledge their divine essence. This type of relation happens only with our whole beings. And when two whole beings meet, healing can happen. According to Buber, "All real living is meeting."[21] The "Yes, and . . ." practice can enable caregivers to expand their capacity for relating to people with Alzheimer's, who are almost always presenting themselves to us with their whole beings, with their divine essences shining through. It's we who need to reach beyond our habits, prejudices, egos, and needs to meet them with our whole beings. When we cross over into their worlds and advance the offers they extend to us, we open the door for true meeting and for healing.

I was leaving the nursing home one night, passing by a group of women residents gathered near the nurses' station. Ellie was there every night when I left, usually slumped over in her wheelchair, asleep. This night, however, she was wide awake and agitated. As I walked toward her, I noticed that she was shaking her clenched fists at me, yelling.

"You can't have him!" Ellie shouted.

This impressive scene implored me to stop. I squatted down to be at eye level with Ellie. Looking into her eyes, I accepted her offer when I said, "Yes, I can't have him!" I advanced the conversation with curiosity by asking, "But, why not?"

Ellie's irate response surprised me: "Because we took vows."

When trying to meet people with Alzheimer's in their world, it's very important to know and play the role you've been cast into. In this interaction, Ellie had cast me into the role of the other woman. I was Jezebel! I got it. But still, she was so very upset. In an effort to create a healing moment, I said yes to being Jezebel and yes to making Ellie look good. These yeses, were actually an effort to be responsible to what was holy in life. In this situation, that was Ellie's emotions.

In relationship to Ellie and her emotions, I chose a life-giving response. Looking again into her angry eyes, I said, "You're right, Ellie. I can't have him because he still loves you. I was wrong, and I'm sorry."

As soon as Ellie heard me say this, she calmed down. Her entire body relaxed. She lowered her arms into her lap and her clenched fists opened. Her anger dissipated. Then she replied, "Well, that's very big of you."

I was so surprised by Ellie's gracious words that my only response was a smile and a grateful heart. "Thank you, Ellie," I said. She took my hands, we looked at each other, and we both smiled warmly.

In this meeting with Ellie, which took only a moment of my time, something very profound happened—for Ellie and for me. Ellie calmed down. She had been angry and agitated, but after this interaction, she was calm. This was the observable outcome. Based on what she said, we can speculate that she felt vindicated over a long-ago wound, and possibly some healing happened for her. But what happened for me was remarkable. From Ellie's response to my apology, I felt deeply forgiven—for every bad thing I'd ever done, actually. This meeting with Ellie felt like "real living" to me even though it happened completely in her world and she thought I was someone else.

By practicing the first rule of improvisation, I was actually manifesting the recommended goal of dementia care described by Tom Kitwood and Kathleen Breden, "to enhance well-being through facilitating a sense of personal worth, a sense of agency, social confidence, and a basic trust or security in the environment and in others."[22] This specific caregiving practice of making our scene partners look good, when implemented, can be healing, as it was for Mom, for me, for Regina, for Ellie. Practicing it gave me repeated experiences of what Buber taught and Foster discovered: Transformation happens in the small corners, in the hallowed everyday, from the yes or the no spoken from our deep center of living.

10 The Sacrament of the Present Moment

One of the highlights of my college experience happened by surprise. New friends had convinced me to attend a concert by a relatively unknown folksinger, John Denver. I'd never heard of him but wanted to become friends with the classmates who invited me, so off I went, reluctantly. The concert was astounding, and we all became instant fans. But the highlight of highlights came after the concert while we were having fries and Cokes at the Bridge restaurant in Dubuque. In walked John Denver, and we got to meet him in person! This moment marked the beginning of a lifelong appreciation for his music and admiration for his spiritual and humanitarian evolution.

More than thirty years later, John Denver's song "On the Wings of a Dream" inspired me as I accompanied Mom through Alzheimer's disease. He sang about dreaming and dying, about awakening to the awareness that "the moment at hand is the only thing we really own." Denver's lyrics remind us of a deep, spiritual truth: What's real in every human life is happening right now—in this moment at hand.

Many of us, however, have come to almost worship our happy and important memories. Just as many of us are haunted by memories of painful experiences and can't move forward with our lives in a healthy way. Still others find our joy and pleasure in dreaming about and planning for the future. We expect a new baby. We look forward to a graduation or a wedding or a vacation. We anticipate buying a new car or our first home. Yet many of us feel worry and dread about the unknowns of tomorrow. Still-unidentified challenges lurking around the next corner make us feel nervous and afraid. Memories and futures, whether embedded in joy or sorrow, have significance in our lives. In reality, though, our pasts are gone and our tomorrows may never arrive.

Everything that's real in our lives is right here, right now. Sometimes we'd rather forget, deny, or avoid the importance of now, especially when the current experiences of our lives are difficult to embrace. Feelings of loss, grief, anger, abandonment, rejection, fear, loneliness, disappointment, and sadness often send us searching for distractions, of which there are many in our busy, modern lives. If we instead choose to accept the present moment, our hearts, minds, and spirits will awaken to the wisdom of putting the past and the future into perspective. Then we can focus our attention, accordingly, on the right now.

"Do not dwell in the past, do not dream of the future," the Buddha tells us. "Concentrate the mind on the present moment." Ancient and modern theologians and spiritual teachers, poets, musicians, and physicians—many of whom have been my life guides before, during, and after Mom's journey through Alzheimer's—have repeated the same message: The present moment is the one that calls for and merits our attention. Now is where we will find reality, connection, meaning, joy, love and, ultimately, God. For those seeking to find spiritual meaning on the journey through Alzheimer's, it's important to mention that *this* moment at hand, the only thing we truly own, is most often where we will experience true meetings with ourselves, others, and God.

Real interpersonal communion, according to Martin Buber, begins in between us—person to person. It begins when human beings relate to one another from the position of I to Thou, rather than relating as I to It.[23] When we relate to others as I–It, we consider them as objects, and this always results in separation, loneliness, and disconnection. *Mis-meeting* and *miscounter* are words Buber created and uses "to designate the failure of a real meeting" between individuals.[24]

In a story from his autobiography, *Encounter: Autobiographical Fragments*, Buber described an I–Thou meeting that happened in a childhood moment while he was petting his beloved horse.

> When I stroked the mighty mane, sometimes marvelously smooth-combed, at other times just as astonishingly wild, and felt the life beneath my hand, it was as though the element of vitality itself bordered on my skin, something that was not I, was certainly not akin to me, palpably the other, not just another, really the Other, itself.[25]

There were no interfering thoughts about the past or the future to distract eleven-year-old Martin. There were no regrets, no worries; there was just now. And in the now, he experienced awareness, presence, and connection. In the fleeting, extraordinary experience of being completely present in that moment, Martin Buber felt life beneath his hand, and he recognized this experience as connection with a transcendent presence: "Other, itself."

Gerald May, who became an important influence during my training as a spiritual director, described an experience similar to Buber's. "I can remember experiencing it in childhood, standing in a field and looking at the sky and just *being* in love.... It was like being immersed in an atmosphere of love, feeling very alive, very present in the moment, intimately connected with everything around me."[26]

Richard Rohr refers to these kinds of experiences, when we find God right in front of us, as "the purest form of spirituality"; French Jesuit Jean Pierre de Caussade refers to these experiences as "the sacrament of the present moment."[27]

"The deepest level of communication," according to Christian theologian and mystic Thomas Merton, "is not communication but communion. It is beyond words, and it is beyond speech, and it is beyond concept."[28]

Often in Mom's presence, I felt Buber's "Other," May's "being in love," Caussade's "sacrament," and Merton's "communion." In moments when I brushed her hair or helped her lick an ice-cream cone, watched her fingers remembering how to make music with piano keys or felt her fingers trying to scratch my back, the communion beyond verbal communication brought us alive. We transcended time and space. We were together and united—being in the now.

Coleen and I became friends at the nursing home. By the time we met, she had been her mother Ilene's faithful companion and advocate on the journey through Alzheimer's for almost ten years. Even after all those years of coming regularly to a nursing home, Coleen still felt particularly alive and connected in the presence of her mom and others with Alzheimer's. When Coleen came to the nursing home to be with her mother, her eyes saw beyond the diminishments and her ears heard beneath the garbled speech. She noticed the hands of residents reaching out to her as she passed by. She recognized humanity in their continuing desire for connection, and she reached back.

A priest-resident of the nursing home who had Alzheimer's, regularly sat at the main entrance, greeting visitors and residents coming and going from the building. Coleen greeted him every time she arrived, and she paused to hold his hand when she left. "The warmth in his hand made me feel good," she said. "Sometimes when you feel somebody's hand, you can feel God in there. This is a presence that is not taken away by Alzheimer's."

Often these transcendent moments seem to happen mysteriously, opening our entire beings to the presence of a life-giving spirit. These sacramental moments, rich with love and presence, are available to us—everywhere, always, in the hallowed everyday experiences. But it's up to us to pause, to be awake and aware, and to open ourselves to receiving them. When we notice and talk about these moments, we often refer to them as peak experiences or moments of grace.

Martin Buber also teaches about the importance of the connection that happens in between us during dialogue, whether in the form of communication or communion. "I have to tell it again and again," he said. "I have no doctrine. I only point out something. I point out reality, I point out something in reality which has not or too little been seen. I take him who listens to me by his hand and lead him to the window. I push open the window and point outside."[29]

Because Alzheimer's has an unpredictable nature with no clear doctrine for pointing us into understanding, it's important to recognize that the dialogue that is taking place all the time between caregivers and people with the disease requires patient, consistent attention. Observant caregivers can't help but notice the ability of people with Alzheimer's to be completely present in the moment. This complete presence is often their contribution to the dialogue. This complete presence is comparable to Buber's pointing finger. People with Alzheimer's are doing their best to show us their reality.

People with Alzheimer's are often, literally, pointing at doors, for which they have a particular fascination. Many will attempt to open every closed door they pass. Dr. Allen Power reminds caregivers to pay attention to behaviors that are commonly and repeatedly expressed by people with Alzheimer's, such as wandering or opening doors. He recommends "curiosity." They are leading us to a window and pointing. But at what? A desire to go home? To be free? To find a loved one? To look at their clothing? To find the kitchen? To go to work? To the bathroom? Where do they want to go? What are they looking for? Pointing to? Caregivers need to assume these actions have meaning, and to seek to know and understand what's beneath them.[30]

Geriatric psychiatrist Pierre Parenteau chimes in, "It's our responsibility to decode what a patient is trying to tell us through his/her conduct. For instance, if a person starts undressing in a place that seems inappropriate, he/she may be trying to tell us that he/she needs to use the washroom." He recommends using our "intuition."[31]

Doorknobs often riveted Mom's attention. She would look at the knob, carefully turn it while intently watching it move, pull the door open, push the door closed; then repeat. If allowed, this activity would go on for a long time—perhaps twenty minutes. This kind of focused, in-the-moment door-opening behavior might disturb some caregivers, particularly if it lasts for a long time, but I was both intrigued and delighted whenever Mom did it. At the very least, it seemed to be good exercise for her arm!

During earlier stages of my life journey, important teachers for me included medical professionals treating stress-related illnesses and spiritual practitioners teaching the techniques and benefits of meditation and contemplative prayer. And now here they were again, offering guidance for the journey through

Alzheimer's. These teachers encouraged me to consider twenty minutes of focused attention on anything—a candle flame, a flower, my breath, even a doorknob—as a highly desirable, health-improving, life-changing skill to acquire and to cultivate. Because one benefit of focused attention can be the deepened experiences of life described by Buber and May, many intelligent and enlightened beings—past and present—have endeavored to attain this ability. Author Henry Miller understood this: "The moment one gives close attention to anything, even a blade of grass, it becomes a mysterious, awesome, indescribably magnificent world in itself."[32]

A doorknob and a door, and what was on the other side, may have constituted a magnificent world for Mom. As I paid close attention to her opening and closing her closet door, and occasionally reaching slowly and deliberately for the hangers inside, she definitely became an awesome, magnificent world for me.

Through her disease and the process of decline that I witnessed on a daily basis, I came to understand that this moment at hand—this fleeting, precious moment with Mom—was the only moment she had and the only moment we had together. Being able to meet Mom as Thou, even as her capacities diminished, and finding joy with her, was like manna from heaven in the desert of Alzheimer's disease.

In praising the ability of people with Alzheimer's to focus their attention so completely, it's not my intention to glorify the cognitive decline that is part of Alzheimer's; nor is it my intention to dismiss the sense of loss, confusion, and frustration that family caregivers inevitably experience over their loved ones' forgotten pasts and their unawareness of the future. Alzheimer's, indeed, creates suffering, and it would be cruel to ask caregivers to deny their suffering.

In reaction to the cries of caregivers with "broken hearts and tired lives" (an apt description), authors Jane Thibault and Richard Morgan ask, "Can we offer any answer, any consolation, any words to sustain the caregivers of parents, spouses, relatives, and friends so that their once-strong bonds of mutual relationship can somehow survive?"[33] My answer to this question is yes; my words of consolation are these: by pointing to the ability of people with Alzheimer's to be in the moment, by raising up the importance of every I-Thou moment, and recognizing the remaining capacity for relational connections, the strong bonds of mutual relationship *can* survive and thrive.

Additionally, caregivers are invited to consider another perspective that may bring some consolation, one that includes the possibility of interpreting the losses and behaviors that are characteristic of Alzheimer's in other ways. At age thirty-seven, Harvard brain scientist Jill Taylor suffered a massive stroke that left her "so completely disabled," that she described herself "as an infant in a woman's body."[34] Taylor's loss of language and executive brain functions was similar to losses experienced by people with Alzheimer's. She describes her experience:

> I met a growing sense of peace. In place of that constant chatter that had attached me to the details of my life, I felt enfolded by a blanket of tranquil euphoria .... As the language centers in my left hemisphere grew increasingly silent and I became detached from the memories of my life, I was comforted by an expanding sense of grace. In this void of higher cognition and details pertaining to my normal life, my consciousness soared into an all-knowingness, a "being at one" with the universe .... In a compelling sort of way, it felt like the good road home and I liked it.[35]

For the reasons Taylor describes, including "being at one with the universe," the desire (by cognitively intact, intelligent, enlightened people) to be present in the moment has been demonstrated for thousands of years. Spiritual teachers and disciples from every major religious tradition have, since ancient times, deliberately sought to experience this state.[36] In the twentieth century, medical practitioners began to recognize that health benefits could be achieved through the focused attention of meditation practice. Decades ago, scientific studies first documented the potential of this practice to reduce stress and improve health.[37] Past studies at Harvard University indicate a correlation between meditation and brain health, including memory retention.[38]

Vipassana, or "insight meditation" (also known as "mindfulness" in our modern times),[39] is a form of meditation from the Buddhist tradition. This practice became an enlightening and healing anchor for me over many years, some of them tumultuous. The goals of mindfulness meditation are to quiet the mind and body and to be present in the moment, noticing, accepting, and responding to what is, right now. Many people think that meditation can be practiced only when they're sitting on a cushion on the floor in a quiet room, with incense wafting through the space and other meditators chanting *om* or another foreign-sounding mantra. What makes mindfulness a special practice is that it can happen off the cushion in everyday activities. The skills learned through sitting and walking meditation can be applied to everything we do, like eating, washing dishes, brushing teeth, etc. As this skill is developed, we can live increasingly in the present moment and participate more fully in everything we do. Zen Master Hiakajo Roshi, who was accomplished in the practice of mindfulness, said simply, "When I eat, I eat. When I sleep, I sleep."[40]

The words of the Buddhist master could also be a description of people with Alzheimer's: When they eat, they eat. When they sing, they sing. When they hug, they hug. When they play ball, they play ball. Buddhist nun Pema Chödrön writes, "If we can experience the moment we're in, we discover that it is unique, precious and completely fresh." This completely fresh moment "never happens twice," she adds. "One can appreciate and celebrate each moment—there's nothing more sacred. There's nothing more vast or absolute. In fact, there's nothing more!"[41]

When we notice that our loved ones with Alzheimer's are intently focused on something, we can consider it an opportunity to pause and join them in the moment, to be fascinated by the magnificent doorknob, drinking fountain, piano keys, or flower—for even a moment. We may be surprised and delighted to discover that we have the potential, right along with our loved ones with Alzheimer's, to be here now and experience a sense of presence, perhaps even peace.

Since the benefits of mindfulness don't require a formal sitting meditation practice, they're attainable even within the overwhelming context of Alzheimer's caregiving. Whenever I allowed myself to fully *be* with Mom during her fascination with doorknobs (or with wiping tables, washing dishes, pushing the button on the TV remote and watching the channels change, or turning the drinking fountain on and off), instead of being impatient and wanting to hustle her off to whatever I had planned, I could choose to pause, to breathe more slowly, and to relax. I began to notice details about whatever she was doing— color, texture, and sound, for example—and to experience my feelings of sorrow and joy as I witnessed her expressing her remaining mental and physical abilities. Often, I felt refreshed when I left the nursing home, as if I'd been on vacation. In a way, I had. My worries, deadlines, fears, and even physical discomforts had all been on hiatus for those hours, because

I had been present and attentive during every moment with Mom.

Before becoming Mom's companion on the journey through Alzheimer's, I'd been practicing mindfulness meditation for more than twenty-five years, and I had learned from Chödrön that "we don't sit in meditation to become good meditators. We sit in meditation so that we will be more awake in our lives."[44] While I sat in meditation for twenty minutes every morning during those years I spent with Mom, many practical difficulties, intellectual challenges, and uncomfortable feelings about our situation erupted during the silence. When this happened, my previous years of mindfulness practice served me well. By staying awake to everything, I was given an opportunity to recognize, accept, and process my feelings about the eruption, to carefully consider alternatives, and then freely choose to move forward toward communion and healing.

Caregivers who are just beginning to focus on being present in the moment will appreciate knowing in advance that courage (to face challenging, unpleasant, and ambivalent feelings, as well as unwelcomed circumstances) and persistence are needed for us to be and stay fully present to what is happening in every moment. People with Alzheimer's do it naturally. Let them be our guides.

11 Gifts from the Alzheimer's Journey

Spiritual practices such as surrender, acceptance, and being present in the moment have their roots in ancient religious traditions. Another practice with spiritual roots, gratitude, becomes especially significant in the context of Alzheimer's care because it encompasses the potential for accepting loss, healing brokenness, and transcending suffering.

As we begin to consider the Alzheimer's journey in the context of gift, poet Mary Oliver offers us a challenging thought to ponder in her poem, "Uses of Sorrow." Like many of Oliver's poems, this one awakened me to new possibilities. She describes receiving "a box full of darkness" from someone she loved, revealing that it took years to understand that "this, too, was a gift."[42]

In this caregiving context, as in the context of any suffering, gratitude probably won't happen automatically or easily because Alzheimer's disease, like no other, can literally bring caregivers to our knees, the posture of surrender. However, being on our knees is not cause for despair. It can actually be where gratitude begins. We are here, in this posture of surrender, because we acknowledge that the external realities and practicalities of the disease are causing us to suffer. We are here, recognizing and embracing our internal realities, the brewing and swirling and festering feelings within us, feelings born of the ways that Alzheimer's has changed and continues to change our lives, including all the ways it causes us stress, drains our energy, and heightens our fears.

"The world is full of suffering," said Helen Keller, shining light on a life reality embedded in most religious traditions. But she doesn't leave it there; nor do the religions. She went on to remind her readers and listeners of another truth; a greater truth, perhaps: the world is also full of the overcoming of suffering.[43] It's this overcoming that reveals to us, and the world, that our suffering and the suffering of our loved ones with Alzheimer's has not been in vain. Holocaust survivor Viktor Frankl knew much about loss, suffering, and overcoming. He reminds us that, above all, what motivates us as human beings is the "will to meaning" in our lives.[44] This meaning, the seed of overcoming suffering, is ours to manifest.

In this lifetime, no person will get a free pass from pain— physical, emotional, mental, or spiritual. All the major world religions speak of this Truth. The foundation of the Buddhist Tradition is that it is in our nature to have pain and illness, to grow old (if we are blessed with old age), to diminish, to die. But the religions also show us various ways through. The metaphor of the "refiner's fire" (Malachi 3:2-3) from the Jewish Tradition is one powerful example. The refiner (any life challenge: Alzheimer's, for example) puts our broken pieces into a crucible, a container that can withstand very high heat, and when the burning process for removing unwanted elements is complete, what remains is precious material. Similarly, the Christian cross is about suffering, and it's also about change.

That's our sacred invitation when we find ourselves in the crucible or on the cross: change

There is no question that Alzheimer's brings unwanted challenges and suffering, into the lives it touches. But with conscious effort, we can develop resilience; we can realize our potential for growth and transformation through painful, refining experiences; we can increase our capacity for accepting what is, the all-important skill for the caregiving journey. And most importantly for our human journey, we can discover our passion for meaning making. These four qualities—resilience, potential, acceptance, and meaning making—will help us to gracefully and graciously make life-affirming choices all along the way, through life and through Alzheimer's, and to recognize the precious material presented to us, in whatever form it takes.[45]

We begin our transformation in the posture of surrender, on our knees, and it is from there that we are invited into a healing process, a process that could lead us from despair to gratitude for what is. We do this by sharing our sorrows with God, or with our own inner knowing, deeply, freely, and honestly. The ancient Hebrew prayer practice of lament can help us. As demonstrated for us in the books of Psalms and Lamentations from the Hebrew Bible, there is a structure to the lament. The first part of the process requires us to express our truth, passionately and without editing. This involves courage. We often prefer not to admit some of our feelings to anyone, or even to ourselves, because we have been socialized to judge as inappropriate what are referred to as "negative" feelings, such as anger, fear, doubt, sadness, guilt, and shame. However, all of our feelings are valid, and they are useful for our growth and healing. Welcoming and embracing our feelings rather than trying to avoid or banish them, to consider them holy messages designed to enlighten and inspire us, inform and guide us—this is a different approach for many of us, and it can be daunting.

When I lead caregiver retreats, participants are invited to identify an experience or feeling that weighs heavily on their souls. Then, in the tradition of lament (and improv), they are given permission to "rant" about their fear, sorrow, heartache, fury, fatigue, grief, or self-judgment for 60 to 90 seconds. Participants must talk fast and spontaneously with no editing. This can be a profound experience of catharsis and cleansing, especially when it's time limited and doesn't allow us to sink into self-pity and wallow there. I've attended Alzheimer's support groups where caregivers complain about their situations, unchecked, for long periods of time. This type of complaining doesn't have wings that will take someone beyond the pain. More often, it has the potential to make caregivers (those speaking and those listening) feel worse. However, a purposeful rant, intended for catharsis, enables the next parts of the lament—praise and thanksgiving—to naturally flow into our hearts.

In the midst of the losses and burdens of Alzheimer's, finding reasons to praise and thank God could seem impossible. But prayer has been known to make the impossible possible. In particular, this prayer of lament has the potential to transform the caregiving experience, and even our lives, if we give it a chance. One of my laments about Alzheimer's (in brief) went like this: "Why me, God? Why did I have to leave my life in Boston and move to Iowa to take care of Mom? Why me? (Grumble. Grumble. Grumble.) Oh, but she said my name today. She knows I'm here! I'm so happy I didn't miss that word, that moment of connection! Thank you for guiding me to come here."

At the caregiver retreats, after the ranting guided by the structure of the lament, I invite participants to pause and recall a time with their loved one when they noticed a moment that felt endearing, connecting, or even humorous, a moment when they felt touched emotionally or flooded with love or joy, surprise or awe. These are the moments that will connect us to our loved ones, other caregivers, and to God. These are the indelible moments that will carry us through this experience with open hearts. When these moments are shared in a group, the energy immediately changes and caregivers feel the connections that are happening within and around them. Often tears of love and joy flow.

Loretta Veney cared for her mother, Doris, who lived with Alzheimer's for sixteen years. In her book *Being My Mom's Mom*, Loretta highlights how humor and laughter created joyful indelible moments for her. She writes, "There is nothing funny about dementia. However, there are moments when situations created by the disease can be hysterical. My Mom is so funny, I've thought about selling a book of her quotes or getting her a show as a standup comedian."[46] In her book, Loretta relays a number of Doris' humorous quotes and includes links to various websites about engaging humor to help with dementia caregiving. Laughter can, indeed, be a buoy on this journey, and most people with Alzheimer's seem to love to laugh. Like Doris, my mom had a special sense of humor, and she could make me laugh like no one else with her storytelling; we laughed together often and with others in all kinds of situations. I remember one lunchtime in the dining room at Mom's nursing home. Twelve residents were eating lunch, and a handful of family members and aides were helping with the meal, when out of the blue one of the residents started to laugh. No one seemed to know why. But her laugh was so genuine, so pure, so infectious that soon those at her table were laughing with her; then a couple aides caught the vibe and laughed along; then I started to laugh, and Mom started to laugh, and then the rest of our table, and the rest of the people in the room all laughed. We carried on with uncontrollable, cheek-aching laughter until the whole room was hysterical with glee, tears streaming down our faces. Without any explanation about what was so funny, this experience, which remains indelible fifteen years later, set the tone for a joyous afternoon for everyone.

As we practice letting go of trying to control what we cannot, accepting what is, and being mindful of what's happening within and around us, our ability to glimpse and touch gratitude, even in the most difficult circumstances, will become enhanced. Being aware of each and every one of Mom's accomplishments, no matter how small, seeing her smile when she recognized my arrival, hearing her say my name or her name, and so many other hallowed little everyday moments in our life together, made my soul sing in thanksgiving.

Benedictine and Zen monk David Steindl-Rast offers a challenge to his students when he shares his belief (inspired by the Gospel of Matthew 7:7-11) that God is benevolent and gives only good gifts. With this theological position as his springboard, Steindl-Rast suggests that we consider being grateful for everything we're given in life, even if we consider it to be something bad.[47] People with Alzheimer's and their loved ones may find this a particularly thorny theological position to even consider, much less embrace.

Alzheimer's a good gift? Most of us, whether we have it or a loved one has it, would consider Alzheimer's a curse. Lynda spent most of her adult life caring for loved ones, first for her mother, who was paralyzed by a stroke; then for her father, who experienced vascular dementia; and finally for her late husband, Richard, who had Alzheimer's. Lynda does not mince words—and speaks for many, I'm sure—when she declares that Alzheimer's is "a very cruel disease." She considers all diseases with symptoms of dementia to be "horrible and dreadful," consisting of horrible and dreadful experiences for those afflicted and caregivers alike.

Jane Thibault and Richard Morgan write that even caregivers of deep faith share Lynda's opinion, and continually ask, "Why has God let this happen to us?" or "How can I go on believing in the goodness of God when I see Mom [Dad] suffering from a disease that destroys her [his] memory and the person I know?"[48] As I pondered these questions in the context of Alzheimer's, I reread the book of Job from the Hebrew Bible. Poor Job. He loses everything that he considers important in his external life: his family, his possessions, his property, his wealth, and even his health. According to ancient Hebrew theology, God only punishes those who have sinned. Therefore, direct witnesses to Job's downfall and misery logically conclude that he must have sinned and so he deserves his current situation as divine retribution.

Rabbi Harold Kushner, author of the insightful book *When Bad Things Happen to Good People*, consoled me throughout my life during numerous times of loss and suffering. Through his reflections on the Book of Job, Kushner once again offered me consolation as I confronted the realities of Alzheimer's disease. Kushner notices that Job is sure of one thing, his own innocence. "Job, for his part, is unwilling to hold the world together theologically by admitting that he is a villain" and conceding that he deserves the suffering he has received as punishment from God. "He knows a lot of things intellectually, but he knows one thing more deeply. Job is absolutely sure that he is not a bad person."[49]

Author Stephen Mitchell, in his commentary on the Book of Job, states that in his suffering, Job represents everyone, "grieving for all of human misery."[50] In the early sections of Job's story, his despair expands because he does not seem to realize, or accept, that wretched conditions and circumstances are a part of our human destiny. For several years, my days were spent in a nursing home filled with people with Alzheimer's who were collectively like Job. They too had lost almost everything of external importance: eyesight, hearing, mobility, limbs, speech, cognition, spouses, children, homes, pets, money and possessions, bladder and bowel control, the ability to feed themselves, the ability to chew and swallow, autonomy, and freedom. Their losses and misery, however, didn't exist solely because of their lives in a nursing home or because they had Alzheimer's. Elders as well as others I know who are healthy, independent, mentally sharp, active, and productive have experienced some of the same losses and pain that Job and the people with Alzheimer's in the nursing home experienced. They have lost spouses, jobs, friends, children, parents, homes, security, social position and respect, limbs, sight, hearing, and teeth. None of us is immune to this pain, these losses, or grief, suffering, and death. The extending human lifespan is currently identified as the greatest risk factor for an Alzheimer's diagnosis. The longer we live, the more we will encounter these unavoidable experiences and losses in our own lives, and we will witness them in the lives of others, of those we love.

The writer of the Book of Job has invited me to integrate the reality about loss and longevity into my beliefs about God and my witness of suffering and death as it relates to people with Alzheimer's and their loved ones—none of whom deserve this disease and the circumstances it creates, but all of whom must endure it. Accepting our inevitable diminishment as part of the human condition may, ironically, aid in alleviating the suffering connected with the diminishments of Alzheimer's. A Buddhist saying illustrates the wisdom beneath this acceptance: "If I break my leg, then I have pain. If I think there is a world where I should not have pain, then I suffer."

Mitchell's analysis of the book of Job helped me to see the intersection of loss, suffering, Alzheimer's, and God in a new way, and to increase my empathy for caregivers, like Lynda, who suffered on the Alzheimer's journey in ways that differed from my own suffering. Lynda and I and Mitchell all agree that every person with Alzheimer's and every caregiver's experience of this disease process will be uniquely their own. "There is never an answer to the great question of life and death," writes Mitchell, "unless it is my answer or yours. Because ultimately it isn't a question answered, but a person. Our whole being has to be answered."[51]

Through their theological inquiries into Job's suffering, Kushner and Mitchell both conclude that God is good, agreeing with David Steindl-Rast. I found Kushner's words to be a guiding light on this subject: "[God] can still be on our side when bad things happen to us... we can turn to [God] for help. Our question, our prayer, and our petition will not be Job's question, 'God why are you doing this to me?' but rather, 'God see what is happening to me. Can You help me?' We will turn to God not to be judged or forgiven, not to be rewarded or punished, but to be strengthened and comforted."[52] It's that firsthand relationship with God that is healing us.

Daisy cared for her mom, Sonia, at home for eleven years. Looking back on her caregiving experience, she realizes that she embodied the guidance offered by Kushner and Mitchell. It was during the caregiving years that Daisy's faith resurrected and deepened in significant ways. As it is for all caregivers, the Alzheimer's journey was a difficult path for Daisy. She had to make so many changes in order to accommodate Sonia's presence in her home and her life, and to adjust to her mother's ever-changing, abundant needs. There were times when Daisy was holding more despair and responsibility than was bearable. It was then that she turned to God in the spirit of lament, with her heart open. She cried alone at night in bed, voicing her sorrows and challenges. Although other people couldn't listen well, or didn't understand, or would give unhelpful advice, or were tired of hearing about it, Daisy trusted that God would always be near, always hear her, always comfort her. Instead of feeling sorry for herself and asking, 'God, why did you do this to me?' Daisy prayed for strength, 'God, just help me through this. I don't want to stop. Just keep working me through this.' In the morning, she would wake up ready to begin again, her body and mind renewed, her spirit ever grateful for the honor of caring for her mother, now, during her time of diminishment.

If caregivers can faithfully practice being mindful and patient, if we can affirm that the Spirit of Life is present in all people and working in different ways to manifest potential and call us toward goodness, and if we can accept the distress that we endure while trying to relieve the suffering of our loved ones, we may find our way *through* the anguish—as Job does, as Daisy and I did—into vast wonder and love. After the intense misery Job experiences while insisting that he does not deserve loss and pain and demanding that things should be different, he finally receives deep peace by accepting and embracing reality.

If we can accept the perspectives about suffering and life offered by Steindl-Rast, Kushner, Mitchell, and Daisy—perspectives emerging from Jewish and Christian traditions–that, through God, all things that happen can help us grow, we open ourselves to surprising possibilities. This opening, however, calls forth another spiritual challenge. If there are good gifts in bad experiences, such as starving children, nuclear menace, natural disasters, wars between peoples and countries, diminishments of aging, and losses from Alzheimer's, Mitchell emphasizes that these gifts are buried somewhere under the devastating rubble of reality.[53] We are required to examine what appears as ruin, searching for strength, longing for comfort, examining the choices we are invited to make between life and death.

Steindl-Rast, acknowledges—even for himself—the difficulty of finding good gifts within hard experiences, the difficulty of even attempting to look for them. He further explains this invitation: "Gratefulness is the full response of the human heart to reality—as it is. Not to this reality or that reality." Anticipating our resistance to gratitude in the face of something that ought not to be there—outrageous words, abusive actions, heartbreaking experiences, or incurable diseases, for example—Steindl-Rast reassures us that he is not instructing us to be grateful for that which has outraged or distressed us. He is inviting us to be grateful in the face of these horrible, dreadful, cruel realities because, by acknowledging them, we are being given the opportunity to do something about them.[54] We who have had the experience are invited to make a healing difference in the lives of people with Alzheimer's, other caregivers, and ourselves.

I was given the opportunity to make Mom's quality of life as good as it could be, to comfort her, and to protect her in small and large ways. These kinds of acts of love, according to Steindl-Rast, are expressions of "thanksgiving for the insights of love's vision."[55] My decision to care for Mom was born of my sense of belonging to her, and her to me. Flowing out of this belonging, the service we caregivers offer to our loved ones is our expression of gratitude for being given the opportunity to serve. "On strong wings," Steindl-Rast writes, "love rises to every opportunity and shows itself grateful for it."[56]

My regular mindfulness meditation practice increased the fruits of my intention to recognize and receive gifts, and to feel gratitude in the midst of Mom's relentless decline. For me, one gift of having a loved one with Alzheimer's grew out of the invitation to slow down. When I chose to walk slowly, matching

Mom's pace, the words of Buddhist teacher Thich Nhat Hanh came to life: "In daily life there is so much to do and so little time. We feel pressured to run all the time. Just stop! Touch the ground of the present moment deeply, and you will touch real peace and joy."[57] I looked—really looked—at the flowers and the birds Mom so loved, examining their intricate details. Doing this heightened my desire and my ability to be present to life and enlivened my enjoyment of every moment. I also chose to speak slowly and simply, increasing the opportunity for Mom to comprehend verbal communication. Consciously choosing not to complete her sentences with words I thought she might say, I waited patiently for her own words to emerge, which were often different from what I would have guessed.[58] I looked closely at her and her world; I listened, carefully, to her.

For both Mom and me, every day was a new day of discovery. Every day, I was given opportunities to notice, accept, and love her, who she was, where she was. Every day brought opportunities to identify and meet her constantly changing needs. Embedded within these opportunities was the merging of love and gratefulness. Observing Mom's declining abilities and opening my heart to her brought me life's greatest gift, the experience of feeling and expressing unconditional love.

Being Mom's legal guardian manifested gifts born of a different kind of loving. The state of Iowa had empowered me to literally *be* Mom's voice. I spoke, not just on her behalf, but I spoke *as* her. As opportunities arose to help her by assertively speaking up or taking action, I was most grateful for this gift of power. When Mom seemed sick, when I perceived her to be in danger, or when I concluded that her needs were being overlooked or neglected, I was not a helpless bystander, fretting and complaining to friends or wishing that things could be different. I could intervene to make things different. I had the power to seek hospice care for Mom, to change her doctor to someone who communicated well with cognitively impaired people, to find out what kind of additional benefits were available to her (speech therapy, for example), to question the nursing home policies and procedures, to recommend interventions, to choose the aides who would work with Mom, to make dietary requests, and much more.

In one instance, when antibiotics no longer worked to cure Mom's recurring urinary tract infections, her doctor researched and prescribed an herbal remedy at my request. This was an unusual protocol for Mom's nursing home, and the nursing staff objected vehemently. It was not, after all, approved by the FDA, the nursing director said in a huff. If there was a chance this herb would relieve Mom's pain and discomfort, I didn't intend to allow the nursing home's objections to stand in the way.

Believing this remedy was in Mom's best interest and knowing that it would not harm her, I did something about it. It was hard and stressful for me to be a thorn in the side of the nursing home administration by being firm about this issue, but I found myself feeling grateful for the opportunity to push beyond my fears of upsetting people and do what was right for Mom. Through the Iowa Council on Aging, I located the nursing home ombudsman, who researched precedence and protocols for administering herbal prescriptions in Iowa. (It happens regularly.) The ombudsman then met with the nursing home administrator and nursing director and ensured that Mom's remedy would be administered as prescribed by her doctor.

After this episode was resolved, I was depleted as a result of the struggle it had become. However, the herb ultimately helped to relieve Mom's infections for almost six months, so the outcome of what was a difficult process for me felt rewarding. The stress and frustration I had endured, and even my subsequent fatigue, transformed into gifts. I felt empowered in my role of guardian, and grateful for the embodied reminder that I had worked relentlessly, and successfully, to relieve the suffering of a vulnerable and helpless being.

Our hardest experiences can be our best gifts because these experiences "make us grow the most," writes Steindl-Rast.[59] However, we don't always appreciate the hard experiences the Universe brings to us, and no one, including Steindl-Rast, expects us to give thanks because the epidemic of Alzheimer's has touched our personal world. He does encourage us, though, to focus our attention on reality, and from there, to try and find something—any tiny thing—for which we can sincerely give thanks. For example, even family caregiver Lynda, who experienced the Alzheimer's journey with and for her husband as horrible and dreadful, reports being grateful for the people who accepted her, helped her, educated her, loved her, and provided examples of good caregiving for her along the way. She also, years later, still feels grateful for the choices she was able to make that helped her loved ones, others on the journey, and herself. She especially feels gratitude to God for the gift of grace that empowered her to make and act on her life-affirming choices.

People living with Alzheimer's, because their emotions are alive and well, will most likely still be feeling gratitude. However, their appreciation for our attention and care will often be expressed in ways that require us to translate and interpret. For years, I observed nursing aides tenderly caring for my mother and many others with Alzheimer's—a mostly verbally garbled or silent population—without expecting or needing a word of thanks. They had learned to feel appreciated by knowing the importance of their work and by noticing the gratitude that beamed forth from their residents through a smile or a touch, from eye contact or a wave.

People with advanced Alzheimer's are those most needing assistance with their activities of daily living. Even though it's generally hard for adults to adjust to needing and receiving help, if this population could speak, I believe most would graciously say words of thanks for the care and attention they are receiving in the midst of an outrageous, unrelenting experience of diminishment. I make this prediction based on my own observations. History, however, also reveals to us that suffering, vulnerable people are grateful for any kindness, and that they can have a life-changing impact on others. In 1889, writer Robert Louis Stevenson visited a hospital in Hawaii specifically for patients suffering with Hansen's disease, more commonly known as leprosy. Six years earlier, Mother Marianne Cope, a Franciscan nun from New York, was asked to establish this hospital, which became known as the Bishop Home. Isolated from the rest of society by law and disfigured by disease, people with leprosy had long been society's outcasts. In caring for this population, Mother Marianne insisted on cleanliness, music, and beauty—to help put a little more sunshine into their dreary lives.[60] I can't help but compare them to the scores of people with cognitive decline who have also been considered outcasts by society.

After visiting the Bishop Home, Stevenson wrote of being "tempted to deny his God" because of the suffering he witnessed. But then he goes on to describe noticing how genuinely the people with leprosy smiled when receiving even small acts of kindness or attention from their devoted caregivers. As the poet looks again, he acknowledges seeing "beauty springing from the breast of pain."

Stevenson's poem "To Mother Maryanne" expresses his recognition of gratefulness as Steindl-Rast defines it, "full aliveness" held together by the heartbeat of this present moment. Stevenson memorializes his own gratefulness for the sisters' ministry along with his awareness of the grateful "innocent sufferers" who inspired him into silence and adoration, and a deepening of his relationship with the Holy.[61]

In my search to understand how people of faith could accept and transcend the losses of aging and Alzheimer's disease, I arrived in my studies at the intersection of Christian spiritual perspectives born of process theology and liberation theology. Process theology teaches that the life-giving energy of the Universe [God] works in relational ways, enlisting others to accompany us, to help us, to guide us to freedom and healing.[62] This theory is popularly known as "God with skin on." Liberation theology interprets the teachings of Jesus in terms of the essential need to liberate the poor and the suffering from unjust economic, political, or social conditions. As I considered the innocent sufferers—Job, the people with leprosy at the Bishop Home, and all those with Alzheimer's in Mom's nursing home and around the world—these perspectives brought me comfort and inspired me. Similarly, I was inspired as I encountered the undeserved pain of people with Alzheimer's and their caregivers. Within these populations I see shining the healing relationship between the Spirit of Life and humanity. This strengthens my belief in the ultimate holiness in all of life,[63] even life with Alzheimer's.

Through my empathic, relational witness of Mom's decline, I felt called to leave my busy life in Boston and to walk slowly beside her on the last steps of her journey "home." Answering yes to this call was an expression of lived process theology: "God's primary avenue to liberation [from the suffering] is through responsive human hearts."[64] My yes to caring for Mom became the greatest honor and the greatest gift of my life. It was and continues to be a meaning-making life experience for me. I have never ceased giving thanks for the opportunity to care for her, for what I learned, and for how I grew more deeply into my own humanity.

The millions of other caregivers who are offering love and care to people with Alzheimer's have also been called, as I was, to serve their loved ones through awareness, relational witness, and responsive hearts. Without question, this call is difficult to receive, and even more difficult to wholeheartedly accept; it is perhaps the hardest experience of our lives so far. If, however, we consider the possibility that there are gifts in the midst of our difficulties, if we look consciously at our frustrations, sadness, burdens, and sacrifices, we will notice opportunities for enhancing our abilities to observe and accept what is, to be present, and to feel grateful. All of this encompasses the heartbeat of the spiritual journey. In these places of loss and suffering—places where we don't expect to find anything of value or beauty—spring the possibility that we can open ourselves to meeting our loved ones with Alzheimer's in mutuality, to receiving grace, and to experiencing gratefulness.

IV

Believing in Relationship

I am losing words.
How shall I describe
the feeling of reaching toward,
reaching out, longing;
how shall I name
what I have loved
and do love,
still love: faces,
flowers, clouds, the long view
across prairie … and lake?
How will I greet you,
how will you know
you are greeted, loved,
and longed-for? Will you
believe me when it comes,
as it will,
that I speak without words,
and forget to hold my arms out
in embrace of you,

who are earth, and sky, and world;
how will I recognize
your embrace of me;
how will we continue
this life's long love,
when I have lost all words?
      —Rev. Libbie Deverich Stoddard

The path of Alzheimer's is vastly unpredictable. Accordingly, as my caregiving companions and I walked along this path with those living with dementia, we were often challenged by what we encountered along the way. We were surprised, again and again, because the path was never quite clear. But our role in the lives of our loved ones was always crystal clear; our role was to love, support, and encourage them every step of the way.

One of the great unknowns on this journey through Alzheimer's is the length of this disease. How long will someone who has been diagnosed with Alzheimer's live? Although it's designated as a terminal illness because there is no cure, Paul Raia invites us to consider Alzheimer's as a disability since afflicted people can live with declining abilities for four to twenty years.[1] Rather than preparing for an imminent death, adapting—day by day—to changing abilities and needs will be required for people with the disease as well as their caregivers and family members.

The long journey home for people with Alzheimer's will eventually lead to a fork in the road. One path leads them into silence, isolation, and loneliness. The other path leads them to a life rich with communication, connection, meaning, and love. Because of the dependent nature of Alzheimer's, especially during the advanced stages, family caregivers and caring professionals will determine which path those afflicted will travel.

My friend Constance, who is over eighty, knows that Alzheimer's and other forms of dementia afflict about 35 percent of people over the age of eighty-five in the U.S. Although she is in remarkably good health, she still fears that she will get this disease. Constance is not alone. The *New York Times* reports that Americans are more afraid of Alzheimer's than of dying.[2] Constance expressed her fear to a friend, who consoled her and calmed her fears by saying, "Well, if there is someone who understands the disease to love you and take really good care of you, maybe it wouldn't be so bad."

Increasing our understanding and our loving will best qualify us to be effective caregivers for, and companions to, people with Alzheimer's on their journeys home. This effort, however, will also enhance our own journeys. Our own healing begins in true encounter with others.

Moving more deeply into the world of meaningful relationships . . . .

12 Emotional Memory

At the doorway of a memory care unit I toured in the Boston area, I was greeted by a sign bearing prophetic words from poet Maya Angelou: "People will forget what you said, people will forget what you did, but people will never forget how you made them feel."

Angelou's words reminded me of an important reality about being human: our emotions matter. They inform our decisions; they guide our reactions; they express our deep truths. Unfortunately, our rational, intellectual, technological, fast-paced world tends to ignore this reality, even for the healthiest of us. The emotions of those who are limited in their abilities to identify and communicate their feelings in traditionally expected ways are even more unacknowledged. However, attentive Alzheimer's caregivers have known for quite a long time that Angelou's recognition is true for *all* people, including cognitively impaired people.

At a dementia care conference, I was introduced to the poem "Heart Memories," written by Louise Eder and published in the Kansas City Alzheimer's Disease and Related Disorders newsletter in 1984. Although I couldn't find out if Louise was a person with Alzheimer's, a family/friend carepartner, or a professional caregiver, the poem reveals her understanding of the retention and importance of emotions in people with Alzheimer's.

I remember you with my heart
My mind won't say your name
I can't recall where or if I knew you
Who you were or who I was.

Maybe I grew up with you or
Maybe we worked together
Or did we bowl together yesterday?
There's something wrong with my
Memory but I do know you—and
I do love you.

I know I knew you
I know how you make me feel
I remember the feelings we had together
My heart remembers
It cries out in loneliness for you
For the feelings you give me now.

Today I'm happy that you have come
When you leave
My mind will not remember that
You were here
But my heart remembers
Remembers the feeling of friendship
And love returned
Remembers
That I am less lonely and happier
Today because of the feeling
Because you have come.

Please don't forget me
And please don't stay away
Because of the way my mind acts.
I can still feel you
I can still remember you with my heart
And a heart memory is maybe
The most important memory of all.[3]

As the theme of "Heart Memories" indicates, some caregivers have known, do know, that it remains possible to connect deeply and maintain meaningful relationships with people experiencing the brain alterations associated with Alzheimer's and dementia. These caregivers have recognized and appreciated the existence and the power of emotions, emotional expression, and emotional memory in people with Alzheimer's. So has Paul Raia. For more than twenty years, Raia, a true innovator in the discipline of Alzheimer's care, provides support to people with Alzheimer's and their families through his work with the Alzheimer's Association in Massachusetts. Before moving to Iowa, I had the opportunity—and great honor—of meeting with him as I was developing Healing Moments programming. Based on his input, I created the "Monarch Moments" services to honor and remember our loved ones with Alzheimer's. From the onset of Raia's work with Alzheimer's, he focused on the emotions and the remaining capacities of cognitively impaired people. Through his commitment to observing the reality of Alzheimer's through "the collective experience of caregivers," Raia recognized that

> the capacity to feel and exhibit emotions persists among people with Alzheimer's disease far into the disease process. What is lost is the insight into what might have triggered a particular emotion or how to control it. The

ability to feel emotions, then, may be our best inroad to the mind of the person with Alzheimer's disease.[4]

Raia's depth of understanding about the enduring, heightened emotions in people with Alzheimer's leads him to echo the tenets of improvisation, and he guides us away from saying no. He explains that when we say no, our muscles automatically tense and the tone of our voice changes, which people with Alzheimer's will notice. Due to their enhanced sensitivity to body language and voice cues, they will instinctively interpret expressions of no as controlling or demeaning, and they will react. Raia reminds us that, because of their limited ability to communicate verbally, "the situation becomes highly emotional."[5] "No," as well as other emotionally charged words uttered without thought, or actions taken without consideration, can deflate or incite people with Alzheimer's. Author Colleen Carroll Campbell shared her observations of this dynamic, which she noticed while caring for her father: "Dad's memory may have been ravaged in those last years, but his emotional acuity was keener than ever. Like an infant reacting to the stresses in his surroundings, Dad's mood was mightily affected by the tone of voice and gentleness or harshness of another's touch."[6]

In our relationships with people who are highly emotionally sensitive, being able to feel and name our own emotions will enhance our empathy, increase our patience with others, and improve our effectiveness as caregivers. At the Healing Moments workshop on Cape Cod where *Still Alice* author Lisa Genova and I met, she was an eager and fascinated participant in the improvisation exercises we offered. During one exercise, when the leader blocked and negated Lisa's offers by saying no to her, Lisa reacted emotionally. She shared her experience with me:

Here is the exercise I remember most. I was asked to say a simple statement, something I believe to be true. I said, smiling, "I have the most beautiful six-month-old boy."

The instructor, looking me straight in the eye and without smiling, said, "You do not have a six-month-old baby. Your kids are all grown. You don't know what you're talking about."

My turn came around again.

"It's a glorious, sunny day outside."

"No, it's not. It's dark and cloudy, and it's going to rain."

Here's what I noticed. Even though I knew this was just an exercise: I didn't want to talk with this woman. I didn't like being told I was wrong, I didn't like the look on her face, and I didn't like her tone of voice. In fact, I felt my emotions stirred by the interaction, like I was readying to argue or fight.[7]

Being aware of our own emotional reactions—in an exercise like this and in life—can help us understand why people with Alzheimer's react as they do. Statements they make, which we consider false, are as true for them, and as important to them, as having a beautiful baby boy was true and important for Lisa. This awareness can be a catalyst for caregivers to change the ways we speak to and interact with people with Alzheimer's. By doing so, we may ease their suffering and perhaps even manage behaviors previously managed with psychotropic medications.

To Raia's collective of caregiver experiences, I add my own observations of Mom's capability to feel and communicate her emotions. During my years in Iowa, it was my practice to spend time with Mom every day, most often in the morning and through her lunchtime. Alternately, I was with her for dinner, followed by an evening walk or an activity. I would usually stay until bath time or bedtime. Sometimes, especially if she was not feeling well, I was with her for both lunch and dinner. Clearly, she had become accustomed to seeing and being with me every day.

On a few occasions, I needed to return to Massachusetts for professional reasons. Intentionally, my trips were short, never more than four days. During my first trip, the nurses charted Mom's emotional pattern. They reported that she was fine the first day. By the second evening, she seemed withdrawn. The next morning, she didn't want to eat. She was lethargic and slept more than usual. No amount of coaxing, cajoling, or entertaining would convince her to smile.

When I returned, I went directly from the airport to the nursing home. It was dinnertime, and Mom was already sitting at her place at the table, which faced the door to the dining room. Always attentive to movement around her, Mom noticed me as soon as I walked in. I stopped, and our eyes met. It took a few seconds for recognition to register, but suddenly her whole face—her entire being—registered joy. She started speaking excitedly in her own language of sounds. She couldn't seem to stop chattering on and on about my arrival. She hugged me tightly, then held my hands and wouldn't let go. An aide had to feed her because neither Mom nor I had a free hand. In my entire life, I have never felt such acclaim. The staff was amazed by this display of emotion, and Mom's joy permeated the entire floor. Everyone seemed filled with happiness that night.

At first, I was sad and disappointed in myself because I interpreted Mom's distress and withdrawal while I was away as my failure to care for her well. I felt I shouldn't have left her. But my absence for four days wasn't exactly the cause of Mom's distress. She missed me, and missing me was a normal reaction for the situation. She was communicating her feelings in the only way she could, sadness manifested as withdrawal. The ultimate cause of Mom's distress was her decline from Alzheimer's and her lost capacities to manage her emotions as they intersected with my absence.

In addition to missing me, perhaps Mom was also feeling afraid that I wouldn't return. Raia explains, "Patients with Alzheimer's disease experience fear throughout their disease course. As they decline and lose capacities, part of what is also lost is the ability to articulate their fears and cope with them. Essentially, what is lost is the person's ability to self-soothe if fears become overwhelming."[8] Without the ability to comfort herself, Mom would have been at the mercy of all sorts of unrealistic fears.

During later trips that kept me away for several days, I arranged for Linda (the reflexologist), hospice volunteers, aides, chaplains, or nurses to spend time with Mom each day. I specifically asked them to do some of the activities with Mom that I did, such as brush her hair, massage her hands, walk with her outside, and take her to Mass and exercise class. Because she could not soothe herself, I asked them to reassure her that I was coming back very soon, and that I missed her too. This external soothing seemed to help stabilize her emotional state while I was away.

Colleen Carroll Campbell's father lived with Alzheimer's for fifteen years. She shares some of her family's struggle: "One of the hardest things about those years—especially for my mother, his faithful exhausted caregiver—was hearing well-intentioned people dismiss the need for her solicitous care or their own failure to visit him by saying that 'he doesn't remember anyway.'"[9] At times, it became necessary for me to defend myself against people with similar opinions, including some members of my own family who denied my mother's need for the care and attention I was giving her. They were convinced that my

BELIEVING IN RELATIONSHIP

daily presence in Mom's life was unnecessary because she didn't remember anyway. Having people question and criticize my good care of Mom was demoralizing and disempowering in the moment. Upon reflection, however, I could only assume that they didn't understand (or were afraid to understand) what it meant for a person to be completely vulnerable, completely helpless, and on their own in a nursing home, completely at the mercy of strangers. I also assumed that they didn't realize how important it is for vulnerable people with Alzheimer's disease to have consistent, loving companionship.

Nearly twenty years ago, Robert, a psychologist from Wisconsin, added his curiosity about the emotions of people with Alzheimer's to the collective of caregiver experiences. His interest in this topic was sparked by an episode similar to the impact my Boston trip had on Mom. Robert's mother, Martha, was eighty-three years old at the time and had moderately severe Alzheimer's disease. She lived in a care facility in a small town in southwestern Wisconsin, and Robert faithfully visited her every Thursday afternoon. There were times when Robert wondered whether his time visiting his mother was well spent. Did his visits actually make any difference to her? He wondered about this because, according to staff reports and his own assessment based on phone interactions with his mother, she forgot his visit by the next day. One Thursday, Robert, swamped with work assignments, decided to skip his weekly visit. The next day, the charge nurse called him to report that Martha was in an unusually foul mood. She was agitated and seemed quite unhappy. They weren't sure why; nothing was different.

Had Martha missed his visit? Robert took his curiosity about this caregiver experience with him to a professional conference. To the good fortune of people with Alzheimer's all around the world, he shared his questions with Daniel Tranel, director of the neuroscience graduate program at the University of Iowa.[10] Generally, scientists aren't all that interested in anecdotal evidence like Robert's story. The world of science had already passed over the anecdotal information expressed in "Heart Memories," published more than twenty years earlier. Science also passed over Raia's writing about the collective experience of caregivers observing emotions in people with Alzheimer's, published a decade earlier. However, Robert and Martha's story made an impression on Dan Tranel. Although it piqued his scientific curiosity about emotional memory in the absence of cognitive memory, Tranel didn't just receive this story as a scientist. He also received it in his heart. Tranel and his graduate students were meeting more and more people with Alzheimer's and their caregivers, and he recognized the pain and the great need of these patient and caregiver populations. The combination of curiosity, heart-listening, and compassion for the suffering propelled Tranel into action via his specialty, neurological research, to address Robert's questions.

Subsequently, Iowa researchers Justin Feinstein, Melissa Duff, and Dan Tranel designed and conducted groundbreaking research into emotional memory. Their findings would change the course of my life over the next several years, identify relational treatment protocols for people with Alzheimer's worldwide, and lead to the co-creation (with me) of caregiver education designed to improve the quality of life for people with dementia, their family members, and professional care providers.

Previous research had studied the impact of emotions on memory, but none had investigated the impact of memory on emotions. The Iowa researchers embarked on their exploration with this question: Can the experience of an emotion persist once the memory for what induced the emotion has been forgotten? The subjects of this initial study were all people who had amnesia due to damage to the hippocampus, a major component in the brain that has an important role in forming new memories and retaining them.[11] Those in the study participated in two experiments. The first was intended to induce sadness as they watched film clips that were exceptionally sad. During the second experiment, which took place at another time, they watched hilariously funny film clips.

The goal of the study was to determine if these people with amnesia would experience elevated levels of sadness or happiness after they had forgotten watching the film clips; if so, for how long after? Analysis of the data gathered from these experiments showed that "both positive and negative emotional experiences can persist independent of explicit memory of the inducing event."[12] Six minutes later, participants had trouble recalling the film clips; some couldn't remember seeing films at all. But thirty minutes later, emotion evaluations showed they still felt sad or happy, often more than participants with normal memories. Those patients with the highest degree of memory impairment retained the strongest emotions.[13] The researchers conclude, "These findings provide direct evidence that a feeling of emotion can endure beyond the conscious recollection for the events that initially triggered the emotion."[14]

Reading this helped me understand an incident that happened with Mom's neighbor, Etty. Each summer at the nursing home, the family of one of the residents brought Shetland ponies that pulled buggies with fringes on top. They took residents, family members, and staff for rides. While Mom and I rode in the buggy, she could not take her eyes, which were dancing with delight, off of that pony. After our ride, she petted the pony and fed him a carrot. I noticed that Mom's neighbor, Etty, rode in the buggy right after we did. An avid animal lover, Etty was obviously cheered to the core of her being by the ponies. Her shining eyes and big smile radiated joy. About fifteen minutes later, I saw Etty upstairs near her room. She was smiling, laughing, and bouncy. But when I exclaimed, "You really enjoyed those ponies, didn't you, Etty?!", her expression changed dramatically. She looked completely puzzled and angry. She stopped bouncing and smiling.

She asked, "What? What are you talking about?"

I felt terrible about interrupting her cheerful pony mood, so I patted her arm, hugged her, and said, "I'm so happy to see you, Etty."

Then I smiled and laughed. She smiled and laughed, and her cheer seemed to resurface as she bounced off down the hallway.

I was shocked by how quickly Etty had cognitively forgotten the pony experience, which had so delighted her. It had just been minutes. Etty's reaction to my question told me that her cognitive decline was progressing. Her short-term cognitive memory could not reach back even minutes, but her emotional memory lingered. This momentary interaction heightened my awareness and alerted me that I needed to adjust my communication with Etty according to her abilities. Because people living with Alzheimer's "display impaired memory for recent events early in the disease process,"[15] this experience reminded me of the importance of paying attention to inevitable changes in cognition that happen throughout the disease.

My introduction to the Iowa study came to me like kismet. On January 1, 2011, my friend and colleague Rev. Esther Hurlburt emailed me a link to an article in *The New York Times,* "Giving Alzheimer's Patients Their Way, Even Chocolate." Esther said the article described state-of-the-art ways to interact with people with Alzheimer's that mirrored what we taught in our Healing Moments workshops. I read the article with great enthusiasm and felt validation for the content of our programming. But it was the results of the Iowa research that captivated my attention on multiple levels. Because people with Alzheimer's and other forms of dementia experience hippocampus damage similar to their study subjects with amnesia, the Iowa researchers projected that their findings could have an impact on people with Alzheimer's and their care. Justin Feinstein, research lead and advanced neuropsychology doctoral student at the time, was quoted in the article. He said, "The results of this study have direct implications for how society treats individuals with memory disorders (such as people with Alzheimer's disease), since events that have long been forgotten could continue to induce suffering or wellbeing."[16] For example, as Robert and I can attest, visits or telephone calls from family members to people with Alzheimer's, or buggy rides, can positively influence their emotional states, and these positive feelings will linger even if the visits or phone calls or ponies are forgotten. On the other hand, neglect from family members and routine neglect and insensitive treatment by staff at nursing homes may leave cognitively impaired people feeling sad, frustrated, angry, and lonely, even though they can't remember why. Since the study results show that these upsetting feelings tend to linger longer than the happier feelings, Feinstein proposed that people with Alzheimer's who are exhibiting behavioral problems could be experiencing sadness or anxiety or anger over an event they don't remember and can't explain.[17]

Five days after reading about Justin Feinstein's 2010 research, Mom died and I entered into a different phase of life, grieving. So it was several weeks before I contacted Justin by email with some questions about his research and a proposal of my own for a joint research study. From his comments in *The New York Times* article, it was clear that he and I and Healing Moments programs were completely in sync about Alzheimer's and emotions and caregiving. By this time, I had been leading Healing Moments workshops around the country for over four years, gathering much anecdotal evidence that our message was useful, often life-changing, for caregivers and their loved ones with Alzheimer's. But I really wanted to know, from a scientific perspective, if the techniques I had developed were truly helpful and ultimately would provide healing for people on this Alzheimer's journey. I wanted to be sure that what caregivers were receiving from me worked; that their time and money was well-spent; that they were doing something that would improve their caregiving lives and their loved ones' lives, too. I was cautious in advertising the workshop, not wanting to promise—or even appear to promise—outcomes that weren't realistic. I wanted to know if data supported universal effectiveness of the unique caregiving techniques that worked for me. Could Healing Moments offer a scientifically informed standard of care?

Justin replied to my email in the Spring of 2011. He noticed the synergy between us regarding Alzheimer's care and was responsive to my inquiries and enthusiastic about my ideas. That first email exchange between us marked the beginning of a years-long collegial friendship and collaboration with the Iowa researchers, who were coincidentally, just down the road from me.

Because the researchers were projecting their 2010 results found in amnesic patients onto people with Alzheimer's, I wondered why they didn't just study people with Alzheimer's in the first place. It turns out that it's hard to get people with Alzheimer's and dementia, or their caregivers, to participate in research. It was easier to recruit the amnesic patients for the pilot study, and those initial significant results would lead to follow up research. Work on that follow-up study began in early 2011, with new doctoral student in clinical psychology, Edmarie Guzman-Velez, in the lead. She had come to Iowa from her home in Puerto Rico, bringing with her a lifelong fascination with memory. She knew some things about Alzheimer's since two uncles were diagnosed with the disease, and she had witnessed her aunts' caring and struggles. However, she was not intimately familiar with the specific and significant aspects of memory loss inherent in Alzheimer's. Justin's study helped her to understand the phenomenon and sparked her interest in the combination of memory and emotions.

Over the next few years, Edmarie Guzman-Velez replicated Justin's study with people living with Alzheimer's as her subjects. Those study results were published in 2014, confirming, she said, "that the emotional life of an Alzheimer's patient is alive and well."[18] Of the results, Dan Tranel, who supervised both emotional memory studies, said, "It's extremely important to see data that supports our previous prediction. Edmarie's research has immediate implications for how we treat patients and how we teach caregivers."

Years later, Tranel and three former University of Iowa doctoral students, now graduated and in professional careers around the country—Dr. Edmarie Guzman-Velez, assistant professor of psychiatry at Harvard Medical School and neuro-psychologist at Massachusetts General Hospital; Dr. Alaine Rescheke-Hernandez, music therapist and assistant professor in the School of Music at the University of Kentucky; Dr. Amy Belfi, assistant professor in the Department of Psychological Science at Missouri University of Science and Technology, replicated the emotional memory study using music that was self-selected by each study subject to induce sadness or happiness. Their results, published in 2020, were consistent to previous findings. The participants with Alzheimer's had impaired memory for having heard the music, but their sad and happy emotions endured for up to twenty minutes. The researchers conclude that familiar music could be a powerful therapeutic tool for inducing feelings of well-being in people with Alzheimer's and dementia.[19]

Again, we are grateful to these researchers for stepping up and scientifically documenting what the collective caregiver community has been observing about music and Alzheimer's for some time. At a conference I attended several years ago, a music therapist showed amazing videos of music being used to manage difficult behaviors exhibited by a man with Alzheimer's. We saw that the therapeutic aspect didn't arise just from familiar music. The energy of the music was also an important factor. The man was angry and physically agitated. In order to calm him, the therapist played music (on her guitar) and sang in a staccato kind of tempo that matched his agitated energy. She was mirroring him, letting him know through music that she understood what he was feeling, and essentially joining him there. Then, ever so slowly and seamlessly, she changed the tempo and energy of the music/song, slowing the tempo, softening the notes and her voice, eventually playing a gentle, relaxing melody. It was fascinating to watch the energy of the agitated man transform to match the energy of the music. Once they connected in the agitation, he began mirroring the music therapist, his energy following the changing tempo of the music. The lesson from this for using music to induce a happy emotional state is to not start with calm or bouncy happy music if someone is angry, sad, or afraid. As with our efforts to verbally and nonverbally communicate and connect with people with Alzheimer's, we want to match their emotions in order to register with them that we understand before we attempt to shift the emotion. We learn from this latest study about memory and emotions, that music can assist us with this important goal.

In May 2023, the FDA approved the first drug for treating agitation in people with Alzheimer's, saying,

Agitation is one of the most common and challenging aspects of care among patients with dementia due to Alzheimer's disease. 'Agitation' can include symptoms ranging from pacing or restlessness to verbal and physical aggression . . . . These symptoms are leading causes of assisted living or nursing home placement and have been associated with accelerated disease progression.[20]

A few weeks after this approval happened, I saw a TV commercial for the drug, an antipsychotic. This approval took place even though side effects for people with dementia taking anti-psychotics include death and a higher likelihood of strokes.[21] The Iowa researchers are showing us that there are alternatives. Meeting agitated people with dementia with music could be a much safer, and maybe even more effective, treatment choice for them.

The collective of caregiver experiences has also known, for decades, about the importance of music for drawing out seemingly unresponsive people with Alzheimer's. There is the famous video of Naomi Feil, founder of *Validation Therapy*, singing to Gladys Wilson, who was withdrawn and virtually nonverbal. Gladys offered repetitive movements as her way of communicating with Naomi, tapping her hand on the chair arm. Naomi matched her own voice intensity and tempo, singing "Jesus Loves Me" to the intensity and tempo of Gladys' movements. Together, their movements, which were at first rather raucous, became slow, peaceful, and sweetly connected. They made eye contact and Naomi began singing (in a whisper) "He's Got the Whole World in His Hands." As Naomi sang, Gladys eventually started singing along ". . . in his hands," matching Naomi's whisper. And then, this previously non-verbal woman with Alzheimer's answered "Yes" to Naomi's questions: "Do you feel safe with Jesus? And with me?"[22]

In 2014, the *Alive Inside* organization produced the documentary "Alive Inside: A Story of Music and Memory," which advocates for the use of music as therapy for people with dementia. They believe all persons with dementia should be given an MP3 player for music enjoyment. We can add this to our list of ways to make a difference! If our loved ones with dementia can't choose their own playlists, we can; the recommended choices are songs from their youth, from teens to early twenties, those formative years when music becomes a part of our being.

When a colleague and I visited an adult day center for people with Alzheimer's, we were delighted by an "alive inside" musical demonstration. One woman at the day center was especially withdrawn and quiet that day, not engaging with us though we tried to interact with her, nor with anyone else. My colleague started to play the piano, offering some familiar songs for the age group. When she began playing and singing "You are my sunshine," this withdrawn, silent woman stood up from her chair and belted out the entire song. Then she sat down. We all applauded, and her previously vacant face burst into a smile.

During her clinical training as a psychologist at the University of Iowa Hospital Neurology Clinic, Edmarie Guzman-Velez's interest in the disease of Alzheimer's intensified. She was meeting face to face with people with Alzheimer's and dementia as well as their caregivers, and she was impressed by the vulnerability, and sometimes desperation, exhibited by the caregivers. They were usually hopeless, confused, frustrated, and even angry. They didn't understand what was happening; they didn't know what to do; they had worked their whole lives, looking forward to retirement, and now this! Edmarie especially took note of the fact that so many of these caregivers cried mournfully in her presence, a complete stranger, understanding from this that their suffering was great.

Aware of nearly two hundred failed pharmaceutical trials, Edmarie and her colleagues were frustrated by not having useful interventions to offer their suffering patients and their suffering families. Not knowing how to help them improve their situations, Edmarie felt the ache of powerlessness. Knowing it would only get worse, she had no idea what to tell them. She gave them pamphlets from the Alzheimer's Association, so at least they could have information about the disease.

Motivated by their findings about emotional memory, Dan, Justin, and Edmarie felt strongly about the necessity to seek out alternative interventions in the form of "new caregiving techniques aimed at improving the well-being and minimizing the suffering for the millions of individuals afflicted with Alzheimer's." Edmarie believed her study results "should empower caregivers by showing them that their actions toward patients really do matter."[23]

We all met in person—Justin, Dan, Edmarie, and I—in September of 2011. Justin had just returned to Iowa from his California internship, Edmarie was in the early stages of her study of emotional memory in people with Alzheimer's, and Dan had been briefed by Justin about our discussions and the Healing Moments workshop for family caregivers, called *Meeting Alzheimer's: Learning to Communicate and Connect.* Dan was on board with Justin's proposal to develop a study about the effectiveness of my unique caregiving techniques, which, when implemented with people with Alzheimer's, Justin considered "holistic treatment." Treatment that could help caregivers create more positive emotions for their loved ones and even learn to avoid causing negative ones, without the side effects of medications. Their hope was to have an effective educational intervention to offer to caregivers in need.

I was invited to make a presentation at the weekly neuropsychology research lab meeting. Edmarie was at that meeting, along with psychiatrists, psychologists, neurologists, professors, and graduate students. I didn't realize at the time how unusual my presence was among this group. Edmarie told me later that it was so rare for a non-scientist to present at a lab meeting; she had never seen this before and thought it was great that Dan was supporting this collaboration. She said that sometimes scientists can be disconnected from the community they're studying, and she believed it would be an incredible opportunity to work with someone who personally went through the caregiving experience and also worked with caregivers. She felt that community participatory research like this, where I would help with the design and execution of the study, was an effective way to help researchers gain trust with potential subjects.

My short presentation at the lab meeting included acting out scenes of real-life interactions with people with Alzheimer's, displaying the impact of reality orientation vs. the improvisation techniques of accepting the offer, playing the role you've been cast into, and making your scene partner look good. As part of my presentation, I said that it was impossible to reason with people who were not able to think rationally, parroting what I had read and learned from experts. After the presentation, one of the scientists challenged this statement, and his comment shifted my thinking. He noticed that in my interaction with Ellie (see page 182), she seemed to be responding quite rationally, highlighting her reply to my apology: "Well, that's very big of you." I was grateful for this expanded way of understanding based on observable evidence (phenomenology), which had been in front of me all along. In presentations, I now say, "It's impossible to reason with people who have lost the capacity to process new and different information that is in conflict with their own reality."

At the lab meeting, I also discussed why caregivers need teaching in the main intervention that has been recommended for communicating and connecting with people with Alzheimer's since the 1990s: meeting people with Alzheimer's in their world, validating their reality, and using therapeutic fiblettes as needed. The reason we need teaching is that this recommended intervention is easier said than done. In workshops or presentations, when I suggest meeting people with Alzheimer's in their world, some caregivers look puzzled, but curious; others look completely bewildered, and I can almost hear them thinking, "Huh? What does *that* mean?" There are others who "get it," but they most often don't know how to do it. And then, of course, there are those caregivers who resist the idea of letting go of their own reality, thinking they are participating in disrespectful deception.

I explained to those gathered at the lab meeting that some exercises we do in the workshop are reflective. Participants are invited to pause, be in the moment, and observe. Other exercises are more high energy. We make eye contact while clapping, mirror each other physically, emotionally, and verbally, and we practice blocking and advancing offers (saying yes and no as we practice fiblettes). Some interactions are playful; some are more serious. For example, during one particularly heart-opening exercise, we appreciate each other, knowing how hard this journey can be for every caregiver. A few of the exercises have been challenging for participants, specifically those in the therapeutic fiblette realm that require imagination. I didn't understand the reason for this challenge, exactly, until one workshop participant explained to me that she hadn't used her imagination since she was in high school, more than fifty years ago. Ah, yes. Rusty imaginations. I added some imagination warm-up exercises to the workshop format. All of these exercises are designed to advance caregivers' willingness to accept what is and develop their skills in the all-important intervention of meeting their loved ones in their moment.

I also shared with the Iowa practitioners and researchers that at first glance the exercises included in the workshop may seem really different, even a little silly. However, they have all been carefully selected to engage, enlighten, and inspire caregivers. Although the exercises are drawn mainly from the craft of improvisation, they coincide with serious treatment modalities such as Habilitation Therapy, Validation Therapy, and Act and Commitment Therapy. What appears as "fun" is actually highly instructive programming. In advertising the workshop, I had not stressed the improvisation aspect since I was concerned this would scare people away. During the workshop, after introducing the idea of improvisation, I always ask participants, "When you heard we were going to be doing some improvisation exercises, how many of you wanted to run from the room?" About 90 percent raise their hands. We all laugh, and I thank them for staying, assuring them that they will not be asked to perform as in "Whose Line Is It Anyway?" The sigh of relief is audible. After one workshop a man from the 90 percent spoke to me and said, "If I had known in advance that improvisation would be a part of this, I never would have come. But, it was terrific. And so helpful. You really hit it out of the park."

My lab meeting presentation received positive feedback, and Dan was ready to move forward. He really liked the idea of a structured workshop for caregivers; one that was short, inexpensive, effective, and easily accessible. No doctor's prescription needed![1] Their previous research into the retention of emotional memory showed caregivers *why* making an effort to connect with their loved ones with Alzheimer's is important. Next, Dan wanted to show caregivers *how* to connect so their efforts would reflect best practices for care; so their efforts would have the most potential for achieving the desired outcome of increasing positive emotions and reducing negative ones in their loved ones with Alzheimer's, essentially improving their quality of life.

Edmarie asked to be part of the study with me and Healing Moments, and she became the study lead. She thought it was "so cool" to be able to work with me, someone from outside the university lab structure who was not a scientist. She liked that I thought differently about things and brought a different perspective from my "on the ground" caregiving experience. Once her emotional memory research data was collected, analyzed, and submitted for publication in 2014, Edmarie and I began our collaboration. We adapted my one-day workshop, which was a very long day, into two days to accommodate for the time needed for participants to complete the required study questionnaires and surveys prior to beginning the workshop. The two-day format also allowed for added technique training, provided time for family caregivers to share their stories and interact with each other (both proved to be essential components of learning), and afforded the opportunity for "homework" so techniques could be practiced with their loved ones and discussed during day two.

Over the next three years, I facilitated numerous workshops to small groups of family caregivers, ranging from ten to twenty participants. In keeping with scientific standards, I followed the exact script for information presented and exercises offered during each workshop. Also keeping with scientific standards, a control group of study caregivers was recruited for each workshop. They completed the initial and follow-up questionnaires and surveys at one, three, and six months, as did the study participants; but the control group was wait-listed to attend the workshop until after their six months of paperwork was submitted. Then the comparison of data was analyzed between the control group, who had no educational intervention, and those who participated in the *Meeting Alzheimer's* two-day workshop.

Mid-way through the study years, Edmarie moved to Boston for her internship year. She continued to oversee the study from a distance, but the day-to-day, workshop-to-workshop management was handled by another doctoral student, Kelsey Spalding-Wilson. It was a joyful experience for me, working with these brilliant, professional, kind, and compassionate young women, who were so obviously dedicated to healing in the world of Alzheimer's. We made a great team, and the study we devised and conducted yielded important results. The data gathered showed that the "intervention significantly reduced [caregiver] perceived stress for up to 6 months, was considered by nearly all respondents to be helpful for managing challenging behaviors ... [and showed] promise for producing lasting improvements in caregivers' psychological health."[24] The data supported the anecdotal feedback I had been receiving for ten years! It showed that if the Iowa researchers' findings about the retention of emotional memory in people with dementia informed and guided caregiver education, their interactions with their loved ones with Alzheimer's would improve, and their relationships could, and would, flourish. We learned from workshop participants' comments that relational flourishing can be promoted by simple caregiver changes, such as "handling" themselves better (vs. handling their loved ones with Alzheimer's), by "slowing down, going with the flow," "stepping into the reality," and by banishing reality therapy.[25] Relational connections can flourish when caregivers refrain from asking questions—especially "Do you remember?", or expecting people in the middle to later stages of dementia to make decisions, even simple ones. One workshop study participant shared with me that he successfully changed his mother's argumentative, disruptive behavior in restaurants.

Instead of asking her what she wanted to order for breakfast—which she didn't know and couldn't say she didn't know—he ordered for her and all was peaceful. "Happier all around," he said.

Promoting relational flourishing can be as simple as removing the word "no" from our vocabulary. Promoting flourishing and enhancing trust will be the natural outcome flowing from the appropriate use of therapeutic fiblettes. Promoting flourishing will also involve accepting that there is no justification for trying to protect an autonomy (such as deciding what to order for breakfast, bill-paying, or more significantly, driving!) that a person living with dementia no longer possesses, and then discerning the right time and the right process for taking the lead.[26]

With their data, the scientists in Iowa have done a great service to people with memory loss caused by damage to the hippocampus, especially those with Alzheimer's and dementia. For many years, Paul Raia has been telling society that we needed this data: "Developing a better understanding of the psychology of dementia—how a person thinks, feels, communicates, compensates, and responds to change, to emotion, to love—may bring some of the biggest breakthroughs in treatment."[27]

Here in Iowa, the breakthroughs have arrived! However, some family caregivers and professionals in the field, feeling that their observations and insights have been overlooked and even diminished at times, reacted with frustration to the attention being given to the data. "We don't need a study to tell us what we already know, what we've known all along!" It's true. Many caregivers, past and present, don't need this evidence. Those who have chosen to become intimately involved with people with Alzheimer's and dementia know that the damage to their brains has not interfered with their heart memories. This difference between validation by data and validation by story, however, reminds me of a comment made by author Joseph Campbell during "The Power of Myth" interviews, first aired on PBS in 1988. Journalist Bill Moyers asked Campbell if he had faith in God. Campbell replied, "I don't need faith. I have experience."[28]

The caregiver collective has experience that has made us believers in heart memories, in music generating aliveness, in the importance of saying yes, in the effectiveness of therapeutic fiblettes. So much of the world, however, does *not* have this experience. And in the absence of experience, doubt and misinformation flourish. Doctors Tranel, Feinstein, Guzman-Velez, Spalding-Wilson, Reschke-Hernandez, and Belfi are not telling caregivers what we already know. They are confirming what we know. In addition, they are telling the rest of the world what it doesn't know, what it needs to know, what it *must* know.

One challenge the dissemination of this data faces is that the collective caregiving experience is a revolving door. Every single day, some caregivers exit the Alzheimer's journey when their loved ones die and others enter the path at the moment of diagnosis. Advocates for people living with Alzheimer's and dementia need to keep this scientific data, which has the power to demand continuing reformation in the field of Alzheimer's caregiving, from being filed away and forgotten so it is readily available for new family and professional caregivers, all of whom need to know. For example, the traditional trend of care, reaffirmed in 2023 by the FDA, tends to medicate behavioral issues (usually to the detriment, and sometimes resultant death, of the person with Alzheimer's).[29] For the well-being of people with Alzheimer's, this needs to change as the first-choice solution. I still feel a chill coursing through my body as I hear my sibling's voice in my memory telling me that the antipsychotic drug given to Mom to stop her likely valid emotional upsets made her "out of it" for a few weeks. A few weeks!

The scientific data from the Iowa research "provides clear evidence showing that the reasons for treating [people with Alzheimer's and dementia-type memory loss] with respect and dignity go beyond simple human morals." [30] Their results describe best practices for care. They are validating the need for that better way I sought all those years ago; they are describing that better way; and their data shows that understanding the emotions of people with Alzheimer's and a shift in interpersonal interactions can be an effective intervention for managing difficult behaviors. Thankfully, caregivers today have more choices and more guidance than I did for finding that better way.

It seems wrong to some dedicated caregivers that data, more so than experience of the individual, should dictate a standard of appropriate care. And so, the caregivers cry out, "Why do we need scientists to tell us that people with Alzheimer's should be treated with respect and dignity?" My voice was part of this cry when I first read the Iowa study. After living the question, however, I eventually found an answer: Because now we caregivers have a type of validation for our experiential knowing that the world values and accepts. Essentially, the studies on emotional memory and best practices have given the individual caregiver experience clout. The next time a nonbeliever—a family member, a friend, or even an uninformed, untrained professional—questions our dedication to caring for our loved ones with dignity, our use of fiblettes, and our commitment to relating to them as valuable members of our lives and our world, we can confidently, powerfully say, "Research has shown . . . ."

The Iowa researchers have given caregivers even more than data and clout. By showing us that one story told to one person can make a world of difference to millions, the Iowa researchers have given us hope. Our voices, our experiences matter.

13 Time Enough

For several summers, in the small Iowa city that I once again call home, caregiver families gathered in the rose garden at the arboretum for a Monarch Moments service. We gathered to honor our loved ones living with Alzheimer's or another disease of dementia, and to remember those who had died after their long journeys. It was a ritual of release. As the name of each loved one was spoken, a chime rang out. The sound united with the wind, and we watched in awe, reverence, and delight as the caregiver released a Monarch butterfly in honor or in remembrance.

At each service, hundreds of butterflies were set free. They dazzled us with their beauty as they filled the sky above during their first flight. Their time for dazzling would be brief, however. This generation of Monarchs lived very short lives—two to six weeks. This fact of nature, of each life ending so soon, evokes sadness in many. But as we contemplate the truth about this natural process of living and dying, the Indian poet Rabindranath Tagore consoles us:

> The butterfly counts not months but moments, and has time enough.[31]

"Time enough for what?" I found myself asking when I first read this poem. The answer surprised me. During their short lives, our Monarchs would have time enough to lay their eggs and to fulfill their destiny: creating the next generation, the migrating generation. They would then miraculously travel from our rose garden in Iowa to the fir trees their ancestors inhabited the previous winter in Mexico. I consider their travel miraculous because the migrating generation of Monarchs doesn't just travel to the same country, the same town, or even the same neighborhood of their ancestors. Relying solely on the guidance of their natural instincts and the instincts of their companions on the journey, they travel to the exact same trees!

The migrating generation needs time enough to make their long flight home and to lay their eggs. So unlike our butterflies, whose lives are fleeting, the migrating Monarchs live eight months or more. Each generation of Monarchs has time enough to fulfill its purpose.

"Time is the most valuable thing we have, because it is the most irrevocable," wrote Lutheran pastor and theologian Dietrich Bonhoeffer from a Nazi prison cell during World War II.[32] Like someone who has received the diagnosis of a terminal illness, Bonhoeffer knew that his days on earth were limited. His precarious state of imprisonment heightened his awareness about the preciousness of each passing moment and the importance of each word he wrote or spoke.

Building on Bonhoeffer's thought, Jewish scholar and mystic Abraham Joshua Heschel believes that "time is the heart of existence." When I was first introduced to Heschel's teachings about time, I felt that he had given me a map for travelling through life in a different way. Like many, I thought that sacred images or sacred places, such as art or churches or nature, were the doorways to experiencing mystery. With Heschel's encouragement, I began to consider the essence of *time* in my quest for God and for meaning in life. "The higher goal of spiritual living," writes Heschel, "is to face sacred moments …. What is retained in the soul is the moment of insight rather than the place where the act took place." He encouraged me to build a "sanctuary in time…where the goal is not to have but to be, not to own but to give, not to control but to share, not to subdue, but to be in accord."[33] Inspired by this possibility, I set out to create such a sanctuary for Mom and me in the sacred time we had left together.

Even now, it remains abundantly clear in my soul that our choices do matter regarding the gift of time we've been given. It became obvious to me that caregiver Daisy also realized this on the Alzheimer's journey with her mom when she said, "Time is everything." I heard the longing in her voice; perhaps longing for more time. Our loved ones with Alzheimer's may live for twenty years with this disease. If we can discover ways to make these additional years of life meaningful for them, and for us, then the longevity medical science gives us can be a blessing. Our own search for meaning remains a mysterious, holy quest whose answer we, and our loved ones, must live into over time.

Whatever gifts, whatever meaning we may uncover on the Alzheimer's journey, and the value of the time we have with our loved ones will vary from caregiver to caregiver, and whatever we each are able to give and to receive in our time enough will sometimes surprise even us.

The "most meaningful present" writer Sherri Edwards received from her mother was "the gift of walking with her on the path of a progressive illness." In their lives it was vascular dementia. Although "shocked to admit this," Edwards was able to move beyond the sense of loss and sadness she experienced, to overcome her struggles with increasing responsibility, and to manage the despair and guilt she felt over neglecting the rest of her life. Having navigated her way through these challenging feelings, Edwards was able to recognize the blessings she received along the way.

Edwards and her mother found purpose and value in their time enough. Even with dementia, her mother continued to be "a teacher, a counselor, a friend," who incredibly still gave her daughter gifts. The first gift Edwards mentions receiving on this journey through dementia with her mother is the gift of *time*. "Many friends have lost parents years ago. Yet here is my mother, who has survived several serious illnesses plus dementia.... I am growing older with my mother right here, and I am grateful." [34]

As Edwards points out, our loved ones with Alzheimer's are still with us. Their very presence in our lives indicates that they have survived the many challenges of the twentieth century— medical and otherwise. As I contemplate the lives of our loved ones with Alzheimer's, I pause and recognize the contributions they have made, and continue to make, to our lives. Many of these diminishing people, now seventy, eighty, ninety, or one hundred years old, showed us how to cross oceans, prairies, and deserts with courage and resilience. Many bravely showed us how to live through wars, holocausts, and depressions. And now, once again they are showing us how to live with Alzheimer's disease. They are lighting the way for us as we travel through this mysterious and treacherous terrain.

Stephen Post begins his book *The Moral Challenge of Alzheimer's Disease* with these words: "Seldom does human experience require more courage than in living with the diagnosis and the gradual decline of irreversible progressive dementia." Post then asks, "How can affected individuals and their caregivers maintain 'the courage to be' before the foreboding specter of dementia?"[35]

Fortunately, many children of people with Alzheimer's have embraced their loved ones and the disease with a spirit born of love, vision, and healing. Many of these family members and friends are coming forward to share their witness of the transforming power of this disease. By doing so, they recognize, reveal, and model the importance of expressing our authentic selves, even when authenticity includes decline from Alzheimer's.

Conventional wisdom, unfortunately, still concludes that Alzheimer's steals personhood along with our opportunities to heal, reconcile, develop, or deepen our relationships with the people who have this disease. However, three of my caregiver companions and I, all children of people who lived and died with Alzheimer's, are honored to share our alternative wisdom about the experience, to express our awe and gratitude for the ways our encounters with Alzheimer's transformed our lives, and to reveal how our time enough strengthened, enhanced, and deepened our relationships with our loved ones and changed our lives forever.

Time Enough for Meeting

For more than fourteen years, Coleen was the primary caregiver for her mother, Ilene. Based on her experiences and observations, Coleen strongly disagrees with those who contend that people with Alzheimer's have forgotten who they are or who we are. Fearing that not enough members of our society have invested the time needed to meet people with Alzheimer's as they are and learn the skills needed to maintain relationships with them, she is concerned for their welfare. Knowing from the beginning that her understanding of this disease would be critical for her mother's well-being, Coleen sought out information. She also attempted to educate her brothers, who mostly avoided the subject. Instead of being angry with her brothers, however, Coleen chose to let them go, and they chose to let her "handle it." In the end, Coleen felt happy, satisfied, and content with her choices.

There were times earlier in Coleen's life when Ilene had guided and comforted her throughout challenging experiences—a painful ending to a serious relationship and the births of her babies, for example. Even while Ilene had Alzheimer's, Coleen continued to see her mother as her guide and comforter. There is a hereditary component for early-onset Alzheimer's, the type Ilene had. "Sometimes," Coleen said, "I looked at Mom, and I saw my future." She saw her mother courageously and gracefully blazing the trail for her. This kind of terrifying awareness, which often sends adult children into avoidance, didn't cause Coleen to turn away from her mother's decline. Instead, she turned toward her mother, growing closer and nurturing their mother-daughter relationship, which transformed into a woman-to-woman bond.

Coleen believes that her fourteen-year journey with her mother through Alzheimer's disease gave her time enough to establish clear priorities in her life. Alzheimer's disease reminded Coleen of her own mortality and spurred her to complete her bachelor's degree in business so she could be satisfied with the contribution she is making to the world.[36] This long journey with Ilene also gave Coleen time enough to learn more about herself. In many ways, Coleen's intimate meeting with her mother through Alzheimer's brought out the best in her, introducing her to an inner strength she didn't know she had. "I'm not that strong," she said. "But when it came to Mom, I just had to be strong. She needed help to have a good quality of life. Not just from anybody—she needed help from me."

Coleen and Ilene's years together on the Alzheimer's journey also gave them time enough for their connection to deepen into a relationship that Coleen considered "very holy." As the disease progressed and their relationship grew more intimate, Coleen, literally "became one" with her mother:

I was her eyes, her ears, her voice. Because I had to 'be' her, our bond became unbreakable, and I truly felt as if I was accomplishing something very important. Although Mom couldn't speak, I knew that she was communicating with her eyes, and this drew me closer to her. No one at the nursing home could hear her or speak for her. She needed me to read her communications through her eyes and to communicate with words on her behalf. I felt strongly about being her caregiver, and it is something I will always be proud of—working on behalf of one of God's children who could not help herself.

There are family members who are "visitors" in nursing homes. With coaxing from Coleen, even her brothers eventually became visitors—and visitors are a good thing. According to an African proverb, "Visitors' footfalls are like medicine; they heal the sick." Coleen, however, was much more than a visitor. She was an active, assertive carepartner for her mother. Indeed, the hands-on care that Coleen gave Ilene—making sure the nursing home aides were respectful of her body, washing her up after toileting, walking with her, holding her memories, feeding her, and spending all night with her in the hospital so she wouldn't wake up and be alone and afraid—was holy work. Once when Ilene fell and was taken to the hospital, Coleen left work and rushed to her bedside in the emergency room. She instinctively knew that her mother would be confused and frightened. "*My* touch is what Mom needed," she says. "She needed *me* there to hold her hand." Coleen also knew from experience that most medical professionals require some clear direction when attending to a person with dementia who can't speak. And Coleen was there, without fail, to provide that direction.

At Ilene's deathbed, Coleen wept. After this long, deeply intimate journey together, Coleen was bereft because she couldn't figure out how to continue walking with her mom as she left this world. Their bond was that strong, that profound.

Throughout the many years that Coleen was a regular carepartner for Ilene at the nursing home, she continued to recognize the presence of God beaming through her mom's eyes and radiating through her hands and the warm hands of the other residents with Alzheimer's. Just as this presence remains recognizable to us, it's possible that the presence of God in our eyes and our hands remains recognizable to them as well.

Time Enough for Discovery and Surprise

If we accept Brother David Steindl-Rast's definition of God as surprise, then Mary Anne encountered God numerous times throughout her mother's diminishment from dementia. After Ione suffered her first seizure in 1997, the diagnosis of Alzheimer's was mentioned. Mary Anne remembers being filled with despair as she considered the possibility that her mother would lose her memory. After years of witnessing Ione's gradual decline, however, Mary Anne was surprised to discover that her fear of having a mother with dementia had been more painful than the reality: "It could have been so much worse. I know Mom had frustrations, but she didn't have pain. Now that I've been through it, I realize it was probably worse for us experiencing Mom's losses than it actually was for her.[37] She didn't seem to know, and she didn't seem to suffer like so many terminally ill people do."

Neither Ione nor Mary Anne ever lost sight of who Ione was. Many aspects of her personality were able to shine through the dementia: "She was always upbeat. She never got depressed. Her unique sense of humor and assertiveness remained." For example: one night at the nursing home, the phone at the nurses' station was ringing off the hook. No one was answering.

Finally, Ione shouted out what everyone was probably thinking: "Answer the damn phone!" When no one came to answer the phone, Ione rolled her wheelchair behind the desk and answered it herself. "Hello," she said, annoyed. "Mom?" asked a surprised Mary Anne, who was the caller on the other end of the phone. "Yes. Oh hello, honey!" replied a delighted Ione.

"Mom always knew her name," said Mary Anne. "She would say, 'I'm Ione.'" Hearing Ione say her own name gave Mary Anne the gift of heartwarming joy, the kind that brings tears to our eyes and reminds us that the Spirit lives *in between* people, even when their capacities decline.

Mary Anne was additionally surprised to discover that focusing on Ione's remaining capacities had the potential to bring joy to them both. Early in her mother's illness, Mary Anne thought that people diagnosed with Alzheimer's didn't have any reason to live. As the illness progressed, however, she noticed that Ione was still experiencing and expressing enjoyment in the company of her family and in eating good food, particularly good desserts! Ione still liked connecting with and talking with others; her failing memory and cognition didn't prevent her from loving her family or enjoying her life in the present moment. She especially enjoyed feeling useful. Mary Anne gave Ione appropriate tasks so she could be successful and feel a sense of accomplishment and meaning: folding towels, snapping beans. Ione was pleased to complete these tasks, always asking for more. This desire to be of service is holy and deserves recognition. Mary Anne was able to see it and honor it. She felt great joy in seeing her mother feel proud and happy in her accomplishments, whatever they were.

As Ione's short-term memory failed, she began to talk more about the past, bringing Mary Anne a gift she never expected. Mary Anne's father had died when she was four, and the loss was so great for Ione that she couldn't talk about him without crying. As a result, Mary Anne knew very little about her father—until Alzheimer's rekindled experiences from the past. Freed from the pain of losing her husband, Ione could talk about him without suffering. These were joyful conversations of discovery for Mary Anne.

The seizures and strokes that continued throughout Ione's long decline raised Mary Anne's awareness that we never know when death will come. During the time enough they had together, living always in the shadow of death's unpredictability, Mary Anne became an assertive advocate for her mother at the nursing home. She insisted that Ione be cared for with dignity and with sensitivity to her individual needs according to the plan of care created by the nursing home staff. Mary Anne was an inspiration for other family members. Through her example, she gave us courage to ask for similar quality care for our loved ones.

The depth of Mary Anne's attentiveness to Ione was touching. "I knew what Mom liked and I wanted things to be the way she liked them," she said. "If this was going to be her last day, I didn't want her to go to bed without her teeth brushed. I wanted the things that mattered to her to be attended to. It was about how well I knew her."

Through the experience of Alzheimer's, Mary Anne discovered how well she knew her mother, and how important it was to know herself. Through Ione's illness and death, Mary Anne found her faith in both God and herself increasing. "I know I can handle more now—without crumbling—than I ever thought I could."

Mary Anne profoundly mourned the loss of her mother when she died in 2008, but while Ione was alive, Mary Anne cherished every moment they had together. "Although our relationship was not the same, I never felt as if I had lost Mom. In some ways, dementia deepened our connection. Because of

Mom's vulnerability, I felt closer to her than I ever had, and my love and respect for her was even greater because of what she was going through."

Trust was one aspect of their relationship that deepened. In certain stages of their disease, people with dementia often become fearful, almost paranoid. Sometimes when Ione's husband Ed would try to give her medication, she would refuse and become very upset. She was convinced that he was trying to poison her. Ed quickly learned that he could call Mary Anne, whose reassuring voice would tell Ione that the pills were safe and that Ed was trying to help her. Ione would hang up the phone and cooperatively take her pills. Sometimes at night, Ione would wake up in utter distress because she couldn't find her kids. Again, Ed learned quickly to call Mary Anne, who, awakened from her sleep would calm Ione. With her sleepy but familiar voice, Mary Anne was able to relieve her mother's anxiety by using a therapeutic fiblette, "Don't worry, Mom, the kids are all here, and I'm taking good care of them." Then they all slept peacefully.

"Mom having dementia wasn't the best thing," Mary Anne admits. "It wasn't something we would ever have chosen, but because Mom had this deep level of trust in me, I was able to be content with the situation. It was such a privilege to be *the* trusted person in Mom's life, and it made me want to be worthy of her trust."

Time Enough for Joy

The Catholic Mass was offered for the residents at Mom's nursing home every day in their chapel. After I moved to Iowa, it took a number of months for me to figure out that Mom attended Mass only when I accompanied her, usually on Sundays. Although the nursing home provided this religious ritual, residents who couldn't say yes when asked if they wanted to go to Mass, or couldn't remember the time and place and get themselves to the chapel on time, were taken only when their families had made prior arrangements.

I had no doubt that Mom wanted to attend Mass whenever it was offered. Through her own words, actions, and initiative—when she still had the capacity to assert her own will—Mom communicated to me that Mass was important to her. During our weeks together in 2004, Mom gathered up her purse every morning, informing me that it was Sunday and time for the 11:00 AM Mass. Before I realized that Mom needed to be supervised, she would leave the house without my knowledge. At first, I would panic when I noticed she was gone. My panic subsided, however, as soon as I figured out she would *always* be found two blocks away, standing at the front door of St. Anthony's Church.

Mom's ability to remember and appreciate her lifelong religious rituals was surviving the destruction of Alzheimer's. She remembered the rosary, which she could also participate in regularly at the nursing home, upon request. At Mass, she looked intently at the prayer book, which I helped her to hold. She especially enjoyed turning the pages when I cued her that it was time. I'm quite sure the familiar words and music of the service were reassuring, as were the taste and texture of the communion wafer. The sight of the priest at the altar wearing colorful vestments, the candles, and the shiny chalices filled with water and wine all mesmerized her.

The Sunday Mass at the nursing home was always crowded to capacity with residents, many in wheelchairs, and a few visiting family members. During the first years after I moved to Iowa, Mom and I proudly walked together to the front of the chapel where Mom could see everything clearly. As her disease progressed and she needed to use a wheelchair for any distance, we sat in the back of the chapel and became part of the sea of others in wheelchairs. Throughout the service, I slowly rolled Mom's chair back and forth in a rocking motion, adding a sense of soothing and comfort to her experience.

As I observed the priest saying Mass, I wondered what it was like for him to prepare a daily homily and preside over a service at which many of his congregants were asleep and most couldn't comprehend his interpretation of the scriptures or the sanctity of the Eucharist. One day I asked him about this, and he replied, "Whenever two or more are gathered in God's name, there is love." The condition of those in attendance didn't matter to Father Ron. The presence of the residents, who would receive what they could receive; the compassion he felt for "his people"; and the faithful leading of the religious ritual he had been ordained to perform nearly fifty years earlier— these were what mattered to him.

If Mom didn't attend Mass, she was in her room alone and sleepy. Sometimes the aides turned on her TV, but rarely was she engaged. And so Mass offered ritual and community, both of which were important and meaningful to Mom and her neighbors. Although Catholicism was no longer my chosen religious tradition, I started taking Mom to Mass so she would have something to do besides sit in her room in isolation. Because I believed this activity was meaningful for her, I deliberately made it a priority in my life. Quite unexpectedly, however, this ritual also become meaningful for me. It was such a surprise one Sunday morning to realize that I was really looking forward to attending Mass with Mom.

Each time we left Mass, I always felt connected to Mom and the other residents, spiritually enriched, and forever enlightened about the surprising journey of life. It seemed that something astonishing often happened at this Mass, and this possibility

BELIEVING IN RELATIONSHIP

kept me alert. One Sunday in the middle of the Mass, a woman whose wheelchair was parked behind a post blocking her view of the priest, shouted out repeatedly, "Where am I? Why am I here? I don't know what I'm doing here!" I was awakened in the moment by the important existential questions this woman was asking. Why have I been created? Why am I here at this time? In this place? These are the most mysterious questions in life, and I had often thought about them myself. Why am I in Iowa? Why am I on earth? This wise woman reminded me to refresh my inquiry.

No one had rushed in to shush the inquiring woman or whisk her out of the chapel for creating a disturbance, and I was so pleased by this. It was a "come as you are, however you are" kind of Mass, and everyone was accepted. Imperfections and irregularities were welcomed, and I felt that I fit right in. Never before, or since, has a church service been so meaningful to me.

Because it was enjoyable and enlightening quality time together, I tried to arrange my schedule so Mom and I could attend Mass together often on weekdays as well as Sundays. On Mondays and Wednesdays after Mass, an exercise class was held in the large space just outside the chapel. The class leader, Dee, was a woman in her eighties. She noticed me at Mass with Mom and kept inviting us to join her class. I knew the class content was way beyond Mom's abilities, but continually rejecting Dee's gracious invitation wasn't feeling good to me. So, one Wednesday, we stayed. Mom couldn't possibly respond to or keep up with the instructions, but it quickly dawned on me that I could assist her. I moved her arms and legs, tapped her feet, stretched her neck and shoulders, and moved from side to side so she would follow me with her eyes. The exercises were set to music and included a combination of old songs such as "My Wild Irish Rose" and the theme from *The Mickey Mouse Club*; more modern songs with movements, such as "YMCA" and the "Macarena," inspiring songs like "I Believe I Can Fly," and my personal favorite, which was just for fun, the "Chicken Dance." It was a marvelous way to take care of Mom's body—to increase her circulation and keep her muscles moving. And I got a real workout too, especially while lifting and rotating her legs. Filled with delight during this class, we smiled, laughed, danced, and waved batons with long, flowing, colorful scarves attached to the ends. For forty minutes, Alzheimer's was forgotten, and movement, joy, and true connection filled our present moments. Instantly, this activity caught fire in my soul, and I deliberately rearranged my schedule so Mom and I could attend the exercise class every Monday and Wednesday after Mass if she felt well enough. For me, this experience seemed like the exercise, socialization, and connection sought by mothers who attend "Mommy and Me" classes with their infants and toddlers. It was fun, energizing, and purposeful. The class provided a full-body workout for Mom, comparable to thirty to forty minutes of physical therapy, gave us both physical and social contact, and created a mother-daughter bonding experience beyond any expectations. At this class, I discovered that play is vital to the soul.

Alzheimer's gave Mom and me more time together. It was time enough to discover how we could smile and dance and exercise together, and how genuinely we could bond through shared joyful experiences. I concluded that nursing homes and senior centers should start advertising exercise (dance, movement, or recreation) classes for aging parents and adult children and really encourage the adult children to come and assist their parents. We can all use a little more high-energy fun in our lives. And there it was—every Monday and Wednesday—just waiting for Mommy and me.

Time Enough for Healing

Carl and I had been ministerial colleagues since the early 1990s, and we had lived in the same geographical area for nearly twenty years. However, my 2003 discovery of his mother's poem "The Wind of the Spirit"[38] was actually the seed of our friendship. A few years later, we connected more purposefully in a peer group of spiritual directors, and our friendship sprouted. When I began the journey through Alzheimer's with my mother, however, and learned that Carl and his mom, Myra, had walked this path before us, an enduring, supportive friendship blossomed.

When I asked Carl to participate in my exploration of the gifts and blessings caregivers receive from their loved ones with Alzheimer's, he agreed to meet with me. He did not agree, however, with my premise that there were gifts or blessings to be found anywhere near Alzheimer's disease. He explained that, throughout Myra's decline, he experienced "terrible pain in seeing her in pain and not being able to change things. It was awful for her, awful for me." Carl claimed there were no moments of joy for him.

While preparing for our meeting to talk about his Alzheimer's experiences, Carl resurrected his journals from the time of his mother's illness as well as his files about her care and her life in various facilities. As he reviewed these old documents, Carl unearthed surprising blessings that had been there all along, just waiting to be discovered. Through the questions I posed to Carl, and through his own reflections on his feelings and experiences during his mother's illness and beyond, he was able to see the journey with his mother differently. He saw how painful this time was for him. He also saw, however, that his mother's diminishment was a call to love. "It was a call I could *not* say no to." "Widen your hearts to us, O Corinthians," Carl eloquently quoted the apostle Paul's second letter. Then he said, "Mom taught me to widen my heart."

Ten years after his mother's death, as Carl read and reread his journals, he realized that his call and the call to many others caring for parents with Alzheimer's is "a precious and unique experience that will be with us for the rest of our lives." As Myra's abilities diminished and Carl's caregiving responsibilities increased, he told me that he had experienced a crisis fraught with stress and spiritual decline. Finally realizing that he couldn't neglect his own welfare, Carl began to pray as never before. Instead of reciting the prayers he had learned from his parents in childhood, he sat each morning with his God, pouring his heart out (lamenting) and asking for help to get through the day. Carl quickly understood that this kind of prayer is not just for a crisis. "This is for a lifetime," he said.

Although Carl and Myra had a "warmly cordial relationship" throughout his life, they were not close. Carl's parents were very busy missionaries in China, and he and four of his five siblings were raised in China by an amah (nanny) from infancy through childhood. "In retrospect," Carl said, "caring for Mother was an experience of resolving a distance I had always felt with her, and I sensed she felt with me. There was not hostility between us. There was distance."

Throughout Myra's illness, Carl grieved. Upon reflection, he realized that his grief went beyond the loss of his mother to Alzheimer's, and ultimately death: "I had a fear of losing a relationship with my mother that I never really had. And so, I wasn't grieving just the loss of our actual relationship. I was grieving the loss of a relationship we never had, and now could never, would never have." Or so he feared at the time.

Carl's journal from a year after Myra's death chronicled his realization of how affectionate he had become with his mother during the course of Alzheimer's. He realized that an intimacy they never shared before had grown between them during those years of her diminishment: "Before Mother's illness, I always gave her a ritual hug when I came and left. We talked about church, sermons, who was doing what. We didn't talk relationships." With reflection, Carl was able to recall many moments of pleasure and connection with Myra during her illness: "I would pray with Mom, sing to her, read to her, and tell her what was happening. During her illness, I felt *deep* pleasure in her company, and *deep* affection toward her. I talked warmly with her. I *felt* I was giving her love. I sat close to her and put my arm around her. I put my head close to her—cheek to cheek. I called her 'Little Mother.' And when I fed her, I always gave her the ice cream first!"

Myra was bedridden and curled into the fetal position for two and a half years before she died. She breathed, ate, eliminated, and slept. Despairing family members repeatedly queried each other and medical professionals, "Why is she still living?" And when she finally did die, Carl's first words when he heard were, "Oh, thank God."

It took more than a decade and an inquiring colleague to spur Carl into reflection about his mother's illness and the years he journeyed with her. In this reflection, he discovered that, in spite of the losses from Alzheimer's, her life had increasing value to him. "What made Mom's life of great value to me was the relationship I had with her during her illness, and what I was learning—even though I didn't know I was learning." Carl laughed as he continued, "A lesson is a lesson whether you know it or not!"[39]

In the time enough Alzheimer's disease gave to Carl and Myra, Carl had the opportunity to show his mother the love he felt he never received from her. In doing this, he said, "I healed myself."

Like the monarch butterflies, we rely on our own instincts and the instincts of our companions for guidance on the journey home. We help each other to get there with dignity by offering encouragement, support, comfort, companionship . . . and love. Although people with Alzheimer's may not remember cognitively that they are on the journey home, they remember with their instincts and with their hearts. And in their hearts, they remember what will help them most along the way. They remember love.

There is *always* time enough for love.

14 The Last Word

When I was writing the first edition of this book, I put off writing about my last experiences with Mom. I knew it would open that wound of missing her. I would relive the pain of losing my mother bit by bit through Alzheimer's disease, and then completely losing her through death.

Over many days, procrastination was my companion. But as I began to write, I realized that remembering and revering all of our moments together, including those of loss and pain, would be the path to accessing and integrating the joy and love we shared. Writing was how I could honor my mother as my important companion, teacher, and guide through Alzheimer's disease, through death, and into my new life.

As I consider last experiences, I think of the poem "How Shall I?" written by Libbie Stoddard, who was my dear friend, colleague, and mentor for more than thirty years. She provided nurture for me when my mother wasn't able to offer enlightening words or comfort. It was Libbie who encouraged me to read *Learning to Speak Alzheimer's*, and when Mom's ability to speak was nearly extinguished, she once again offered guidance. Thinking of Mom and me, Libbie wrote "How Shall I?" (page 215) and sent it to me as a birthday gift.

Mom and I lived each day with the questions Libbie's poem asked us to consider, unsure of the answers, but open to living into them, as poet Rainer Maria Rilke suggests:

> I beg you . . . to have patience with everything unsolved in your heart and try to love the *questions themselves* as if they were locked rooms or books written in a very foreign language. Don't search for the answers, which could not be given to you now because you would not be able to live them. And the point is, to live everything. *Live* the questions now. Perhaps then, someday far in the future, you will gradually, without even noticing it, live your way into the answer.[40]

Many of the young women working in Mom's nursing home were having babies. The older women's daughters were having babies. Through many pregnancies, many births, and many babies' visits to Mom's floor, I witnessed the process of life beginning, while at the same moment in time, I was also witnessing the process of life ending.

When a baby is expected we celebrate the first movement inside the womb, even placing our curious, excited hands on the mother's growing belly. We anticipate that awe-inspiring moment of birth, sharing each new development with amazement and joy. The sonograms are passed around the lunch table. Detailed birth stories are gaily shared. There are stories of difficult labor and the baby's first breath signaled by the first cry. Thus begins the long list of firsts to be recognized and celebrated: first smile, first word, first tooth, first step ... .

Through all of these stories of firsts, I found myself comparing the attention lavished on children at the beginning of life with the withdrawal of attention from elders at the end of life. We anticipate and celebrate the first word. Parents want to be present when that first precious word is spoken, and the nursing home's working moms lamented with misery if they missed this or any other firsts. Their instinct to love almost demanded that they be present to witness that first miraculous word.

What about the last step, though? The last word? The last smile? What about the continuing cycle of growth that leads us to death *from* this life instead of to birth *into* this life?

Carl noticed a distinction between joy and pleasure during the journey through Alzheimer's with Myra. He didn't feel joy with her because exuberance was not present. New mothers are, indeed, often exuberant, uninhibitedly enthusiastic. Carl recognized, however, that he did feel pleasure and satisfaction in his mother's presence. Similarly, the last step, the last word, the last smile will perhaps not elicit enthusiastic feelings, but neither should they inspire absence. They could actually be the most valuable, the most memorable, the most healing, and the most surprisingly inspiring moments of our lives.

The process of dying to this life is guided by an instinctual growth process that inevitably leads us to "lasts." These expressions deserve honor and respect as they invite us into the awe-inspiring potential for transformation. Mom's last word embodied this potential. The last word I heard Mom speak was on my birthday during the summer of 2007. For Mother's Day that year, I had sent her a framed picture of us taken in the front yard of our house when I was two months old. She was holding me. Her advocate at the nursing home wrote me a note sharing Mom's reaction to the photo. "I could tell she enjoyed it," the advocate wrote, "as her eyes were on the picture for a good long time while holding it." By the time my birthday arrived in August of that year, I was with Mom in Iowa. I took the picture down from the wall in her room and showed it to her. Mom immediately took it from me and held it tightly with both hands. She looked at me, then at the baby in the picture. These were long, intent gazes. Mom looked at me again, her inquiring blue eyes meeting my matching blue eyes. Then she clearly said my name: "Jade."

Until that moment, I wasn't sure if Mom realized I was her daughter. Her last word, however, connecting me to the baby picture, told me that she knew I belonged to her. Even in the later stages of Alzheimer's, some part of Mom's brain could still make a relational connection, and with her remaining capacity, she spoke one last word so that I would know she recognized me. What a gift I was given, the forever cherished memory of hearing my mother's last word! Of course, I didn't know at the time that it would be her last word. But there were even greater gifts to be received from the experience. On the surface, there was the heart-opening gift of knowing that Mom's last word was my name and that she knew me. But on a deeper level, this one word strengthened my faith in my mission. Mom knew who I was. She knew I was there with her on this journey. I hoped, believed, that in knowing her daughter, Jade, was with her, Mom felt safe, secure, comforted, and loved as she walked deeper into the mystery of Alzheimer's disease on her way home.

Later that summer, Mom demonstrated one way we would live into the answers for questions from "How Shall I...?" On a Saturday morning, two of my cousins came from out of town to see Mom and me. Although Mom had not seen them for a few years, she seemed to recognize their voices right away. Knowing how much Mom loved this duo and how much she enjoyed hugging, I helped her to stand up from her recliner chair. Pat and Lucy lined up to give Mom a hug, and I stepped out of the way, partly sitting, partly leaning against the heating and air conditioning unit in her room. First Lucy and then Pat:

Mom hugged them and she smiled. Then, taking me completely by surprise, she turned around, facing me. She walked a few steps toward me and opened her arms, inviting me into the best hug ever. She smiled; I was teary. Then, realizing that Mom had just demonstrated her remaining ability to initiate and express affection, I smiled, and we hugged and laughed together in a moment of pure joy.

My earliest teacher about Alzheimer's, Joanne Koenig Coste, writes, "The emotion behind the failing words is far more important than the words themselves, and needs to be validated. Assume the patient can still register feelings that matter."[41] Mom showed me the truth of this statement.

Encouraged by this experience, I trusted that together we would discover how her love and her needs would be communicated. Along the way, professionals in the field of Alzheimer's care gave me insights, researcher Stephan Millett, in particular. He identifies people with Alzheimer's as "semiotic subjects,"[42] indicating that they are proficient at using signs and symbols for communication purposes. We must learn to translate. As we open our minds and hearts to a new type of communication process, we might be surprised by the possibilities that remain.

While I was wondering about how Mom and I would communicate without words, I encountered the work of Stephen Levine, Buddhist teacher; groundbreaking practitioner and author in the field of loss, dying, and grief; and colleague of Dr. Elisabeth Kübler-Ross, the psychiatrist and pioneer in the field of death and dying who developed the Five Stages of Grief model. Levine reminded me that, "from the day we are born, we communicate without language."[43] In their book *Who Dies? An Investigation of Conscious Living and Conscious Dying*, Stephen and Ondrea Levine brought to my attention a term that helped me understand and embrace the living answer to how Mom and

I could communicate when her words were lost: *heart speech*. Describing heart speech as words and feelings arising within us that may or may not be audibly expressed, Stephen Levine first used this phrase to describe a style of communicating through presence and intuition with people in comas and people who are close to death. As he sat at bedsides, silently experiencing and expressing understanding and compassion, restless patients would become calm, tears would clear, eyes would meet in knowing awareness, and peace would enter the space. Levine describes his experience as sitting quietly and sending love and understanding through his heart. He does not claim that the ill or dying person picked up the silent words in his heart through some kind of telepathy; however, he believes, and experienced, that the "attitude of love and care generated an acceptance of the moment" that brought forth an atmosphere of peacefulness.[44]

When the Levines first began implementing their skillful practice of heart-speech in hospitals and hospices in the 1970s and 1980s, many of the nurses began to try it. They said it "changed their relationships to many of their patients and their painful job in general. They had another tool to open to another, and perhaps transmit that openness." Other nurses came forward to express "how wonderful it was to hear someone speak of a technique that they had intuitively been employing for some time."[45]

Through his decades of experience in the world of death and dying, Levine concludes that people who may seem disengaged and unresponsive, especially as their verbal abilities decline, "often are reachable through heart speech and... trust in the depth of our connection as human beings."[46] My own trust in my connection with Mom inspired me to believe that communicating with her in sincere and meaningful ways was still possible.

Earlier in my life's journey, I worked in human resources for a large financial institution. My job included communication training for managers. There I learned that a required aspect of effective communication is reception. For communication to actually take place, the message must be received. I taught managers how to effectively encode their messages so their communications would have a better chance of being received and understood by their employees.

Now that Mom had lost all words, the writings of Allen Power, Stephan Millet, Pierre Parenteau, and Stephen and Ondrea Levine were teaching me how to communicate with her—to both send messages and receive messages so that our process of communicating would be effective. They respectively recommended curiosity, noticing and interpreting signs, intuition, and heart speech,[47] all of which seem like reflections of the first rule of St. Benedict, which was inspired by the Book of Proverbs: "Attend with the ear of your heart."[48] This ancient invitation is being re-extended to us by modern prophets.

Mom was already proficient in heart speech, as is often the case with people in the dying process who are nonverbal and/or living with more active intuitive right brain function due to stroke or disease. Stephen Levine writes, "Somehow, it seems, many who are seriously ill are sensitive to such deep touching."[49] I was the one who needed to learn. At first, I tried being chatty with Mom, telling her the details of my day. She sat quietly and without expression through this process, which felt somehow empty to me. It seemed that reception was missing, and being chatty quickly became tiring and dull for me. I assume it had the same effect on Mom. She did, however, respond joyfully to the sound of my voice, so I often read and sang to her. When I talked to her, I used simple words and phrases with a positive tone and musical inflection. I intentionally maintained physical contact with her during our interactions. My words were always affectionate and encouraging, and my touch was tender and loving. I was sending Mom the feelings in my heart.[50]

When I began to use words more sparingly, I felt energized by my interactions with Mom, which would not be surprising to Stephen Levine. He already knows that the intuitive process of heart speech, which sends truth and love directly from one heart to another, is "of considerable value to the sender of such wholehearted blessings."[51]

Levine's description of heart speech as "meeting deeply in the heart" expressly identifies this kind of communication as relational and reinforces the idea of being carepartners with people with Alzheimer's. We connect with "another silently, intuitively, feeling as one might when singing a child to sleep. We speak into another's heart as an expansion of our own continued healing."[52] People with Alzheimer's are communicating with heart speech all the time. Although they "have lost all words," and can no longer comprehend all of our words, they can transmit and receive the attitude of love and care and acceptance.

Once I had learned to communicate with Mom using heart speech, we sent each other reciprocal messages of love, care, and acceptance every day, often through a look or a smile or a touch. Practicing this kind of communication for over three years, I came to realize and benefit from the healing it made possible. Stephen and Ondrea Levine explain, "When you speak from the heart you send love, not your needs or desires for people to be any way other than they are."[53] Stephen Levine reminds us, "We love what is, instead of what might be."[54] Or in the circumstance of Alzheimer's disease, instead of what was. Loving what is can truly be a challenge for caregivers. I've heard family members say that they don't visit their relatives in decline because they want to remember their loved ones how they "used to be."

As Mom's disease progressed, our power struggle over my life choices had effortlessly faded away. Those things I had done that hurt, frustrated, and angered her had silently been removed from her consciousness. It didn't seem to matter to Mom what I ate, what God I believed in, whether or not I avoided alcohol, if I had a schedule to keep, or if I wanted to meditate and exercise every day. She had lost the capacity to criticize, judge, and reject me, and in the absence of my fear of these capacities, I no longer felt defensive around her. I knew that Mom didn't exactly choose not to criticize, judge, or reject me. This knowledge, however, did not rob me of the experience of feeling totally, wholeheartedly accepted and loved by my mom, just exactly as I am, for the first time in my life. In Mom's present reality, I was her faithful, kind, loving, and protective companion. That's all that mattered to her. I felt so accepted and appreciated by her that the wound caused by knowing there were times she was not proud of me, times I had disappointed her, and times I was not who she wanted me to be began to heal in the presence of a mother who loved me now.

My acceptance and my receptivity were also needed to activate the healing power of heart speech. Through my academic study of Alzheimer's and my personal experiences and observations, I had learned about the process of decline determined by Mom's disease, and I was able to fully accept her increasing limitations. While learning and accepting, I had developed realistic expectations of Mom. I had completely let go of expecting her to be the kind of mother I always wanted, and I accepted the kind of mother she had now become. Once I did so, I was able to notice that she had, in many ways, become the mother I needed.

My acceptance and my now realistic expectations of Mom had opened the door for me to recognize her as the one person in the world who could never disappoint me. I didn't expect, demand, or want her to be anyone other than who she was at each moment. I gracefully and gratefully received what she could give, and I didn't ask for or need more.

From this new perspective, I could see how much Mom was still able to give me, including important things that a daughter needs from her mother. Because Mom's diminished capacities kept her in one place all the time—her nursing home—I received the gift of being able to trust that she would always be available and receptive to me whenever I needed my mom, like when I was sad or stressed and needed a hug or a smile from someone who cared. She was always happy to see me, always. She was an attentive audience whenever I needed to talk, never interrupting me and hijacking the conversation (the pattern she had perpetuated throughout my life). And she let me know how important I was to her through looks, smiles, touches, and sounds—her perfect version of heart speech.

Even though she perhaps lacked the ability to formulate an intention to mother me in these ways, Mom's presence still gave me the experience of being mothered. Sometimes I actually sat on her lap. Although I weighed less than a hundred pounds and Mom was still quite robust at the time, I always kept one foot on the floor, making sure to hold most of my weight off her. I also used this foot to rock the wheelchair slowly back and forth. Mom had her arms tightly around me, and I imitated the voice of her baby doll, softly saying, "Mama, Mama." I was inspired to say these words often, believing they were a comfort, believing that if Mom could speak, she would be saying, "Mama, Mama," to me. I'm not sure which one of us was healed more by what felt like an experience of mutual mothering. The look on Mom's face at these times seemed peaceful and content. This deep connection between us was made possible by the grace of her diminishment and her increasing ability to experience the world by functioning and communicating through the intuitive, emotional right side of her brain.[55] These changes had inspired us both to open our hearts to the flow of love. We had both grown into the most accepting, most loving, and most nonjudgmental people we had ever been—our best selves.

Although Alzheimer's was the catalyst for the changes within us and the deep connection growing between us, our acceptance of and love for each other was no less real or profound. What Mom gave me, and what she received from me, was enough to create a heartfelt and strong bond that we both recognized and cherished.

Many family members suffer from believing that Alzheimer's is a kind of death before death, feeling that their loved ones with Alzheimer's are already gone. I didn't experience this particular suffering because I recognized so many signs of life through Mom's efforts at self-expression. I later learned that, throughout the human development process, we all, including people with Alzheimer's, possess an innate drive to maximize our potential.[56]

At the end of my seven-week visit during the summer of 2007, I returned to Boston for a semester of school and to prayerfully consider moving to Iowa. In October, Mom's social worker informed me that she had a bad cold, was weak, and wasn't walking. They speculated that this would mark the end of her ability to get out of the wheelchair, and I was sure I had accompanied Mom on some of her last steps. She surprised everyone, however, by expressing her potential. By the time I returned in December, she was walking again!

Mom had always been physically active, doing yard work, shoveling snow, painting the exterior of her house by herself, and walking a mile to and from work every day for more than twenty years. Knowing that being active was important to her, I wanted to preserve her physical abilities and help her continue to find enjoyment in using her body for as long as possible. A year after I moved to Iowa, a hospice physician informed me that I had been successful. Mom had been a hospice patient for a year and was being "graduated." Not only had she not died but, even as Alzheimer's had predictably progressed, her physical condition and capabilities had improved. The doctor remarked that, given the progression of her disease, now in the end stage, Mom would have been bedridden and completely helpless if I hadn't been there every day, walking with her, engaging her in activities, helping her maintain her skills (such as feeding herself), and giving her loving attention. I hadn't realized that my efforts to enhance Mom's quality of life would support her desire to maximize her potential in such a significant way.

Everyone was amazed by Mom's remaining capabilities. A few times, during the last years of her life, she was hospitalized for infections. Because I didn't want her to forget how to walk while she was in the hospital, each time I requested a physical therapist to come daily to help Mom get out of bed and walk with her. "Seriously?" the nurses always asked. "Seriously," I replied. And when Mom walked through the hallways and smiled wide at them, the very surprised nurses instantly fell in love with her. Heart speech was working its magic.

As the disease progressed and Mom no longer qualified for physical therapy or rehabilitation programs offered by the nursing home due to Medicare limitations, we were on our own. I asked for and received permission from the nursing home to take Mom to the physical therapy room and use some of their equipment. There were toys for hand dexterity and strength, balls for catching and throwing, and our favorite, the portable stairs. I would push this big platform into the middle of the room and position Mom facing the stairs going up. I stood on the other side of the up and then down stairs and asked her to come to me. At first, she needed coaching about holding the rails, lifting her right leg, pulling herself up, and lifting her left leg. And then, up she went. She was better going up than going down, but if I asked her to look at me, instead of the steps, she sailed down the three steps with ease. We practiced stairs on Sundays after Mass while most other residents sat alone in their rooms waiting for lunch. Mom's legs got stronger, she walked confidently without assistance, and she so enjoyed the big hug waiting for her at the end of the stair climbing.

One day, Mom and I were taking a ride in the nursing home minibus to see the sights around town. Bus rides always ended with an ice-cream cone from the Dairy Queen, and this was a treat for all the residents. Mom loved the bus! She even enjoyed the rides when the destination was the doctor's office. During the months I was away coordinating my move, the staff transferred Mom into the bus by having her sit in a wheelchair and then ride up on the mechanical lift. I agreed to their process. As we walked out the front door toward the waiting wheelchair, Mom let go of my hand and walked, with intention, directly toward the open door of the bus. She had seen the stairs! Without any assistance or direction, she put both hands on the rails and lifted her right foot onto the first step. There she paused. I'm sure the staff was thinking, "Oh no. What do we do now?" I went and stood behind her, coaching her as I had in the physical therapy room: "Pull yourself up with your arms, and lift your left leg up." She followed this instruction and climbed the rest on her own. Up all the steps she went into the bus. The staff and the residents already on the bus applauded. Mom radiated smiles and pride!

Eventually, our stair-climbing practice ceased. One Sunday, Mom could no longer climb down the stairs. She was stuck at the top, seeming to panic about what to do. Her panic was, perhaps, a reflection of my own. Realizing she was stuck, I knew I needed to get help, but I didn't want to leave her alone, fearing she would move and fall. So I asked Mom clearly to stand still and wait for me to get back. Thankfully, she did. I rushed out and found a nursing aide, who helped me to get

Mom down the steps. But Mom was scared, a clear indication that the stair-climbing activity was now beyond her ability.

Then came the time when walking to and from the dining room was too exhausting; then she could no longer walk with just one person assisting her; then she could walk only to the doorway of her room. These would be her last steps. And then, about a week before she died, she could no longer stand on her own. Through observation and acceptance of Mom's decline, I adjusted my expectations according to her abilities and held the memories of each last gently in my heart.

The aides at the nursing home who were Mom's most beloved caregivers also witnessed Mom's drive to maximize her physical potential. In the telling of the endearing stories of her accomplishments, we all became closer. As Mom's hands became more constricted and clenched, the occupational therapist brought palm guards to keep her fingernails from damaging her palms. One day, her aide Alexis was trying to get Mom to relax her hands and open her fingers enough to put on the palm guards. Trying to get Mom's clenched fists to open was challenging and time consuming, and the aides needed to be careful to avoid hurting her fingers. The occupational therapist had taught us all how to do the necessary hand massage that would relax her clench, but this took a long time. Having other tasks to do, Alexis became exasperated and finally wailed, "Oh, come on, Jeanne. Help me out here. Open up your fingers." And open them she did. No one had thought to ask Mom to do this. She opened them every day after this, very slowly, upon request.

A few weeks before Mom died, she caught a cold and her breathing was labored. We went briefly to the emergency room for a breathing treatment to make her more comfortable. The ER staff at the hospital was always remarkably kind to Mom. They treated her as they would any other patient, which, sadly, isn't consistently the case with medical and hospital personnel encountering people with dementia. Even though Mom was severely impaired by Alzheimer's and clearly not feeling well during the last ER visit, she was still able to surprise the doctor. The nurse was taking Mom's blood pressure from her left arm, and Mom was watching her intently. The doctor stood on Mom's right side, and from this position, with her looking away from him, he said her name, "Jeanne." Slowly, she turned her head, looked right at him, and smiled. I could see the surprise in his eyes, which matched his exclamation. "Wow!" he said.

People with Alzheimer's possess the drive to maximize their remaining potential, and there will be countless opportunities for caregivers to nurture that drive. We just need to pay careful attention to them and give them chances to surprise us.

Mom and I communicated through heart speech until she drew her last breath. She was in the hospital over the Thanksgiving weekend, and although she recovered from the condition that took her there, I knew we were at the threshold of her departure from this world. Before returning to the nursing home, we waited together for the van to come for us. We sat quietly holding hands, looking out the window. During this contemplative time, I realized that it would be helpful to know what Mom needed from me to get ready for her journey into the next life.

When I got home that night, I contacted a local holistic healer who I experienced as an intuitive and loving person. I asked her to come and sit with Mom, to see if she could receive any clarity about what else Mom might need from me at this time. The healer said she was open to doing this but didn't feel she was the right person. Feeling let down at a time of need, I was upset. I didn't feel confident in my own intuition about something this important, so I tried to find someone else in nearby Madison, Wisconsin, without success.

Almost rebelliously, I decided to do it myself. I put on our favorite soft music. I held Mom's hand and asked her through heart speech, "What do you need, Mom, to get ready to go?" Intuitively, I received her reply: "I need to feel wanted." Given Mom's life story of abandonment, this reply didn't surprise me at all.

From that day until the moment she died, I let Mom know with my words and my actions that I loved taking care of her, loved being with her, and wanted her to be a part of my life. I didn't want to confuse her or delay her journey, however, so I also let her know that Jesus wanted her too, and that it was OK to go to him.

On Christmas Eve, while I was brushing her teeth, Mom looked up at me with eyes overflowing with trust. I was so moved that I couldn't hold her gaze. I gathered her up into my arms and held her close, telling her with my heart that I would do my best to be worthy of her trust.

Two days later, I asked her again what she needed. I sensed her reply: "Will you stay and wait with me?" I felt chills throughout my body. Her request reminded me of Jesus' request of Peter, James, and John as he prayed in the Garden of Gethsemane for the cup of suffering to be taken away from him. Jesus "began to be distressed and agitated. And said to them, 'I am deeply grieved, even to death; remain here, and keep awake.'"[57] Mom was confirming the insight of Thibault and Morgan: When people with Alzheimer's are dying, nothing is more important "than family members sitting with them, holding their hands, and praying with them as their spirits leave this world for the next."[58]

"Of course, Mom," my heart replied to hers. "I promise I will stay and wait with you." I reassured her of this every day with my words as well as my presence.

I sent a note to the holistic healer, thanking her for paying attention to her hesitancy to help me. I was pleased to let her know that the right person to listen to Mom was me.

Eight days later, I arrived at the nursing home in the morning. Mom looked beautiful, wearing the snowflake turtleneck I had given her for her birthday. Her hair was brushed and gleaming. Colorful clips decorated her hair, and a white beaded necklace completed her ensemble. We hugged and smiled, and off we went to exercise class. As I moved her arms and legs as instructed by Dee, the class leader, Mom was attentive and joyful. I helped her kick the colorful beach ball, and this made her smile. She ate a little that day, although she had made it clear a couple weeks earlier that food was no longer of interest. She was rapidly losing weight and becoming physically weak. She hadn't walked for a few days. But her eyes, her smile, and her spirit were shining brightly.

That night after dinner, I hugged Mom good night, and wheeled her to the bathtub room. At the door, I leaned over, looking deep into her eyes. The connection between us seemed so strong, I decided to see if she would give me a kiss, like she used to. (Months earlier, to my sadness, she had stopped responding to my request for a kiss.) I looked into her clear blue eyes, touched her hand, and slowly, clearly said, "Kiss." Like I used to, I demonstrated how to kiss. I put my finger to my lips, puckered, and kissed. Never losing eye contact, I said it again, "Kiss." Then I put my lips to her lips, and without hesitation, Mom kissed me good night. It was the last kiss. My eyes filled with tears; I hugged her again. "I love you, Mom. I want you to be with me."

It was hard to leave her that night. It was always hard to leave her. By the time I got home, I was elated. I felt high on life, literally. Mom and I had shared such a great day. I thought we would have many more. Maybe weeks. Maybe even a month or more together. I felt gloriously happy.

That night at 1:56 AM, my phone rang. I was awake instantly. The nurse on the other end of the phone recited incomprehensible medical details: heart rate, respiration, nonresponsive, mottling. "Should I come now?" I asked. "Yes," she replied. "Come now."

If ever I wanted to run away, it was now. How could I let her go? How could I be there witnessing her nonresponsive face, a death mask? I had never been with someone at the moment of death, and I was scared. Scared of death, scared of loss.

But I went. I kept my promise to Mom. I stayed, and I waited with her.

During the next fifty-eight hours, the web of relationality I had woven around Mom over the previous four years teemed with life, bringing guidance, companionship, and comfort. The nursing home carepartners were attentive to us both. Mom's dearest companion aide, Kathy, brought her a rosary bracelet to wear, and this bracelet is now my most cherished piece of jewelry. The hospice nurses were ever-present, monitoring and relieving Mom's perceived pain and distress, and consoling and guiding me through every aspect of this unfamiliar experience. Other family members with loved ones at the nursing home, our long-time companions, kept a vigil at Mom's door. The hospice chaplain was there; my cousin, Father Ron; and my pastoral friends, Rev. Diane and Marilyn, all came—and stayed. They prayed with us. Our hearts were touched, and our needs were filled.

Although Mom appeared unresponsive, our connection remained intact. We listened to music. I sang, prayed, and gently massaged her. I brushed her hair. The aides made space for me in her bed, and I snuggled close and held her, through the night and through the day. I tenderly stroked her face. She loved this most of all. I told her those truths still unsaid. Our hearts spoke of love and leaving.

Before I left Massachusetts, I had asked my spiritual director, Sister Catherine Griffiths, what she believed happened when someone died. She shared her interpretation of one of Julian of Norwich's revelations. God told Julian not to fear death, because as we breathe our last breath out, God will come in upon it, and it will become one breath, the Breath of God.[59] I wanted to be with Mom, holding her for her last breath. I wanted to be next to God, breathing in, becoming part of that One Breath.

Three mornings after Mom kissed me goodbye, the hospice nurse, proficient in heart speech, told me that although Mom was torn about leaving her life with me and moving on, today would be her last day. I reassured Mom about my love, and about how much I wanted her to be in my life. "But Jesus wants you too. And it's OK to go to him now." For almost four years, I had been holding Mom's mortal being close, and now I needed to gently let her immortal being go. As I cried about having to let go of my mom, both my faith and my friends accompanied me tenderly across this threshold.

Two of Mom's relatives were coming from out of town to say goodbye. The hospice nurse, knowing my desire to be with Mom to receive her last breath, suggested that the others visit for only fifteen minutes. We all agreed, but I was distraught that Mom might die while I was away from her bedside. My friend Rev. Diane had attended at the bedsides of many dying people. She counseled me, "Just ask her to wait for you." I did this. I held Mom. I told her who was coming and that I would give them some time alone with her. "Wait for me to come back, please. Wait for me." Fifteen minutes later, I returned to Mom's bedside. Within a few minutes, her breathing became labored. Another fifteen minutes, and God and I became one with her last breath.

I wept. And then there was a vision of me walking with Mom on a long journey that led us to a dock stretching far out into the ocean. A large cruise ship was there—waiting. This was as far as I could go with Mom. She boarded, and as the ship sailed away, she waved goodbye to me from the deck. Then she was gone—out of my sight, off on this new adventure.

The last word. The last step. The last kiss. The last breath. The last goodbye.

I am so grateful and happy that I did not miss them.

V

Looking Back, Walking On

For all that has been—Thank you.
For all that is to come—Yes!
—Dag Hammarskjold

On Thursday, January 6, 2011, my mom went on to her new life. At the same moment, we both stepped across the threshold of new worlds.

Some who knew me through my caring of Mom remarked that she was my "whole world." That assessment wasn't exactly true since my life at the time was rich with purpose and meaningful relationships in addition to my care of Mom. What was and is true, however, is that my mom unquestionably became the love of my life. Most people, me included, look for this kind of fulfilling, intimate love in a romantic relationship. So imagine my surprise to find it in relationship with an old woman with Alzheimer's disease!

In many ways, Mom became my soul mate. Through Alzheimer's, she taught me the most important lessons for living—not at the beginning of my life, as one might expect of a parent, but at the end of hers. Mom taught me how to love with my whole heart, how to organize my life around what really matters, how to be a better person, and how to accept and appreciate what is. As David Steindl-Rast proposes, Mom gave me the opportunity to say a "limitless 'Yes' to everything as it is,"[1] including pain, loss, hardship, death, challenge, joy, discovery, surprise, healing, and love. Saying that limitless yes has been the most transforming experience of my life.

Catholic priest Ronald Rolheiser defines *soul mate* as "the one who takes you home."[2] If this is a true definition, perhaps Mom was able to recognize me as her soul mate. Tenderly, I carried her to the threshold of her new world. At Mom's funeral Mass, my cousin, Father Ron, delivered the homily. It was when he spoke about noticing how much Mom smiled when I was with her that I realized the actual purpose and holiness of my caregiving mission. Ron said, "When Jeanne was smiling, we knew she was not suffering either physical or emotional pain. Her smile indicated that she was going beyond herself; she was interested in her surroundings, and she was connecting with others."

I had come to be companion and advocate. I didn't realize that I would be enabling connection, maximizing potential, and relieving suffering. When Ron's words helped me to realize what I had done, I wept.

After Mom died, I missed caring for her. I missed (and still miss) the flowing love we shared every day. I miss her hugs and kisses. I really miss her smile. In the midst of all the missing, however, I'm grateful to have had the time and opportunity to be Mom's companion and soul mate on the journey. Being the one to relieve her fear, pain, and suffering, even a bit, and being the one to take her home was such an honor.

Although I was her companion, Mom was really the guide on the journey. She was showing me and all those she encountered along the way how to live life and how to approach disability and death with acceptance, dignity, and joy in the remaining moments. Because of her cognitive decline, Mom's walk toward death seemed instinctual. She seemed to gracefully lean into it, without resistance, and hopefully without fear.

Looking back, I appreciate all those who encouraged me to pay attention to Mom's guidance and showed me how to allow Mom's wisdom about life and death to shine forth. Walking on, I realize that my experience of caring for Mom is still lighting my way. My learning in the school of life and love, by looking at the world through the lens of Alzheimer's disease, did not end when Mom died.

My world looks different now, and new . . . .

15 Forgetting, Forgiving, Reconciling

Six weeks after I officially relocated my life, including my car and all my belongings, from Boston to Iowa, Mom became very sick with the flu. It was serious, and she was accepted into the hospice program. On April 2, 2008, the nurse called me at 7 AM to report that Mom's fever had risen to 104 degrees. The hospice nurse and Mom's parish priest were called. I went to the nursing home immediately, climbed into Mom's bed, and snuggled next to her. I held her, rocked her, and put ice packs on her forehead. We all thought she would die that day, and I experienced the fullness of human sorrow.

I felt sorrow for the many ways Mom had harmed me, for the close relationship I longed to have with her that had never been. I felt sorrow because I had not been able to do more to protect Mom and nurture her during this time in her life when she was so vulnerable. I did what the system allowed me to do. I did what my physical and emotional limits allowed me to do. I did my best, but oh, how I wished I could have done more for her. I felt sorrow because I never apologized to her, and she never apologized to me. I felt surprising sorrow because I had discovered how much I loved being with Mom, and all of what we now shared would be gone—too soon.

My friend's first grandson, Gabriel, was born that day in the early morning hours. I got that news as I was rushing out the door to be at Mom's bedside. Gabriel begins. Mom ends. That's what I thought the day would be about. In the midst of this extraordinary day of birth and death, joy and sorrow, ordinary things were also happening. Mom and I listened to music as we often did. The birds outside were singing. The nursing home's cleaning woman vacuumed in the hallway outside Mom's door.

On that sorrowful, joyful, extraordinary, ordinary day, I suddenly felt the presence of God surrounding Mom and me. During one seemingly miraculous moment, which I was fortunate to notice in the midst of an intense swarm of emotions, I realized that I had forgiven my mother. It was as if her whole life flashed before my eyes, and my heart suddenly knew her, and embraced her. I felt the life-filled breath of love flowing from my heart to her heart and back again. And I forgave her for everything.

Because this day of Mom's death was inevitable, people had asked me how would I feel, and what I would do if Mom died shortly after I moved to Iowa. In all my decision-making, I had to consider this possibility. My answer to them, to myself, was, "I don't know." On that extraordinary ordinary April day, however, I lived into knowing. If Mom had died only weeks after my cross-country relocation, I would have had no regrets about rearranging my priorities, letting go of my professional opportunities and aspirations, completely changing my life, and moving to be with her.

There I was, twelve hundred miles away from everything that was familiar to me, forgiving and loving the one who had harmed me throughout my life, the one who had betrayed and abandoned me during many of my times of great need. In spite of her failings, I was at her bedside. I had not forsaken her. My choices and my feelings in the context of our fractured relationship were hard to understand at the time, even for me. But I knew one thing for certain: I had no regrets.

In my heart, the forgiveness I felt for Mom on that April morning was complete, arising spontaneously and effortlessly. It was just miraculously there, unbidden. I spoke of this experience often, and always with awe. Many reacted to my story of forgiveness with skepticism.

"Really? Forgiveness just happened?"

"Really," I would reply. "It just happened."

So it seemed, at the time.

Usually, when I'm presented with an important life lesson, or I'm working through an issue, my mind grasps what's happening long before my emotions do. Throughout my journey of personal and spiritual growth, my learning process has been what people commonly describe as "understanding it with my head, but not feeling it in my heart." The process for forgiving and reconciling with Mom happened in the opposite order—I felt it in my heart first. Although I recognized it at the time, I didn't have enough intellectual knowledge of true forgiveness to be able to articulate how it had actually happened.

A ministry course in the psychology and theology of forgiveness, which I took during the last months of Mom's life, enlightened my understanding somewhat. But the final piece of the forgiveness puzzle came into my heart on Thanksgiving Day, almost ten months after Mom died. My Thanksgiving tradition includes writing a letter reviewing the highlights of my year to enclose with my holiday cards. In what seemed like an effort to procrastinate from writing my annual letter the year Mom died, I spent a lot of time looking through a file of old correspondence. It turned out this was really preparation for the letter. Tucked away in that file were all the letters Mom wrote to me on her teeny-tiny stationery in 2003 and 2004. I had not seen those precious letters, which chronicled her decline and expressed her appreciation for me, for seven or eight years. Accidently unearthing those treasures brought into full awareness my understanding of how the forgiveness I felt and the reconciliation that Mom and I experienced actually happened, and more importantly, how it began. The seeds were in those teeny-tiny letters from her, which I had allowed to be planted in my soul. They grew and grew, eventually into full bloom.

Earlier in my life, focusing attention, time, and energy on forgiving Mom for not protecting me from my father and for abandoning me when I most needed her help had not been a priority for me. Healing from the severe wounds of my childhood had appropriately been my focus. The writings of modern spiritual teachers and professionals working with childhood abuse survivors had urged me over the years not to forgive too quickly.[3] They describe the road leading to true forgiveness as long and arduous.[4] Later in my theological studies, I learned that numerous scholars echo this advice and this wisdom.[5]

During the last months and weeks of Mom's life, I studied and contemplated forgiveness in my ministry class. Challenged by the continual questioning of the skeptics, I was specifically seeking to understand my spontaneous experience of forgiveness.

I was especially surprised to discover how strongly my intellect resonated with forgiveness as it's understood through the lens of the Jewish tradition, even though I had been raised in the tradition of Roman Catholicism. According Solomon Schimmel, Professor Emeritus of Jewish Education and Psychology at Hebrew College, a victim who has been unjustly injured is entitled to feel resentment "and the perpetrator has incurred a moral and/or legal debt to the victim, such as to apologize, make reparations or be punished." An abuser is not forgiven until reparation is made and forgiveness from the injured person is formally requested.[6] Judaism's interpretation was a comfort to me, letting me know that my anger and resentment toward my parents were justified, and that I was not a bad person for feeling as I did throughout much of my life. After all, my parents had not acknowledged my wounds and losses, nor had they asked for my forgiveness.

Although I didn't focus on forgiving Mom through the decades of my healing process before Alzheimer's touched our world, I intentionally kept communication open with her. Occasionally, I traveled to Iowa to visit her, truly hoping that one day she would see me, that she would recognize my hurt, be accountable, apologize, and make amends somehow. Unfortunately, our dueling priorities and lifestyles often collided, and after these visits with Mom it took weeks to recuperate and regain my sense of self-worth. "Why do you keep going there? Why do you put yourself through this?" friends asked. I wasn't sure. It seemed that, somewhere in my heart, a painful hope for forgiveness and reconciliation was springing eternally.

When Mom was diagnosed with Alzheimer's, my hope for an apology from her vanished, along with my hope for feeling forgiveness or having a meaningful relationship with her. I lamented, miserably, the fact that Mom would no longer be able to admit what had happened, to say she was sorry, or to make amends. Every possibility I could imagine for forgiveness and reconciliation was lost along with Mom's cognitive abilities. It seemed that hope was over. However, as I grieved this loss of hope, the words of Brother David Steindl-Rast resurfaced, encouraging me to let go of expectations and to remain open for surprise.

In that "Refiner's Fire" of Alzheimer's, where the flames were burning away feelings I no longer needed and purifying my soul, I looked for insights about forgiveness. Observing Mom, myself, and other caregivers—especially my friend Mary Kay—from within the fire, I saw an intricate and complex web of impressions and emotions. I realized that our ideas about forgiveness are influenced by personal histories, often misunderstood or misinterpreted theologies, and hearts longing for connection. In the context of Alzheimer's care within Mary Kay's life, Mom's life, and my own, several specific concepts relating to forgiveness caught my attention and I decided to explore them.

Unforgiveness

Psychology professor and researcher Everett Worthington, Jr., instantly expanded my understanding of forgiveness by introducing me to the word *unforgiveness*, which he describes as a "jumble of emotions," including "resentment, hostility, hatred, bitterness, simmering anger and low-level fear." He goes on to say, "*Fear and anger, immediate responses, are not unforgiveness.* Unforgiveness must ripen through rumination .... It takes time and reflection to develop unforgiveness." Comparing the jumbled feelings of unforgiveness to "a hot potato," Worthington acknowledges the discomfort we all feel in this state and our desire to "unload it" as soon as we can. The emotional discomfort felt by many, heightened by the moral obligation imposed by some religions to forgive even unrepentant abusers, may lead us into forgiving too soon. Our efforts to relieve ourselves of this emotional burden include several strategies: "forbearance, successful revenge, seeing justice done, giving up the right to judge, telling a different story, and accepting the transgression."[7] Some of these strategies are born of denial and some of them are healthy coping techniques. However, only the complete process of forgiveness, which includes embracing our feelings rather than rapidly unloading them, will lead us into healing.

Forgiving God

Worthington's insights were in the forefront of my mind when my friend Mary Kay revealed to me her feelings of unforgiveness toward God. She was furious at God because her mother, Marie, had Alzheimer's. She harbored feelings of anger and bitterness and had completely lost her faith. Marie was a lifelong, devout Catholic, and according to Mary Kay, her mother, like Job, was completely innocent. She *did not* deserve this horrible illness in the first place, and having it linger for this length of time (almost two decades) was unacceptable, unforgivable. As revenge, Mary Kay had disconnected from any sense of spirituality.

When we all met, Marie had been living in the nursing home for more than fifteen years. She was Mom's next-door neighbor there, so I got to know her well. She didn't walk or talk; she couldn't stand or move her legs, although she could move her arms a little. I had seen her take a tissue and try to wipe her runny nose. This seemingly small effort at self-care was a large accomplishment for Marie, and quite touching and endearing to those observing this act with their hearts. Marie did make some sounds, and she ate well, especially when one of her daughters patiently fed her. It was hard for Marie to hold up her head, so mostly she was lying in her bed or sitting slumped in her wheelchair looking at the floor. "This is not living," lamented Mary Kay, her youngest daughter.

Feelings of unforgiveness toward God because of Alzheimer's were not an isolated experience happening in Mary Kay's heart alone. Surely, there are millions of people of faith who don't understand why the all-powerful God many of us learned to believe in as children allows so much suffering. Not understanding can implode into helplessness and subsequent rage when suffering enters our own lives, as it does with Alzheimer's. We are powerless to stop the losses, the decline, the financial burdens, the difficult choices, and the emotional and physical challenges.

In the circumstance of Alzheimer's, we have no place for blame, if not God. Unlike diseases caused by smoking, for example, where we can point to tobacco companies and blame them for our pain, there is no identified cause for Alzheimer's. We can't even blame the sick person who chose to smoke for exercising their free will in reckless ways. We don't know, for sure, what to do, or not do, in order to avoid Alzheimer's. This not knowing leads many to point at God and rant.

Certain theologians, however, look at suffering, such as Alzheimer's, and conclude that God is compassionate but has limited power and is, therefore, not responsible for causing disease. Accepting this perspective would require a complete theological overhaul for many people of faith. Some caregivers, therefore, might find more comfort in Jon Levinson's conclusions. A modern Jewish theologian, Levinson directs our attention to the varied ways that God is still "engaged in combat against powerful forces of chaos and evil in the world." Looking through the lens of the Hebrew Bible, he concludes that the vastness of God's omnipotence "has not yet fully manifested itself."[8] This interpretation holds possibility for God's current and future intervention.

Clearly, God *is* in combat with the powerful force of chaos that is Alzheimer's disease. Armies of physicians, researchers, caregivers, family members, creative and talented advocates, authors, news reporters, and even politicians have been deployed to active duty by internal calls for compassion, care, healing, activism, and love. In Mary Kay's present, however, God's army was not saving her mom. In the cauldron of unforgiveness for this injustice, she could not forgive God and she suffered.

Forgiving Ourselves

For two years, Mom and Marie lived next door to each other at the nursing home. Before Mary Kay and I officially met, she had seen me in Mom's room. Wheeling Marie down the hall, her first glimpse was of me washing Mom's feet. Mom had an ingrown toenail that was infected, and the foot doctor had prescribed warm water soaks in Epsom salts twice a day. Knowing that this added task might overburden the aides, I did this care myself. When Mary Kay saw me, I was sitting on the floor in front of my barefooted Mom in her wheelchair. While one foot soaked, I massaged the other. During this treatment, Mom was in heaven—I could see this in her eyes. I was relaxed and grateful for the opportunity to do something tangible to help her. Partly because of Mary Kay's negative impressions of older people's feet, she perceived my foot-washing as an extraordinary act of caregiving. Over time, Mary Kay observed that I was a daily presence in Mom's life. She admired my commitment, but comparing her own caregiving to mine, she felt inadequate. One day she confessed to me that it was "just too hard" for her to see her mom in this condition. She shared her harsh self-judgment for not being emotionally strong enough to visit daily, as she had when Marie was in the earlier stages of the disease. I noticed, however, that Marie had the Cadillac of wheelchairs, researched and ordered by Mary Kay. And every Sunday morning, without fail, she and her sister took over the nursing home beauty shop and washed and styled their mom's hair. Mary Kay's jumble of emotions was caused by love. She loved her mother so much and wanted to do more for her.

As we became friends, Mary Kay shared more of the complexity about her feelings of distress over Marie's illness and her unforgiveness toward herself. "I know that not going is selfish," she said. "Not going doesn't benefit Mom in any way. It benefits me." She paused thoughtfully after she made this statement, and then added, "Only in the short term does it benefit me not to go. But I know I'll feel guilty for the rest of my life because I didn't spend more time with her." Hoping to plant seeds of self-acceptance and self-forgiveness that would sprout within her, I consistently and compassionately acknowledged Mary Kay's struggle and reminded her that she was truly doing her best under difficult circumstances.

Mary Kay really was doing her best as a caregiver for her mother and was surely worthy of forgiveness. This I know because I witnessed her earnest engagement in both external and internal struggles. For her mother's benefit and her own, Mary Kay continued to challenge her emotional limits. She sought out information by attending workshops and reading many books; she reached out for strength from others by courageously sharing her feelings. She began to recognize that small expressions of compassion—such as hugging her mother or scratching her back—could relieve their suffering and heal them both. She told me about a quiet, gentle time with her mom when she scratched her back and they listened to music together, and I could feel Mary Kay transcending her pain in the holiness of those moments. In these acts and this transforming realization, Mary Kay was manifesting one of Jacqui Lewis's fierce love principles: "What hurts you hurts me, what heals you heals me."[9]

The realization that one moment of connection with her mother made a difference beckoned Mary Kay to step out of her own suffering and toward her mother's bedside more often. This, I believe, is a shining example of God's power in combat with the chaos of Alzheimer's disease—manifesting itself in and through Mary Kay. In the glow of light from the holy moments, Mary Kay told me that she felt strong, proud, and forgiven.

Through the conventional lens of conquering disease, it appeared that God was failing in the battle against Alzheimer's. However, imagining Mary Kay and Marie basking in the light of connection and comfort, of suffering lessened through love, what I saw was a clear victory for God.

Healing Wounds from the Past

Mom was seventy-five the first time she told me how angry she was at her mother for abandoning her when she was sixteen. I was astounded by this emotional revelation at what seemed to be a late date. She had told me many times about Grandmother Philomena dying during routine gallbladder surgery as a result of physician error, but her anger was always directed toward the surgeon, toward all doctors by association. When Mom revealed her anger about being abandoned, I validated her and tried to engage her in a conversation about her feelings. Quickly, she employed a coping strategy and minimized the loss. A few years later, she brought it up again. And again, I invited her to talk about it. She didn't minimize it this time; she just didn't say more. Perhaps it was too painful for her.

Possibly Mom's anger over this abandonment continued to fester within her soul, and she carried this heavy baggage into the world of Alzheimer's as she continued on her life journey. She may, however, have forgotten her anger. Or maybe what I hoped for actually happened. During her last years with advancing Alzheimer's, Mom had regressed to an infancy-like state, and I hoped she thought I was her mother. Social worker Naomi Feil says that a "mother's hug creates warm, safe feelings," and that a mother's face becomes recorded indelibly in the infant's brain.[10] Every day, Mom saw my loving face and received my warm hugs. I hoped that her feelings of loss and anger were replaced by the comforting awareness of being loved and safe. I hoped that, in her soul, she knew she was not abandoned, that, within her heart, the pain she felt because of her mother's death was healed, or at least lessened, and that her dear mother was forgiven.

Forgiving Each Other

Being human, we all hurt each other, often unintentionally. Authors Robert Browning and Roy Reed observe that we "repeatedly fail to treat each other as sacred, and instead tend to use one another in order to deal with our anxieties."[11] It was important for my own healing process to acknowledge that I had also hurt Mom in countless ways. Many of the choices I considered healing and life-affirming for me had disappointed and threatened her over the years. In my thirties, I sent her justifiably angry letters, the kind that therapists working with abuse survivors suggest we write as catharsis without actually sending them. I know the pain these letters caused her was searing. So it's likely that Mom also felt the jumbled emotions of unforgiveness toward me. This could explain her frequent angry outbursts and her passive-aggressive behavior toward me throughout much of my adult life.

Being with Mom at the threshold during the early stages of Alzheimer's, how I wished I had been able to ask her for forgiveness earlier in my life. When we began this journey together, I believed that receiving forgiveness from her would be impossible. Eventually, however, it seemed that Mom must have forgotten her resentments toward me, since our unfolding and evolving relationship felt unburdened by my past failings. The damage to Mom's rational thinking somehow freed her and allowed her to engage and communicate with me differently. The bond between us was growing stronger based on the ways we validated each other in the present.

During those first years of the disease, something was happening that didn't take root in my consciousness at the time. Although neither of us had apologized, Mom must have instinctively moved on to the next step in the forgiveness process, which therapist Terry Hargrave refers to as "rebirthing" a relationship.[12] Through her actions, her remaining words (in the teeny-tiny letters), and her heart-speech, Mom was continually planting seeds for reconciliation. Janet Ramsey reminds us that although it's possible to feel forgiveness (an internal process) without engaging the person who caused the injury and without receiving an apology, it takes two for the embrace of reconciliation (an external process) to occur.[13] In spite of her cognitive limitations, Mom reached out to me. She was initiating the embrace. I wasn't consciously aware of this until I re-read her teeny last letters on that Thanksgiving Day almost a year after she died.

Forgiving Abusers

During the process of healing from childhood sexual abuse, which began in earnest when I was thirty-four, I experienced lingering and sometimes overwhelming feelings of unforgiveness toward Mom, including justifiable feelings of anger and resentment, because she had not protected me from my father's abuse and because she had abandoned me, seemingly for life, through alcohol use and denial. I was therefore so surprised to spontaneously feel forgiveness for Mom in 2008 at what I thought was her deathbed. Upon reflection, I realized there was nothing spontaneous—that is without effort—about it. For more than twenty years, I had been actively, although unwittingly, suffering and struggling through the hard work of therapy to attain a feeling of forgiveness toward her. Robert Enright considers forgiveness to be a moral choice born out of the struggle and suffering I was enduring, and he once again evokes the metaphor of the "Refiner's Fire"[14] to describe this process. That April morning, when I recognized the feeling of forgiveness alive in my heart, I chose to say "yes." And finally, those burdensome feelings of unforgiveness were completely burned away. What was left was love. I felt lighter. I felt kinder. I felt healed.

If forgiveness of an abuser becomes part of the healing process, according to sexual abuse counselors Ellen Bass and Laura Davis, it happens at the end of the process, only after the survivor has "gone through all the stages of remembering, grief, anger, and moving on."[15] Early in my healing, I had been warned that forgiving, and especially forgetting, wounds caused by an unrepentant abuser could be dangerous, and that *trying* to forgive could result in a "futile short circuit" of the process. Stressing the importance of safety for victims, the work of Janet Ramsey helped me understand what forgiveness is and is not and how to protect myself:

Forgiveness is not forgetting. Remembering the harm helps you stay safe.

- Forgiveness is not minimizing.
- Forgiveness is not justifying or condoning.
- Forgiveness is not an event. It's a process.
- Forgiveness is not an act of willpower. It is not something we can command.
- Forgiveness is not universal. It's not even a goal for some.
- Forgiveness is not reconciliation. We have to stay far, far away from some people.[16]

Safety and trust were qualities I needed and sought in relationships. Sadly, I hadn't felt either with Mom for most of my life.

Concentrating on my own healing, I focused necessary attention on forgiving myself. Schimmel explains that sometimes abuse victims and survivors feel guilt-ridden and ashamed, harboring an inward anger that manifests as depression, even though there is no moral or rational reason for feeling this way.[17] Abused children are at particular risk for this dynamic, and abuse counselors stress that self-forgiveness is what's most important for our healing.[18] When I began to feel forgiveness for myself, for my own human failings, it just naturally extended itself to other people in the world. I started to understand humanity's limits and longings. I became able to see when somebody was doing something "right." During those early years of Alzheimer's, Mom was doing something very right, something very relational. And I was able to relationally respond to her humane, loving actions.

From remnants of my Catholic upbringing, I had concluded that forgiveness was not a cognitive, willful process. In the Christian context, one can take concrete steps toward forgiveness; however, the actual experience of feeling forgiveness is a grace-filled process, "a gift from God, and a sign that God is present with us." Ramsey highlighted, for my consideration, the "impossibility of forgiveness," concluding that to forgive "is not a human achievement." She talked about some highly unlikely situations in which severely injured people manage to forgive—extramarital affairs, for example. "But people do it," she said, showing the "openness for Spirit to enter the human experience. God creates the condition. We have to choose—and take radical responsibility for what we do in this world."[19]

The process for healing from abuse and the processes for experiencing forgiveness and reconciliation are similar.

They all include a "deep remembering" of the wound and acknowledging feelings, including hurt, anger, hate, and shame. The processes for forgiveness and reconciliation, however, add steps that take the abuser into consideration, inviting the wounded person to seek to understand who the abuser is and to see if empathy is possible.[20] Through hearing Mom describe the pain she felt over losing her driver's license and her autonomy, through witnessing her losses—the labored writing on the teeny stationary, for example; through noticing her growing dependency and confusion; and by being a part of her proud efforts to stay engaged in life and to stay in relationship with me, I recognized her vulnerability. In my own therapy, I had explored what it was like for me as a vulnerable child, helpless and afraid, with no one to protect me. And I could empathize with Mom's experience of being powerless in the presence of Alzheimer's.

"To understand everything is to forgive everything," said the Buddha. This guidance supports the modern theorists, such as Everett Worthington, who believe the key for opening the heart to forgiveness and reconciliation is empathy.[21] Each person sincerely attempts to understand the other's experience and perspective. There were things I came to understand that helped to deepen my forgiveness of Mom. For example, throughout my adult life, I learned by painful experience that trying to get people intent on being abusive to stop is practically impossible. Maybe Mom had tried to stop my father and failed, just as I had failed to stop abusers. Maybe she had tried to protect me, but times were different then. A year before I moved to Iowa, I learned that relatives had been aware of my father's abuse. Although my aunts and uncles took precautions to protect their own children, they didn't help Mom protect me. She was alone in an abusive situation, probably doing what she could to survive, possibly drinking to drown the pain she felt for not protecting me.

Reconciliation

A key element for reconciliation to occur is commitment. Each person refuses to give up on the other, no matter how long and difficult the process may be. Mom and I never gave up on each other.

What seemed like a miraculous event, my spontaneous forgiveness of Mom, was actually the convergence of my healing process and our unintentional steps toward reconciliation. For more than five years, through the progression of her illness, we had been creating a hopeful future for our relationship that was comprised of trust and peace.

For me, this creating process involved remembering and reflecting on Mom's helpful presence as well as the wounds she inflicted. In many ways, Mom had not protected me and she had not met my needs, but in some important ways she had done both. For example, she had been especially supportive after my two broken engagements. The first time, when I was twenty-two, she comforted me with wine and cigarettes. This showed her intention to ease my pain, although her valiant effort wasn't especially helpful. (I got very sick.) It was, however, what she knew how to do at the time. After the second broken engagement, which happened when I was fifty, I didn't even tell Mom until two months after the fact. I feared she would criticize and blame me, according to the pattern that had been established after I separated from her and her alcoholic lifestyle. Instead, hearing that I would lose my home along with my relationship, Mom surprised me by inviting me to move in with her. Although this breakup happened as Alzheimer's was beginning to manifest in Mom's brain, she was still able to express concern for my financial and physical well-being. Even more remarkable were her expressions of concern and empathy. Mom met my heartache with compassion and told me about the pain she had experienced when she was abandoned by her true love sixty years earlier. I didn't know this about Mom, and in this moment, our hearts embraced in mutual understanding.

My relationship loss became legally complicated due to jointly owned property and contractual agreements, and unfortunately, it dragged on through the court system for years. Even though Mom's cognitive abilities kept declining during this time, she continuously showed a sincere interest in and sensitivity about my struggle. I had never before received this kind of attention from her. As her thinking weakened, it seemed as if her feelings were becoming stronger, as was her attentiveness to others and to details of personal interactions.

Immersed in the devastating aftermath of my broken relationship, my mind wasn't registering Mom's support as an indication that she had forgiven me; nor was I cognitively recognizing her extended hand as a gesture of reconciliation. My heart, however, must have been receiving her messages loud and clear. I realize this now, because when the time came for me to meet Mom's needs, to take radical responsibility for my actions in the world, and to decide what to do when she was abandoned and alone in a nursing home, I chose our relationship—with my whole mind, heart, and soul.

Throughout the seven years between Mom's diagnosis and my decision to move to Iowa, we had been co-creating a powerfully developed sense of affiliation with each other. We had actually been rebirthing a lasting, trusting relationship. Although I was not being deliberate and was not conscious of my intentions, and I assume Mom wasn't either, we had been living out what Browning and Reed identify as our "basic human desire for attachment,"[22] a desire clearly not deterred by Alzheimer's disease!

According to Professor Earl Thompson, the process of reconciliation is more than dialogue; it necessarily includes action. He continues, "For true reconciliation to occur, the people *must* be changed. They *must* break with the past and move toward a new future of amendment and restitution."[23] Mom and I were both changed; I by my healing process, and she by Alzheimer's. Her past was gone, forgotten. I haven't cognitively forgotten the ways Mom wounded me in the past, and if necessary or useful, I can tell the story in detail; however, my lifelong painful feelings of abandonment and betrayal *are* forgotten. My feelings of hurt and anger have been displaced, and I'm now surrounded by warm feelings of being loved, accepted, and taken care of by my mom. The feeling of being safe in the arms of a loving, protective mother—forever—is what I hoped I could give to her, how I hoped to heal her soul from the wounds of a lifetime of abandonment. Surprisingly, this is exactly what she gave to me. This is how she healed me. I hear an echo of Jacqui Lewis' message, "What heals you heals me."

Mom's and my openness to forgiveness and our actions toward reconciliation miraculously triumphed over extreme familial abuse and Alzheimer's disease. Martin Buber explains how this can happen: "In the beginning is the relation."[24] Mom recognized our relationship and she reached out. I reached back, discovering that in the beginning, at the end, and during every precious moment in between—longing, loving, living, being, and truly meeting each other, who we were, where we were, how we were—it was all about relationship.

16 Nourishing Compassion

We need one another. From birth to death on our journey through life, we will always need one another. At certain times, however, this need is more apparent and crucial than at others. Writer George Odell illuminates some of these certain times:

> We need one another when we mourn and would be comforted.
>
> We need one another when we are in trouble and afraid.
>
> We need one another when we are in despair, in temptation, and need to be recalled to our best selves again.
>
> We need one another when we would accomplish some great purpose, and cannot do it alone.
>
> We need one another in the hour of success, when we look for someone to share our triumphs.
>
> We need one another in the hour of defeat, when with encouragement we might endure, and stand again.
>
> We need one another when we come to die, and would have gentle hands prepare us for the journey.
>
> All our lives we are in need, and others are in need of us.[25]

There is no question about this need. We humans are an interdependent species, more critically dependent on others for care and love than any other beings. According to author Karen Armstrong, "Our brains have evolved to be caring and to need care—to such an extent that they are impaired if this nurture is lacking."[26]

One way we receive this needed nurture, all throughout our lives, is by a relational process called mirroring. Expressed consciously or subconsciously, mirroring is an effective way to communicate and connect by repeating the words we've heard, or by copying body language, vocal tones, or the energy and attitude of another person. It's long been known that for humans to develop positive self-esteem and a healthy identity, we need to experience this mirroring from outside ourselves. Psychotherapist Christine Louis de Canonville explains that "in the early stages of an individual's life, the soul is not capable of self-reflection or self-monitoring We need mirroring from birth. Infants need their emotions mirrored back to them, especially love, by caring eyes, voices, and touch. This creates an experience of oneness for new human beings and helps us begin to feel safe and protected in the world. "It is through loving, compassionate mirroring that the child senses that they are accepted, good enough, valued, treasured as a worthy individual, and loved."[27] In her book *Fierce Love,* Jacqui Lewis writes about the importance of mirroring for developing self-love. She says that when children are ignored and don't "have a mirror showing them their beauty, creativity, and value" they become anxious, "looking around for a mirror that doesn't exist."[28] Early mirroring is considered vital for building self-confidence as well as self-worth. Without this, a child experiences a kind of abandonment and could develop what's known as a narcissistic wound. Those with this kind of wounding can find it difficult to feel good about themselves[29] and can experience significant feelings of disgrace and shame, perhaps lasting a lifetime.

People with Alzheimer's are emotionally fragile like young children and infants; they are therefore vulnerable to this kind of wounding to their sense of self-worth and to feeling painful shame and anxiety when their emotions are not acknowledged and validated, or when they feel unloved. Therefore, the caregiving technique of mirroring is highly recommended for use with them. It's as vital for enhancing the sense of well-being and self-identity for people with Alzheimer's as it is for young children, especially when they feel and express difficult emotions. The intense emotions of people with Alzheimer's can be one of the biggest challenges for caregivers; therefore it's advisable to take note of social worker Danielle Maxon's "4 Easy Steps" for mirroring the intense emotions of children, which include a reminder to "take a step back" emotionally and observe what's happening and then to "match and reflect." If a child is screaming, she suggests using a louder voice with a more intense tone; if a child is barely whispering and seems sad, she recommends matching that soft tone and emotion. Most important is to remain calm. Through the focused attention that happens with mirroring, we are communicating with our eyes, facial expressions, body language, and tone of voice that "all of your feelings are ok; you are wonderful just the way you are; you are not alone in the world. I see and understand you."[30] This process, developed with children in mind, is equally effective with adults, including our loved ones with dementia, in a variety of situations, and is especially useful as verbal and language skills diminish.

When we consciously mirror another person, especially our loved ones with Alzheimer's, we are nurturing them while also nurturing our own capacity for empathy. When we mirror another person, we are invited to observe, to receive/replicate, and to (hopefully) empathically understand the information that is being communicated to us, quite often nonverbally. This relational activity can also provide an opportunity to practice making eye contact with our loved ones and to notice the truth that is revealed through their eyes. Eye contact can help to reassure our loved ones that they exist. It's likely that we'll notice our loved ones with Alzheimer's doing a really good job of making eye contact with us, letting us know that we exist for them!

Mirroring is a staple in every curriculum for improvisation training and can even be used as a technique for beginning a scene on stage: one actor walks on the stage and does jumping jacks, for example. The second actor walks on and does the same, then the third. The first line emerges from the mirrored movement; when one actor says, out of breath, "How did I ever let you young ones talk this old grandpa into coming to aerobics class!?" And instantly, everyone, audience included, feels the connection and knows what's happening.

Of all the improv exercises I've encountered and studied, mirroring has the most capacity for increasing empathy, inspiring compassion, and enhancing connections with our loved ones with Alzheimer's. The mirroring exercises I teach through my *Meeting Alzheimer's* workshops give caregivers an embodied experience of acknowledging and respecting another person's feelings, making nonverbal, empathic connections, and letting others know we get it, that we understand. As caregivers, it's important to remember that people with Alzheimer's have intact emotions and that they can recognize, receive, and respond to an emotionally empathic reaction from us. It's also important for effective caregiving to know that people with Alzheimer's will mirror us, including our facial expressions, our movements, and our emotions. Knowing this can be a helpful tool in maintaining their moods and enhancing their participation in activities of daily living. They will mirror us as we brush our teeth, set the table for dinner, prepare meals, fold laundry, rake leaves, dust, dry dishes, etc. We can use this technique to keep them busy and happy in their feelings of usefulness and self-care.

Mirroring Exercise

The mirroring exercises from the *Meeting Alzheimer's: Learning to Communicate and Connect* workshop can easily be practiced at home with a partner. Begin by facing each other and making eye contact.

1. The first part of the exercise will be about body mirroring. And I invite the person in your partnership who has the longest hair to be the one to begin the movements—arms, legs, head, bending, turning—all of which should be slow and easy to follow. After 30 seconds; switch leaders for another 30 seconds of body mirroring.

2. The second part of the exercise involves facial mirroring—yes, you get to make funny faces! And your partner will mimic them. Again, begin with eye contact; always keep eye contact. Again, the long-haired partner starts making the faces. After 30 seconds switch leadership.

3. The next part of the exercise is vocal mirroring. Make eye contact; the long-haired partner begins making sounds, any sounds, which the partner mirrors. After 30 seconds, switch leadership. Done in a large group, this can sound a bit like feeding time at the zoo! But do feel free to express any sounds during this part of

the exercise, even using your "outside voice."

4. The last part of the mirroring exercise is emotional
   mirroring, first with facial expressions only. After
   making eye contact, the long-haired partner begins
   and expresses an emotion with facial expressions,
   choosing between sad, angry, afraid, or happy. The
   partner mirrors. Continue offering emotional
   expressions for 30 seconds, and then switch leadership
   for another 30 seconds. An advanced form of
   emotional mirroring is to add body movements
   and vocal expressions to the facial movements. For
   example, an angry face could be accompanied by
   a stomping foot and a loud sound of "Harrumph."

Note: If you don't have a partner to practice with, you
can literally practice in front of a mirror. This practice
will help caregivers to recognize body language, facial
expressions, and sounds of the various emotions your
loved ones with Alzheimer's will be expressing. And
caregivers who already have practiced mirroring these
emotions will better know how to respond.

The end of life—our own future mirrored to us by our loved
ones with Alzheimer's—is a particularly vulnerable time, when
those who are leaving us need our greatest care. I remind you,
however, that one of the challenging realities we meet when
our loved ones are diagnosed with Alzheimer's is that the length
of time we spend with them on the journey to the other side
of this disease could be quite long. Although Alzheimer's is
technically a terminal diagnosis, it's not a sentence of imminent
death. Acknowledging this, some researchers and caregivers

have described Alzheimer's disease as death in slow motion. David Shenk explains it eloquently:

> As the disease relentlessly progresses toward the final dimming of the sufferer, it forces us to experience death in a way that is rarely otherwise experienced. What is usually a quick flicker, we see in super slow motion, over years. It is more painful than many people can even imagine, but it is also perhaps the most poignant of all reminders of why and how human life is so extraordinary. It is our best lens on the meaning of loss.[31]

This chronic disease of progressive losses reveals what it means to live and love to our fullest potential, including our potential for feeling empathy and expressing compassion. Although the words empathy and compassion are often used interchangeably, their meanings are not the same. Empathy is actually an instinctual feeling that allows us to be aware of other people's emotions and to know on a deep level what they're experiencing. It's this instinct that moves us to cry during movies. Compassion is our response to feeling empathy, creating in us a desire to help or connect in some way.[32] Empathy can blossom into compassion, and compassion, at its best, can manifest as acts of kindness, simple or grand.

In her poem "Small Kindnesses," Danusha Laméris reminds us that simple acts of kindness, such as saying "bless you" when someone sneezes or "thank you" to the barista who hands us our coffee, helping a person pick up spilled groceries, or smiling at someone and having them smile back, although brief moments, could be "the true dwelling of the holy, these fleeting temples we make when we say, 'Here, have my seat,' 'Go ahead —you first,' 'I like your hat.'"[33]

People with Alzheimer's are continually changing, continually dying, as we all are. As I exquisitely learned, however, they aren't gone until they have taken their last breaths. From within their long journeys toward death, people with Alzheimer's continually extend invitations to us to grow emotionally, to love them through all the changes of their lives, and to be kind, perhaps kinder than we have ever been. Every day as I walked down the hallway of the nursing home, I noticed these invitations. When they saw me, people with dementia extended their hands and pleaded for connection—for a touch, a hug, a glass of water. Many simply pleaded, "Help me." Stephen Post, in his book, *Dignity for Deeply Forgetful People*, encourages caregivers to meet these simple requests in some way, saying that "patience and a kind voice" have the greatest potential to relieve anxiety. He considers even the simplest acts of kindness, such as a smile, a reassuring pat on the shoulder, or a touch of the hand, to be meaningful expressions of interconnectedness that will make a difference to people with dementia.[34]

From the beginning of my journey through Alzheimer's with Mom, I experienced the reaching and pleading of those afflicted with this disease as an opportunity to broaden my worldview in order to make a place in my heart and in my life for "the other," which Karen Armstrong identifies as an important attitude for fostering our feeling of compassion.[35] While observing the care provided to residents by some of the nursing home staff, I noticed the many ways they manifested compassion as Armstrong defines and describes it:

> Compassion impels us to work tirelessly to alleviate the suffering of our fellow creatures, to dethrone ourselves from the centre of our world and put another there, and to honour the inviolable sanctity of every single human being, treating everybody, without exception, with absolute justice, equity, and respect.[36]

"Caregiving," writes Stephen Post, "is so fundamental and so basic to human well-being and security that it must be at the core of any acceptable theory of justice or politics." He emphasizes caregiving as especially important due to the lack of current breakthroughs for prevention or cure of Alzheimer's. Right now, caregiving is all we have available to relieve the suffering caused by diseases of dementia. Stephen continues, "Caregivers need an ethic that actually focuses on providing care—on the cultivation of relationships, on noticing expressions of selfhood, on kindness, and on concrete need—that leaves no one behind . . ."[37] No one.

Anyone who has spent time in nursing homes observing aides and nurses caring for the residents, particularly residents who are completely helpless, will be able to readily distinguish the compassionate professional caregivers who work tirelessly to alleviate suffering and honor the sanctity of every person from those whom author Sam Keen identifies as "care-sellers."[38] Although I don't harshly judge the care-sellers (everyone has to work for a living), they give only the services they are paid to give and perform their tasks from a rational perspective. Alternatively, the compassionate caring that Armstrong describes is given for free, from the heart. Bioethicist Jeffrey Bishop claims that the act of true, heartfelt caring originates in the bodies and souls of the caregivers, from that instinctual place that defines empathy, and will be directed by our bodies and our souls at the bodies and souls of those who need care. Compassionate caregivers take away pain, not with pills but with the offering of self.[39]

When Mom's nursing home policies evolved, allowing me to choose her primary care aides, I chose Julie to care for Mom during the morning shift, which began at 5:30 AM. This remains one of my life's best choices. Julie had been working with the elderly for her whole career, over thirty years, because she cared. I saw that Julie's caring for my mother (and all her residents) was what Bishop calls a "fully embodied activity" that came from her empathic desire to help.

The most important gift any of us can receive at times of loss, pain, or need is steadfast presence. "Caring is messy," says Bishop, "and inefficient."[40] End-of-life incontinence, believe me, is messy. And because this mess requires immediate attention, it undermines a caregiver's efficiency. No matter how big the mess, however, Julie never retreated from my mom. She was there six mornings a week, before many of us were even out of bed, attending to Mom's needs—whatever they were.

Julie's full-time schedule required her to work five days a week. However, understanding how important consistency was to her residents, all of whom had Alzheimer's or some other form of dementia, she regularly signed on to work an additional day. This consistent, compassionate, patient care—demonstrated by Julie's commitment, her kindness, and her attachment to the residents—was part of what made Mom's nursing home experience and Julie's work successful. Personal attachment to residents, according to Bishop, is the key element that prevents burnout.[41] Instead of dreading coming to work, resisting the physical demands, and avoiding the incontinence messes, Julie signed on for more of this.

Compassion should not be confused with pity, says Armstrong, because it is not about feeling sorry for those in need.[42] "True compassion," according to Buddhist teacher Pema Chödrön, "does not come from wanting to help out those less fortunate than ourselves, but from realizing one's kinship with all beings."[43] Other spiritual teachers echo this definition. Armstrong writes, "Compassion means to endure with another person, to put ourselves in someone else's shoes, to feel her pain as though it were our own, and to enter generously into his point of view."[44] Richard Rohr says, "Love is recognizing oneself in the other."[45] Marcus Borg adds the element of being inspired by the feelings into action: "Compassion thus means feeling the feelings of somebody else in a visceral way, at a level somewhere below the level of the head; most commonly associated with feeling the suffering of somebody else and being moved by that suffering to do something. That is, the feeling of compassion leads to being compassionate."[46]

Although Julie didn't personally identify with the complete vulnerability of her residents, she told me that she did identify them with her own mother, who had suffered for a long time and died a few years earlier. Julie had cared for her dearly as well. Many of the aides and nurses who were freely giving compassionate care echoed Julie's experience of caring for the residents as if they were "their own." Borg tells his readers that, in the Hebrew language, the singular form of *compassion* is translated as "womb." Being compassionate, therefore, "has nuances of giving life, nourishing, caring, perhaps embracing and encompassing."[47]

Both Bishop and Rohr speak about the connection between care and relationship. According to Bishop, babies *require* warm caring and friendliness in order to survive.[48] In his discussion of the "True and False Self," Rohr acknowledges that we are social creatures. In order to be truly loved, we need to be vulnerable with another and allow ourselves to be seen in our "littleness." "Someone else," Rohr says, has to recognize our vulnerability and "acknowledge us as beloved."[49] This was Julie's specialty. Her skills of observation were acute—she saw Mom's vulnerability which Mom and all the residents had no choice but to reveal. She listened well to my descriptions of Mom's needs and desires and fulfilled them with joy. And she helped Mom to feel good about herself. During the last two years of Mom's life, when Julie accompanied her to the bathroom for toileting, washing, and tooth-brushing, Julie sang to her the 1974 hit song "You Are So Beautiful to Me." Imagine beginning every morning with someone singing, "You're everything I hoped for.... Such joy and happiness you bring," and feeling that you are beloved on this earth. This is an example of loving mirroring at its best. After singing to Mom, Julie dressed her in a coordinated outfit, brushed her long hair and spritzed it with water to bring out the natural waves, decorated her hair with colorful or flowered clips, and then chose a necklace to complete her ensemble. Six days out of seven, when I arrived to spend time with Mom, she had already been awakened and cared for by a person who was the embodiment of compassion. Witnessing and appreciating this care, I concluded that Julie was another of Mom's soul mates, compassionately guiding her home.[50]

Julie was a big part of our carepartnering circle, and her care extended beyond Mom to me. Because she had cared for her own sick and dying mother, Julie could identify with my fears, worries, and struggles. She knew that Mom's quality of life and well-being were important to me and made extra effort to ensure that my needs and wants for Mom's care, as specified in the care plan, were met. What Julie received from me, which Mom couldn't give her, were regular expressions of gratitude for her attention to details and her gentle kindness. While Julie was singing, Mom did tend to look at her through starry eyes, so Julie knew Mom appreciated her. But hearing "thank you" every day from families and knowing that their efforts are noticed gives nursing aides an energy boost. Being appreciated gives everyone a boost.

Julie wasn't working the morning Mom died. As soon as Mom was gone, however, a close coworker called her, knowing that Jeanne's life and death mattered to her. Julie dropped what she was doing when she got the call and came immediately to the nursing home to be at Mom's bedside and say goodbye.

She also came to comfort and share her grief with me. She felt the loss of her friend and companion Jeanne. Julie was grateful that she wasn't working that day, so she was able to experience the fullness of her grief without needing to attend to other residents.

This experience of loss is the challenge for compassionate health care workers in nursing homes who become personally attached to those destined to die soon. But that's their job, to get people ready to die. Person after person after person, these compassionate caregivers must say goodbye to their friends and feel the loss when they leave this world.

Julie sat beside me at Mom's funeral and held my hand.

As I've talked with other family members who have loved ones with dementia and other diminishments living in nursing homes, some have said something like, "I don't visit Dad at the nursing home because he wouldn't want anyone to see him like that." I wonder if this is really true. Diminishment is indeed hard to experience and hard to witness, but if we put aside our own vanity and egotism, is that what people really want? Is that what *we* want—for our imperfect humanity, our "littleness" to be invisible to those we love? As writer Mary Vineyard says, "It takes radical and radiant humility to accept our helplessness and bow to the necessity of being cared for by family members and strangers."[51]

In the humbleness of my humanity, I know it would be painful for me to be sick, confused, vulnerable, unable to speak or walk, and left alone in a nursing home, helpless to fend for myself. Because it would be devastatingly painful for me to be abandoned at my time of greatest need, I chose not to inflict this pain on my mother. It was compassion, informed by empathy, that brought me to her side. At the time, however, I wasn't consciously aware that my choice to protect Mom from abandonment reflected the Golden Rule as it was originally taught by Confucius in China over twenty-five hundred years ago. This first version of the Golden Rule invites us to "look into our own hearts, discover what gives us pain, and then refuse, under any circumstance whatsoever, to inflict this pain on anybody else." About a hundred years later in India, the Buddha introduced a practice of meditation on the "four elements of the 'immeasurable' love that exists within everything." The Buddhist tradition describes compassion, one of these four elements, as the determination to free those who are suffering from their pain. These ancient teachings agree that compassion is not only natural to humans but what Armstrong calls "the fulfillment of human nature."[52]

Around 300 BCE, Confucian philosopher Mencius was the first to challenge humanity to cultivate what he called our natural "shoots" of compassion, claiming that once cultivated, our compassion will then acquire a "dynamic power of its own." According to Armstrong, human beings have always been prepared to work hard to enhance a natural ability. Consider the evolution from the self-protective running and jumping skills of our ancestors to the graceful physical abilities of ballet dancers or gymnasts that result from years of dedicated practice. This demonstrates the irrefutable reality that, if we persevere, we can acquire an ability that at first seemed impossible. "In this same way," Armstrong says, "those who have persistently trained themselves in the art of compassion manifest new capacities in the human heart and mind; they discover that when they reach out consistently toward others, they are able to live with the suffering that inevitably comes their way with serenity, kindness and creativity."[53]

Ancient sages, prophets, and mystics from all religious traditions did not regard compassion as an impossible dream. They worked as hard to implement compassion in the difficult circumstances of their lives as our social structure works today to identify the cause of and find a cure for Alzheimer's disease. Although Armstrong believes that compassion is intrinsic in all human beings, she also believes that each of us needs to work diligently to cultivate and expand our capacity for compassion.

I've become convinced that this disease of relentless diminishment has come, seemingly as a scourge upon the world, to remind us that the human well of compassion will never run dry, and that, in fact, the more we draw on it the more we have. Taking our inspiration from the ancient sages, we caregivers need to remind society that nourishing our shoots of compassion as earnestly as science searches for cures is an important manifestation of our humanity. According to Marcus Borg, this reminder to society would be a faith-filled response, since this was also the work of Jesus. "For Jesus," Borg writes, "compassion was more than a quality of God and an individual virtue: it was a social paradigm, the core value for life in community."[54]

Almost eighteen months after Mom died, I attended the "Joy of Caring Conference" at a local university where I met Jeffrey Bishop. During one of his presentations, he introduced participants to an icon from the Greek Orthodox tradition, the *Dormition of the Theotokos* ("The Falling Asleep of the Holy Mother of God"). In this stunning painting depicting Mary's death, Jesus stands behind her human body holding a baby, which represents Mary's soul. Because icons present an experience artistically, through pictures rather than words, they are emotionally evocative. Just as one of the contemplative spiritual practices recommended by St. Ignatius of Loyola encourages us to place ourselves in the Gospels as we read them,[55] I placed myself into this icon. In my imagination, it was I who was given the blessed opportunity to tenderly hold my mother's spirit, literally as an infant, during those last years when Alzheimer's progressed to the late and end stages. Mine became those gentle hands O'Dell described, gentle hands to prepare Mom for her dance with death.

This tender holding of Mom's body and soul in my hands over several years was cultivating my compassion and motivating me to be kind, even if I didn't fully realize it at the time. Almost two years after Mom died, an encounter at the nursing home made me aware of how much my compassion had grown. I had not been back there since cleaning out Mom's belongings from her room and saying goodbye to the staff. Although many family members do return as volunteers after their loved ones die, I couldn't bring myself to return. Then a friend had knee-replacement surgery, and after leaving the hospital, he was transferred to Mom's nursing home for rehabilitation. I seized the moment and went one morning to join him for Mass and then to see about helping with the exercise class Mom and I had loved. As I stepped into the elevator on my way to the chapel, I saw a resident in her wheelchair. She was leaning over the side of her chair, drooling. She was still wearing her pajamas, which had remnants of breakfast smeared down the front. Her hands were nervously rubbing the arms of her chair; she was making garbled sounds as her pleading eyes darted between me and the man running the elevator. This was a remarkable moment for me. Earlier in my life, I would have felt disgust, horror, judgement, or fear while observing this woman; perhaps I would have fled from the nursing home the instant the elevator door opened. On this day, however, after years of nourishing my "shoots" by caring for Mom, the only feeling I noticed was compassion for this woman overflowing in my heart. This feeling nudged me to be kind. I knelt down, touched her hand, smiled, and said, "Good morning. It's so nice to see you." Oh, and how she smiled in return. After this encounter, I returned to the nursing home as a volunteer, helping to lead the exercise class. Apparently, I make it fun for the residents. At least this is what Katrina, one of the exercisers, told me.

And then I noticed another shift in my capacity for compassion. I was walking in the late afternoon as I usually do, and I unexpectedly remembered a childhood experience that I have always considered to be one of Mom's terrible parenting moments.

It was a Saturday evening during the summer when I was five. My parents were getting ready to go out for the night to play bridge with their friends. This every-other-Saturday night ritual was the extent of their social life. I had gone to the store with older neighbor kids to buy candy. As we walked home through an alley shortcut, I stumbled on the loose gravel, falling and cutting my leg on a piece of glass. It was a long, deep cut. Blood gushed from the wound and I was hysterical. When the neighbors brought me home to Mom, she was furious. Dad quickly exited from the bloody, emotional scene and went to pick up the babysitter. Mom sat me on a wooden chair in her bedroom and hurriedly tried to clean and bandage the cut as I screamed and sobbed and squirmed. Mom's voice was harsh; her handling of my wounded leg was rough; her facial expression was mean. It was not the mirroring I needed at the time. Somehow the bandaging was accomplished, the babysitter arrived, and my parents went out to play cards.

Mom must have harbored vivid memories of this night, as I did, and presumably she felt guilty about it. For decades after the event, she brought my attention to the three-inch long scar on my left leg, saying she should have taken me to the hospital for stitches. It was this scar, and this scar alone, she said, that would prevent me from being Miss America. Hearing this as a young person, my fragile self-esteem was maimed.

Historically, in my memory of this story, there was cruelty layered upon cruelty. I interpreted Mom's behavior to mean that playing cards was more important than caring for and comforting her injured and terrified child. But as I re-remembered this story with enhanced compassion, I could see it from different perspectives. I saw my Mom's life as wife and mother in the 1950s. The era and these roles were limiting for creative, enterprising women, stifling and depressing for many. Since she accepted her expected roles of wife and mother reluctantly, Mom didn't have an especially happy marriage or fulfilling life.

It was their one night out. Mom's one night in fourteen away from the demands of children and housewifely duties. This night out was important to my parents. They hired a babysitter and took time and effort to get ready. Dad wore a suit and tie. Mom wore a fancy dress, nylon hose, high heels, and a necklace with matching clip-on earrings. She was looking forward to being free from responsibility and having fun with friends when her clumsy, crying child threatened to spoil her reprieve.

With my enhanced compassion, this story became more expansive for me. It's larger now than the pain, fear, and hurt feelings I experienced. In the context of Mom's unhappy life, she didn't see me fully. Overwhelmed by the prospect of disappointment or concerned about the cost of a visit to the emergency room, Mom didn't realize how her words and actions would wound me.

Through most of my life, Mom didn't see me. However, my increasing capacity for compassion, which developed more so over my years of caring for her, helped me to see her—and to continue seeing her, with fresh eyes, even after her death.

After all my years of observing and studying about Alzheimer's disease, I've concluded that we really need the ones who are slowly declining from this and other diseases of dementia. Dying people have a purpose beyond showing us how to fight to conquer every disease. They are giving us countless opportunities to acknowledge and enhance our natural human tendencies toward compassion, and to practice being loving and patient and kind. They are encouraging us, needing us, to nourish our innate compassion into its full dynamic power. On this topic, poet Naomi Shihab Nye writes, "Before you know what kindness really is you must lose things." People living with Alzheimer's and dementia have certainly lost things, and they, therefore, will innately recognize our kindness. As caregivers, if we can allow this disease of such tangible loss to transform our sorrow, we will emerge from the refiner's fire knowing in our souls the truth of the poet's words: "Then it is only kindness that makes sense anymore."[56]

Author Martha Beck points out that, when frightened, all mammals except humans will seek a safe place. Humans seek a safe person.[57] I was Mom's safe person during her certain time of need. Compassion had made it possible.

17   Re-imagining Survival

Dementia care support in Dubuque County, Iowa, began in 1996 when Franciscan Sister Michelle Nemmers, fueled by a passion to learn more about this cruel disease and to help those afflicted, partnered with a local social worker; together they staffed the original office of the Alzheimer's Association. Over the next two decades, many thousands of family members, myself included, sought information and guidance from this office. Considering the geographic location, which includes one small city and surrounding rural areas, this number is stunning. Recent statistics from 2020 indicate that the county prevalence rate of dementia for people 65 and older is 11.1 percent, "slightly above the statewide average . . . . though it is also among the highest prevalence rates in Iowa counties with the largest numbers of people 65 and older."[58] Even more stunning than prevalence and statistics is that only a handful of people helped by the Association returned there as volunteers. Dubuque's annual Walk to End Alzheimer's attracts a small percentage of the thousands of residents, past and present, touched by the diseases of dementia. Compared to the numbers of participants and contributions received through similar fundraising programs for other diseases, such as for breast cancer, diabetes, or heart disease, the Alzheimer's effort has miniscule support.

It's the same all across the country: fewer volunteers and participants, and less financial support. Hearing this sparked my curiosity. "Why is this the case?" I asked the Alzheimer's Association staff member who shared this news with me. She answered without hesitation: "Because there are no survivors."

This reality, so bluntly stated, gave me pause. Although I had gone to the Association's office to talk about volunteering and leading programs for other caregivers, this prospect of no survivors made me want to run away and never return. My heart cried out, "It's so true!" Alzheimer's, like life, leaves no survivors. Accordingly, there are no victory celebrations honoring those who have fought the good fight against Alzheimer's disease and won.

For a brief time following this conversation, the idea of no survivors, which I accepted as the truth of Alzheimer's, seized my heart, seemingly choking my open-heartedness toward this population. It guided me away from the disease and the diminishments, and I got lost. Eventually, as I allowed myself to wonder more about surviving and Alzheimer's, I began to realize that my automatic reaction reflected what I consider the conventional wisdom of our society. Because our primary focus is on conquering disease, the scientific, medical, and most common understanding of the word *survivor* is often used in its narrowest meaning: "one who remains alive."

Christian theologian Marcus Borg, through his discussion of alternative wisdom,[59] and Buddhist nun, Pema Chodron, who encourages us to use the life we already have to make us wiser rather than more stuck,[60] encouraged my heart to beat once again in solidarity with people with Alzheimer's and their caregivers. If we look at Alzheimer's disease through the lens of alternative wisdom—which Borg notes is often the place of wondering for philosophers and spiritual sages, not scientists[61]—the concept of survival reveals a goal more consistent with healing than with curing. Through this lens, *to survive* means "to continue to function or manage in spite of some adverse circumstance or hardship; hold up; endure." According to this definition, people with Alzheimer's could be considered the ultimate survivors. Every single day of their long journeys, Alzheimer's survivors face loss and adversity. And every single day, for up to twenty years, they endure, adapt, function, and live to endure, adapt, and function another day. Their survival is marked by resiliency, compensating for losses, reconfiguring life and relationships, healing, and transforming.

When this understanding of survival is embraced by caregivers, we also do more than just get through it alive. We grow, we become wiser, and we can actually thrive, making room in our lives for all that is real. Borg describes a purpose for the wisdom we will acquire: "It speaks for the nature of reality and how to live one's life in accord with reality."[62]

As I continue to seek meaning in my life, I return to the world of Alzheimer's. I return to this world where people are authentic, where they are meeting reality with honesty and resilience, and where they are surviving every day. I return because it abounds with opportunities to make a difference and with wisdom to help me find my own way home through this mysterious maze of my mortal life. I return to the world of Alzheimer's because connecting with people who have no hope of conquering their diseases, as well as with caregivers who are seeking ways to care for and connect with their loved ones, I feel awash in the presence of God. I recognize and feel the Spirit of Life and Love manifesting all around me as longing for connection, and manifesting within me as compassion, respect, kindness, and gratitude for those who still have much to show me about living. Through my relationship with Mom, which inspires me even after her death, I continue to make discoveries that encourage and enlighten me as I walk on.

A few months after Mom died, I attended a six-week grief support group offered by a local hospice organization. The group was a safe, helpful way to explore my feelings of loss in the company of others who respected my process. One woman in the group shared that, on her husband's birthday, she and her children took helium balloons to the cemetery and released them as they sang happy birthday. I began this ritual immediately.

On Mother's Day, on Mom's birthday, and on the anniversary of the day she died, I bought a single balloon displaying an appropriate message for the occasion, careful always to choose one that was biodegradable, and attached a small card with my thoughts about this day and my wishes for Mom on her journey. I took the balloon and card to the cemetery, released the balloon, and watched it rise and float on the air, south down the Mississippi River.

The balloon always floated south, it seemed, and I solemnly watched until it was gone from my sight. I was careful not to blink or to glance away at anything else even for a moment, so as to prolong my sensory connection to the balloon and its message for Mom. I imagined it would reach her.

On the second anniversary of Mom's death, I watched as the balloon rose high, floated far away on the wings of the wind, and then disappeared from my view. Although the small speck eventually moved out of the range of my vision, I knew with my whole being that it was still there, still floating, still on the way to its unknown destination. In that fleeting, extraordinary instant, I felt connected to Mom in her new world, to the whole universe, and to whatever lies beyond it. At that moment, a passage from Paul's second letter to the Corinthians (4:18) from my morning reading returned to my consciousness: "For what can be seen is temporary; but what cannot be seen is eternal."[63]

Walking home from the cemetery that day, I wondered, "What else exists beyond the reach of my five senses, beyond the comprehension of my mind?" Savoring this expansive moment of deep encounter, I also wondered when the next unexpected mystery of life would cross my path. Over the years, I've come to accept that some mysteries will no doubt be sorrowful; others will be joyful or glorious or luminous. Or like my journey with Mom through Alzheimer's, some future life mysteries might contain all of these elements. Walking on toward healing and wholeness, I know that wherever my path leads me, Presence, wonder, and trust will always be my faithful companions.

18 Companionship on the Journey

My spiritual direction training through the Shalem Institute was, in the early 2000s, considered unique. It was a distance program. This was before online education was a standard way of learning, before Zoom, before COVID-19. The majority of the work was done in our home locations, and each year the class met in person for an eleven-day residency immersion experience. The first-year residency took place at the Bon Secours Retreat Center in Maryland near the Shalem offices and included a 72-hour silent retreat. I've never been overly good with this kind of long-term silence. I'm not alone in this, I know. What often happens is that emotional pain, in the form of sadness, fear, worry, shame, self-criticism, anger—those feelings we've been trying to avoid—bubble up to the surface, begging for our attention and making us feel uncomfortable. It happened that way for me at Bon Secours, and I experienced this as suffering. I was on a retreat. I wanted peace, not this!

It was a frigid February day in Maryland, so I didn't go outside, which could have been a comfort, I think, or possibly a distraction. Instead, I spent most of the time alone in my room, starkly aware of the miseries of my life, miseries that I was seemingly helpless to end. Sitting on the edge of the bed with my head in my hands, suffering, something unexpected happened. I looked up, and there before me on the wall was a crucifix. I thought of Jesus as he died on that cross and said to myself, "Now, there's someone who knows something about suffering." I slid from the bed onto the floor, onto my knees, and burst into tears. This moment of acknowledged suffering became, for me a threshold where the worlds of conscious human suffering and the Divine touched.

How could suffering have anything to do with God? Many of us likely wonder about that in times like these. "God isn't to be found in the suffering, but in the question," says renowned yoga and meditation teacher, Sopurkh Singh. It's the wondering that takes us across the threshold, into the place where we start our wrestling to find God. It's a step forward on our spiritual journey.[65] There, in my moment of misery with Jesus on the cross, I took a step forward. I knew right then, and have never forgotten, that I am not alone.

During this first Shalem residency, I had not yet spent those two weeks in Iowa with Mom (that experience was still five months into my future) so I didn't know how much she needed me, and my challenges on the Alzheimer's journey were not yet a large part of my life. My emotional turmoil at the time of the residency had to do with my life circumstances, still surrounding the end of my engagement: the losses, the practicalities, the financial burdens, the lawyers, not knowing what was next, my perceived powerlessness—all terrifying. My belief that it didn't have to be this way, shouldn't be this way, actually shouldn't be happening to me at all, was the Job-like source of my suffering on that day.

While I was still in that relationship-ending turmoil, a friend from my twelve-step program observed what he referred to as my greatest strength: the ability to ask for and accept help. That personal strength had guided and benefitted me through one life-challenge after another; but nowhere in my life had this strength been more needed or life-giving than on my journey with Mom through Alzheimer's disease.

As cognition declines, people with Alzheimer's—along with their family caregivers—tend to become isolated for many and varied reasons, including shame about diminished capacities, possible rejection by frightened family members and friends who don't know what to do or say, confusion about what's happening, frustration, fear, and pure exhaustion. Looking back at my own experiences, I realize that companionship can be a determining factor as to whether caregiving will become a burden or a blessing, and that God's work, manifested in relational ways by enlisting others to guide and help us, is real.

As professors, colleagues, and friends listened to me and read about my caregiving experiences with Mom throughout the years, they noticed that something seemed to be missing. I wasn't suffering in the ways they expected I should be. They didn't understand. Since other family caregivers talking about and writing about Alzheimer's often seemed burdened and in great pain over the stresses and losses inherent in the disease, I didn't really understand myself. Because I wasn't suffering like other caregivers were, I thought maybe I was doing something wrong—*until* I started making the list of my companions, teachers, and guides on this journey.

I had come to Iowa—alone—to be with Mom. Having been away from my hometown for thirty-two years, I didn't know anyone except Mom. I knew, however, that I needed help—to learn about the disease, become an effective caregiver, address my fears, find a place to live, meet compatible people, develop a support system, take care of myself, find spiritual inspiration, and make sure Mom had the best care and the best quality of life possible. So I reached out. I asked for what I needed—and I received information, guidance, companionship, and support beyond anything I could have imagined. I didn't want Mom to suffer with this disease any more than was absolutely necessary. Surprisingly, my efforts to relieve her suffering also relieved my own suffering on many levels.

With gratitude for each and every one of my companions, teachers, and guides, I share my list as an acknowledgment of their contributions and as encouragement for all Alzheimer's caregivers to ask for what we need. Help is available... just waiting for us to seek, to ask, and to find.

The companions, teachers, and guides who helped me to see the Spirit of Life shining through Alzheimer's include:

- authors and poets
- musicians and singers
- mystics and theologians—ancient and modern
- professors at Andover Newton Theological School, Weston Jesuit School of Theology, and Boston College
- healers of all kinds—counselors, spiritual directors, doctors
- spiritual directors' peer groups in Massachusetts and Iowa
- my centering prayer group
- friends and colleagues whose parents and spouses also had/have Alzheimer's
- daughters, sons, and spouses of nursing home residents
- many friends—old and new friends, near and far-away friends
- my very good friend at the nursing home, Homer, who shared the experience with me on a daily basis for almost four years
- church services
- my lawyer, Werner Hellmer, a wise and trusted advisor for more than six years

- Mom's doctors—Dr. Angela Kelley, the primary care physician, who could see Mom's worth and dignity; Dr. Allen Meurer, the physician who examined Mom regularly at the nursing home, came to see her on her deathbed, and cried with me; and all the doctors in the emergency room who always treated Mom with the same respect and care given to every other patient
- carepartners at the nursing home—the nursing aides, especially Karen, Julie, Angela, Angelic, Roxanne, Tracey, Kim, Al, and Dawn; the nurses; the social workers; the speech therapists; the occupational therapists; the food service staff; the administrator; the activities staff; and the advocates, especially Jan
- emergency room and hospital staff
- hospice staff—especially Kelly, Amy, Cindy, Stephanie, Penny, Ashley, and Harold
- Alzheimer's Association staff in Iowa and Massachusetts
- my newly found, dear cousin, Ron
- the Sisters of St. Francis and the staff at the Shalom Retreat Center, who welcomed me to Iowa, made a home for me, and prayed with me, especially Sr. Margaret, Sr. Kenneth, Sr. Carol, and Sr. Marie Therese
- The nursing home residents, especially the dear ones with Alzheimer's
- Mom, my most faithful, my most beloved companion

I specifically want to acknowledge and express my appreciation to the following individuals who personally guided me and supported me throughout the journey, and who helped me mold and fashion this book:

Sister Catherine Griffiths, my beloved spiritual guide, was the one clear, unwavering voice encouraging me to follow my call to care for my mother.

Lindsay Brennan worked for the Alzheimer's Association in Massachusetts during my journey. As I wandered through the mysterious, sometimes thorny maze of Alzheimer's caregiving, she provided compassionate care and patient guidance, even after I moved to Iowa. Lindsay recognized the unique vision of my Healing Moments approach to caregiving and wholeheartedly encouraged me to share my vision with others, as did Melanie Chavin from the Illinois Chapter.

As I was searching for a better way to care for Mom during the earlier stages of her illness, Joanne Koenig Coste and Dr. William Berlingieri taught this curious, eager novice so much about effective caregiving. Thanks to their observations and learning about the disease, I was able to step off the high dive into the ocean of Alzheimer's care, feeling confident and competent. For generously sharing their wisdom, Mom and I are forever grateful.

Learning the craft of improvisation from David La Graffe and Will Luera transformed my life. My inspiration to transfer the skills of improvisation into Alzheimer's caregiving also transformed Mom's life— from potential isolation to a life rich with connection. And now, as I pass on the skills I learned from David and Will to other caregivers, the ripples in the pond started by their gems of knowledge and joy grow larger and larger.

Dr. Brita Gill-Austern was the midwife for this work. She and other professors in the Doctor of Ministry Program at Andover Newton Theological School, Dr.

Earl Thompson and Dr. Jennifer Peace, gave me the
opportunity to creatively integrate my personal journey
with my academic endeavors. What a gift this has been
for my heart, my soul, and my life journey!

On the journey through Alzheimer's and after, I was
blessed to encounter other family caregivers who
embraced me with their open, loving hearts. Carl,
Coleen, Marta, Mary Anne, Mary Kay, Stephen, Daisy,
Loretta, Lynda, and Sondy agreed to explore their
experiences and feelings and share them with me for
this caregiver resource. Their perspectives enlarged my
own and helped me to see and hear, with amazement,
the miracles that are around us always. Caregiver Betsy
Peterson also generously shared her story with me as
well as her comfortable and beautiful home during my
trips to Boston.

My colleagues in the Healing Moments for Alzheimer's
Ministry—Rev. Esther Hurlburt, Rev. Darrick Jackson,
and Rev. Laura Randall—have been my committed
travelling companions. They have given my ideas wings.

My soul's companions—Arlene, Bonnie, Carla, Carolyn,
Diane, Janaan, Karen, Kelly, Marie, Mary Anne, Sr.
Mary Owen, Nancy, Sheila, and Shirley—encouraged
me through the challenging twists of this project and
embraced me at every celebration. Their presence in
my life has taught me much about myself and much
about friendship.

Barbara Day brought expertise and graciousness to the technical editing process, and words will never express the magnitude of my appreciation for her skill.

Mary Benard, director at Skinner House Books, believed in this project from the beginning. Her contributions and the contribution to the creation of this book by the Skinner House staff past and present, Marshall Hawkins, Betsy Martin, Kate Bates, Joni McDonald, Suzanne Morgan, Kiana Nwaobia, Pierce Alquist, and Larisa Hohenboken, have been deeply appreciated.

To Rev. Libbie Stoddard and Gary Whited, my mentors and guides for more than thirty years, I am most grateful. I owe much of who I am now and what I have accomplished in my life to them. They saw my potential and believed in me, encouraged me, and loved me during all those years when Mom couldn't. Unquestionably, their presence in my life aided my healing and made it possible for me to care for Mom when she needed me.

Although I'm sad my mom had to take the path through Alzheimer's disease on her way home, I am eternally grateful that she reached out to me during her time of need and let me know that my presence in her life was helpful and healing. It was through her decline and resulting vulnerability—and through her initiative—that our relationship was restored. I hope that the stories of Mom's courageous meeting with Alzheimer's, her willingness to humbly ask for help (something she had never had to do before), and her ability to recognize kindness will be endearing and inspiring to others. Mom would be so happy to know that, through her example, our experiences together, and my writing, she has been able to help someone else in need.

If we let them, people with Alzheimer's can make a difference in our lives!

VI

Resources for Caregivers

Teachings come from everywhere when you open yourself
to them.
That's the trick really.
Open yourself to everything, and everything opens itself
to you.

—RICHARD WAGAMESE

Reflection Questions

When did the relationship shift so that you took on the role of caregiver? Was there a defining moment?

What are some moments in your role as caregiver that have brought you joy?

What moments with your loved one with dementia have brought you a sense of fulfillment?

What have you learned about life and love?

What has been your most valuable lesson?

What has been your greatest challenge?

What has been your greatest loss?

Even as your loved one's capacities have diminished, what has made their life valuable . . .

> to them?
> to you?
> to society?

What has surprised you about the quality of your relationship with your loved one even as the dementia has progressed?

What has surprised you most about your loved one's remaining capacities?

What aspects of your loved one's personality have been retained?

What has motivated you to alter your life to care for your loved one?

What have been some of the most remarkable experiences with your loved one?

Why?

How have you grown spiritually throughout the course of your loved one's illness?

Spiritual Practices

The most important aspects of any spiritual practice are making the time and following through on a commitment to do it, no matter how we feel and no matter how challenging the circumstances become. It's about showing up, with our hearts open to receiving grace, guidance, and support.

Alzheimer's caregiving provides an opportunity for spiritual practice that will ultimately benefit both the caregiver and the care receiver. As a place to begin, I suggest that the most important spiritual endeavors for Alzheimer's caregivers are prayer and the spiritual practices of acceptance, mindfulness, and self-care.

Prayer

Over the years, as I worked on healing from my history of abuse and addiction, the Serenity Prayer by Reinhold Niebuhr[1] had become important to me. When Alzheimer's became a part of my life, I altered this prayer in ways that supported my process. I offer my adapted prayer as a sample to other caregivers. Use this prayer, find another one that's meaningful to you, or create your own:

God, grant me
the Serenity
   to accept the things I cannot change:
   the predictable, relentless diminishment that is
     Alzheimer's;
   the ongoing losses;
   the mysteries embedded in this disease that
     continue to elude explanation and cure.

God, grant me
the Courage
   to change the things I can:
   my attitude, my reactions, my expectations, my
     priorities.

And grant me the wisdom to know the difference between what I can and cannot change.

God, may I open my heart to the peace that passes all understanding.
May I care for and comfort my loved one with patience and compassion.
May I be Hope.

Amen.

Prayer for Help. Caregivers need not hesitate to pray for help. I've heard it said that the simple prayer, "Help me," is one of the truest prayers we can say. Perhaps repeating this prayer will allow caregivers to realize that needing and receiving help are necessary for sustaining life. None of us can get through this life—or Alzheimer's—alone.

Prayer of Gratitude. Meister Eckhart, a German Christian mystic living in the thirteenth century, wrote, "If a man had no more to do with God than to be thankful, that would suffice."[2] Every day, even the difficult ones, it has become a powerful practice for me to notice one thing for which I feel gratitude. One thing: Today I am grateful to *not* have a headache. David Steindl-Rast says, "It's not the happy people who are grateful. It's the grateful people who are happy."[3]

Prayer for Gratitude and Acceptance. Dag Hammarskjold, a twentieth-century Swedish diplomat with a spiritual worldview, offers care partners what I consider the most healing prayer of all. The prayer includes an apt expression of feelings shared by many people with Alzheimer's and their caregivers and goes on to address both memory and hope:

> For all that has been—Thank you!
> For all that is to come—Yes![4]

Acceptance

Research has identified acceptance as a coping technique that significantly reduces caregiver stress and distress. It's, therefore, imperative to become informed about Alzheimer's disease so you know what to accept and how. Make the time and find the courage to listen to CDs, watch films and YouTube videos, read books, attend support groups and seminars, and connect with other caregivers as well as Alzheimer's organizations that provide education and support. Understanding the disease and how it's intersecting with your loved one's personality, and knowing that people with Alzheimer's are doing the best they can 100 percent of the time, will ease your need and desire to control what can't be controlled or to change what can't be changed. Caregivers need not be alone on this journey. Seeking companions and accepting help could transform a potentially burdensome experience into a blessing.

Mindfulness

Pay attention to your loved one and yourself. Enhance your outer and your inner vision. Mindfulness will help you know what you need, how your loved one is doing, and what needs and wants are being expressed. People with Alzheimer's aren't the best reporters of how they're feeling or of any medication side effects, whether they've had lunch, if their shoes hurt or their pants are too tight. Being able to notice and interpret sounds, facial expressions, and mood changes is a critical skill for caregivers to learn. In the early stages, when people with Alzheimer's are aware of their diminishing capacities, they may intentionally disguise their vulnerabilities. For example, instead of acknowledging that they don't understand what you said, they may laugh or respond in a way that seems appropriate. Mom had a default word: "Right." Whenever she was asked anything, she just replied, "Right." This disguise could be interpreted as agreement.

Because our emotions and reactions make a lasting impact on our loved ones, even after they've forgotten our visit, being aware of how we speak and behave, mirroring their emotions, and being positive (smile and don't forget to breathe)[5] will improve our interactions with people with dementia. The quality of their lives, and ours, will also improve.

Self-Care

Caring for a dependent adult with dementia is a challenge to our minds, bodies, and spirits. In order to minimize exhaustion and resentment, receive this responsibility as a call for mandatory self-care as well as an invitation to evaluate and rebalance your lifestyle and priorities. Consider adjusting to your loved one's pace. Slow down. Our culture seems to be addicted to noise and speed. Slowing down and paying attention to little things can provide a respite. Notice the birds and the flowers, and listen carefully and patiently as the person's words become harder to speak. (Breathe. Smile.)

Becoming the caregiver for a person with Alzheimer's is a perfect time to learn meditation, to practice centering prayer, or to begin walking or exercising daily. It might seem impossible to add self-care to an already busy life, now made busier because of the time and attention needed to care for a person with Alzheimer's. It's not impossible to add self-care, but doing so requires a willingness to change priorities. Alzheimer's disease radically shakes up our existing patterns. If we keep our minds and hearts open, adjusting our priorities to meet the new, ever-changing needs of our loved ones—and ourselves—can be life-giving!

One important reason that my relationship with my mother after the onset of Alzheimer's brought me such deep healing was that Mom made no demands on me. Of course, as the disease progressed, she couldn't make demands on me or on anyone. This circumstance allowed me the opportunity and the control I needed to meet my own needs while simultaneously doing my best to meet hers. Because Alzheimer's caregiving can be physically, mentally, and emotionally exhausting, even when our loved ones are in nursing homes, I learned that self-care is the most critical practice for caregivers. There were possibly times, many of them, when Mom needed me by her side or wanted me there for company, but because she couldn't communicate this to me, I wasn't tormented over the choice of meeting her needs or my own. This free practice of self-care, unimpeded by pressure from someone else to be or to do more than I could, greatly enhanced my ability to be present with Mom and increased my joy in taking care of her. Sometimes it's actually the hardest choice to take care of our own needs, particularly when another's seem greater or more important.

We need to give ourselves permission to set and maintain healthy boundaries. For example, a man at a workshop shared how frustrated and exhausted his mother was becoming because his father, who had Alzheimer's, was constantly calling her from the nursing home and demanding that she come to pick him up and take him home. This is an opportunity for the wife to take care of herself by screening her calls and talking with her husband only once a day, if that's what she can handle. It sounds radical, I know. But talking with him once from a joyful place will be more helpful to everyone than reluctantly taking eight phone calls a day, arguing about whether she will pick him up, making up stories about the car being in the shop, and feeling frustrated, angry, and resentful.

To acknowledge and ask for help is also a practice of self-care. When a loved one is in great need, it seems wrong to focus on ourselves. The stress of long-term caregiving can put caregivers' health and well-being in jeopardy, however, so giving our needs importance—not through a selfish motivation, but from a place of self-love—will benefit everyone.

Caregivers Making a Difference and Finding Meaning (with Links)

As Brother David Steindl-Rast suggests, Alzheimer's disease gives us countless invitations to do something about it and to receive the gift of knowing that what we do can make a difference for our loved ones with dementia, for other caregivers, and also for ourselves.

The gratitude I feel for the opportunity to share my discoveries from the journey in this book and in the workshops and presentations I offer is ongoing, as is my gratitude for those caregivers who made a difference for me. Through their devotion, care, activism, and advocacy, caregivers who have gone before us are contributing to the healing of our loved ones; they are showing us how to transform our pain and suffering into love, passion, and gratitude; and they are contributing to the healing of their communities as well as the wider world.

The Epistle-writer, Paul, in his Letter to the Romans (Romans 12:6) tells us that "we have gifts that differ according to the grace given to us." The difference-making/meaning-making caregivers whom I have been blessed to encounter and to know have demonstrated countless ways of overcoming suffering and loss by sharing their unique gifts of grace with the world. They are beacons of light for all those who want to follow them. Based on my own experience, I predict that these caregivers will be the most essential teachers for others on the journey. These caregivers are not merely teachers who impart information or knowledge to dispel ignorance. They are practitioners. They are influential mentors. They bring lived experience as well as the commitment to teach by example, practicing what they preach. What their words and actions preach is about loving kindness, about showing us that the time and effort we devote to caring for people with Alzheimer's is time and effort well spent, time and effort that can change their lives, and ours.

Seeking and finding opportunities to do something that will make a difference—in our own lives or the lives of others—is the most effective antidote to feeling helpless, the most effective antidote to suffering, the most fruitful way to experience healing, and the most direct path to finding meaning and purpose in the challenges of life. Using what we learn through our difficult experiences to enlighten, encourage, and assist others is the most powerful prescription for transforming heartbreak into gratitude. For example:

Write and tell your stories. We can all be guides for the caregivers who will come after us, just as the caregivers you've already met in these pages have been for me: **Joanne Koenig Coste**, **Elliott Stanley Goldman**, **Olivia Hoblitzelle**, **Arthur Kleinman**, and **Michael Leach**. These authors all have memorialized their life-transforming experiences born of caring for their spouses with Alzheimer's, and they have been like found treasures for me and thousands of others.

Enlighten and inspire family caregivers and professional care providers. You've also met **Stephen Post**. He is a grandson, who during his youth, was a regular nursing home visitor with his grandmother, Nellie, who had Alzheimer's. Stephen specifically recalls providing her with feeding assistance, and the tenderness and wonder this evoked in him. Years later, professional opportunities took Stephen, along with his tenderness and wonder, into clinics and homes working with people with Alzheimer's and their caregivers, eventually leading him to become an internationally renowned thought-leader, author, and presenter in the Alzheimer's field. Stephen's words of wisdom, born of experience, present us with the possibility of transformation happening through caregiving: "Dementia breaks into the previously routine lives of individuals and families, like a tidal wave disrupting everything in its path. The person with dementia is eventually swept away, while caregivers look back and feel forever changed by their experience."[6] Reflecting back on these words, they were a prophesy for my life, possibly for every caregiver's life. (stephenpost.com)

Neuroscientist **Lisa Genova** felt despair and frustration about not being able to connect with her Nana Angie in meaningful ways on the Alzheimer's journey. Even the knowledge she had gained from her neuroscience studies and Alzheimer's research did not prepare her to "be" with her grandmother relationally, to understand her, or to have empathy for her. Lisa's quest for empathy led her to write *Still Alice*, a fictional story that has had far-reaching impact.[7] Lisa's use of fiction to engage and enlighten readers about such a difficult subject was remarkably effective for me. Even after discovering ways to connect with Mom using improvisation and beginning to offer Healing Moments workshops the year before I met Lisa, I was, on a personal level, still terrified and mostly avoidant about the hard facts of Alzheimer's disease. It was something about the fictional aspect of *Still Alice* that gently opened my mind and bolstered my heart, giving me the courage to delve more deeply into the subject of Alzheimer's.

Remarkably, it was on this quest for empathy for her grandmother that Lisa also discovered her life-purpose as a neuroscientist-novelist. She has written five best-selling novels that engage and inform readers about little-understood neurological diseases. Lisa's first nonfiction book, *Remember: The Science of Memory and the Art of Forgetting*, was published in 2021. Community service inspired this volume. In her presentations over the years Lisa was constantly fielding questions from frightened dementia caregivers about "forgetting due to owning a human brain versus forgetting due to memory impairment." And so, *Remember* is Lisa's gift, born of her graces of listening and responding through her writing, to all of us who worry about our memories as we age, to all of us who are scared to death of having Alzheimer's. (lisagenova.com)

Expand the World of Caring. **Lynda Everman**, as the founder and convener of the Clergy Against Alzheimer's Network, also known as the Faith United Against Alzheimer's Coalition, invited religious leaders and communities into the caregiving effort. She also addressed the spiritual needs of caregivers with one of her book projects, *Seasons of Caring: Meditations for Alzheimer's and Dementia Caregivers*, which contains more than 100 comforting and enlightening meditations by clergy and faithful caregivers from various religious traditions. (usagainstalzheimer's.org/networks/faith)

Kathy Good, caregiver for her husband, Dave, is, at this writing, director of the Family Caregivers Center as well as the DeWolf Family Innovation Center for Aging and Dementia, both in Cedar Rapids, Iowa, both affiliated with Mercy Hospital. During her caregiving years, and still, Kathy is passionate about supporting caregivers because she knows their needs are great.

Even as a professional social worker, Kathy felt overwhelmed and didn't know what to do when Dave was diagnosed with Alzheimer's. When talking about her caregiving years, Kathy uses words that are surely relatable to many dementia caregivers: "distraught," "overwhelmed and alone," "agonizing." Because of her personal experience, she felt an easy "Yes" arise when Tim Charles, the then CEO of Mercy Cedar Rapids, asked if she would develop a Family Caregivers Center. Being a realist, Kathy knew firsthand that nothing she or a caregivers center could do would make the experience of caregiving *easy*. But she felt inspired to take on the hopeful mission of doing everything she could to make it *easier*.[8] (mercycare.org/services/the-chris-suzy-dewolf-family-innovation-center-for-aging-demen/ and mercycare.org/services/family-caregivers-center)

Lori La Bey journeyed through Alzheimer's with her mom, Dorothy, for nearly thirty years. Early in her caregiving experience, Lori was "shocked at the lack of resources, products, tools, services, and educational support available to families and professionals. Given the pain she saw and felt, she left her career of twenty-five years as a residential realtor, specializing in the senior market, which she loved and never saw herself leaving. She was now committed to making a difference in shifting dementia care from crisis to comfort around the world."[9] This commitment led her to become the founder and director of the *Alzheimer's Speaks* website, which was launched in 2009 and has continually offered a full section of free educational resources. The award-winning *Alzheimer's Speaks* radio show was launched in 2011 and by 2022 was still named the #1 Alzheimer's podcast. In 2020, Lori began a collaboration to develop Dementia Map, a free global resources directory for those diagnosed with any form of dementia, family members, and professionals providing care. (alzheimersspeaks.com and dementiamap.com)

After a lifetime of learning about all aspects of dementia care through a lifetime of family and professional caregiving roles, **Terry Skoog** recently began offering individual consultation to families living with dementia all across the country. This newly minted profession of dementia support consultant—also known as Alzheimer's coach—is so needed, and so appreciated, and it is making a healing difference one person with dementia, one family, at a time. (skoogdementiasupport.com)

Engage your community. I had been a guest on Lori LaBey's *Alzheimer's Speaks* podcast, but it was a joyful surprise for me to meet her in person here in Dubuque when she was the keynote presenter at a local dementia conference. Her ideas and suggestions inspired and motivated me and others to make a difference in our community. One suggestion was to start a Memory Café. In 2013, Lori launched what is believed to be the first Memory Café in the U.S.; we followed her lead, and in 2017 started "A Place for Friendship: Dubuque's Memory Café." We offered this supportive, entertaining social activity for people with dementia and their caregivers until the COVID-19 pandemic caused a pause in 2020. Lori made a lasting difference in this one small Iowa town, and she continues to do so all around the world! The Dubuque Memory Café was revived in 2024 and now meets twice monthly. (memorycafedirectory.com)

Steve, caregiver for his wife, Nancy, attended one of my *Meeting Alzheimer's* workshops, after which he encouraged his granddaughter, Becky, owner and director of *Above & Beyond Home Health Care and Hospice* in Monticello, Iowa, to sponsor a workshop for their local professional and family caregivers. Above & Beyond offered a free dinner for all participants before the workshop, which was also free. They registered nearly 100 people. Monticello is a very small town, and after the workshop I thought, "Wow, this whole town is going to have really good care for their loved ones with dementia." On Steve's recommendation, Becky was able to provide a needed and meaningful community service. (for more information about this workshop: jadeangelica.com)

Visit and support your friends and family with Alzheimer's. Marilyn and her husband, Joel, shared a short journey through Alzheimer's. One morning, during the early to moderate stage of the disease, they were exercising at the gym when Joel collapsed due to a massive cardiac event. He died a few days later, surround by family and song. Marilyn was grief-stricken by this sudden loss, but also thankful to know that Joel and she were spared that long goodbye many caregivers endure. After Joel died, Marilyn did not flee from Alzheimer's. On the contrary, she stepped up to be the primary companion and local eyes and ears for the far-away daughter of her closest friend, also named Marilyn, who was diagnosed with Alzheimer's. When the Memory Café in Dubuque was operating, Marilyn had attended with Joel. After he died, she attended with Marilyn.

Share whatever helped you with other caregivers. "Mother taught me," **Loretta Veney** said, "if you find something that works to help you, share it with other people." And so she did: Legos. Loretta got her first set of Legos when she was five, and these blocks became a way for mother and daughter to connect and communicate for a lifetime, including during the Alzheimer's journey. At first, Loretta used the Legos as a communication tool with just her mom, but in 2010 she put their Legos story and photos of some of their creations out onto social media. People were interested in learning more, so Loretta developed Lego kits and took them to various care centers to share with people with dementia. Since then, she has developed Legos puzzles for people with dementia, a specific Memory Café kit, and she recently launched a new "Inspiration Kit." The purpose of using Legos with people with dementia, Loretta says, "is to hear all voices." As she develops new programming, she has also discovered that inviting caregivers into this "serious play" experience can help them to resolve conflicts. (lorettaveney. com/lego-themed-events)

Don Wendorf, a retired psychologist, is also a musician, lyricist, and author; he was caregiver for his wife, Susan. Throughout the dementia journey, Don wrote rhyming verses about his experiences and feelings. He often sang these verses to himself while doing caregiving tasks or self-care (running, for example) and discovered that the lyrics and melodies brought him comfort, became a safe place for him to go in his mind, and kept him alive during the most difficult times. Don has shared this method of comfort with other caregivers through his book, *Caregiver Carols: A Musical, Emotional Memoir*, as well as several pieces he set to music and performs during his various talks. (Don Wendorf, Youtube)

Don also shared his gifts of grace by contributing one of his poems to *Seasons of Caring*, and he met Clergy Against Alzheimer's convener Lynda Everman. While connecting about this project and through their other work together in Clergy Against Alzheimer's, Lynda and Don became close. They are now married, living in Alabama, and Board members for the Cognitive Dynamics Foundation. Together, Lynda and Don are carrying out their dual missions of raising money to end Alzheimer's and caring for those currently on the journey. They are of like minds when it comes to the evolution of their advocacy: It started off with seeing a need and then seeing an opportunity to help in some way. "It's a leap of faith as you respond even if you don't know the territory or how to act," they said. Not really knowing where they will be taken, they start where they are; they meet others who show the way; they learn; and they grow, usually in ways never anticipated. Two of the places their advocacy has taken them are into editing multiple religious-themed resources for dementia care and presenting together at conferences around the country.

Enlist the arts! **Michael Verde**, Director of Memory Bridge, produced a documentary film, *Love Is Listening: Dementia without Loneliness*, in honor of his grandfather. This beautiful, evocative, enlightening film was screened at various film festivals (including the Julien Dubuque International Film Festival) and is raising awareness about the importance of engaging relationally with people with dementia. (memorybridge.org)

Inspired by my journey with Mom, *Healing Moments for Alzheimer's* produced a radio play, *The Forgiving and The Forgetting*, designed to teach our unique caregiving techniques and to instill hope that meaningful relationships remain possible. (The Forgiving and the Forgetting--Healing Moments, Youtube)

Margi Buhr is the Director of Education at the Dubuque Museum of Art and has engaged her workplace to help make a difference. Inspired by her mom, Rose, a lifelong teacher and lover of art who died from Alzheimer's, Margi developed the museum's In the Mind's Eye (ITME) program for people living with dementia and their caregivers. ITME, modeled after the Arts & Minds initiative, co-founded by **Carolyn Halpin-Healy,** which began at the Metropolitan Museum of Art in New York City and has expanded to museums across the country. The program provides meaningful art-centered activities that create positive cognitive, emotional, and social experiences. Participants look at and discuss art, engage in an art activity, and build a new community of friends. (for more information: mbuhr@dbqart.org; artsandminds.org)

Enlighten the world with your discoveries from the journey. **Dan Potts** is a neurologist, an author and co-author of multiple books on caregiving, and co-founder, with art therapist

Angel Duncan, of Cognitive Dynamics. His father, Lester Potts, was a lumberman. Lester spent his working life cutting trees and was proficient with a saw. Before being diagnosed with Alzheimer's, he had never picked up a paint brush. After being diagnosed with Alzheimer's, Lester attended an adult day program where, during an activity, someone gave him watercolor paints, a brush, and a piece of paper. The result was the creation of a stunning collection of paintings that surprised everyone, particularly Dan, who was personally and professionally intrigued by the expression of his father's uncovered talent as his cognitive abilities declined. Lester's remarkable collection "has been shown from Beverly Hills to Paris, has been the subject of research, and appears in articles, textbooks, devotional books, and documentaries." Lester's last painting was of a saw. (cognitivedynamics.org, lesterslegacy.com)

Fundraise. My neighbor **Terry Willenborg** wanted to do something to honor his grandmother, Mary, who had lived and died with Alzheimer's. A competitive runner, Terry decided to host a fundraising run for Alzheimer's. He launched his 5K event in 2013, attracting 124 runners and raising $2,400 for the Alzheimer's Association. By the eleventh year, this community event included running and walking categories ranging from 5K to a half-marathon, a team relay, and the Ainsely Angels, an organization that pushes disabled individuals in chariots to help them feel involved in events. More than 340 participants were registered, and $15,000 was raised. Terry's fundraising total to date is $89,000. When I recently asked him about his ongoing passion for this event, Terry said, "Having lost my grandmother from Alzheimer's, it feels good to give back and remember each year why I do this event." Fueled by his passion, he expects to be organizing this event for another forty years at least! (Alzheimers5k.com)

Get involved in lobbying efforts. On their journey together, **Kathy and Dave Good** were committed advocates for the greater well-being of all those touched by Alzheimer's or other forms of dementia. In 2009, they were invited by the Alzheimer's Association to submit testimony about their experiences and needs to the Social Security Administration "to encourage them to name Alzheimer's as a Compassionate Allowance." Dave's testimony was so compelling that it appeared on the Social Security website. The words of Kathy and Dave and many others ultimately helped to make this lobbying initiative successful! As a result, the applications for Social Security disability benefits by people with early-onset Alzheimer's are expedited for consideration, and if they are awarded benefits, the two-year waiting period for health insurance through Medicare is waived.[10] This change represents a monumental support for people with Alzheimer's and their families.

Even before her husband Richard died, **Lynda Everman** began investigating the possibility of an Alzheimer's postage stamp. She soon partnered with another caregiver, **Kathy Siggins**, whose husband, Gene, also had Alzheimer's. Together they launched a campaign for the issuance of an Alzheimer's awareness and fundraising (semipostal) stamp. It took 27 years of combined effort, tens of thousands of letters to Congress and the U.S. Postal Service, and incredible tenacity and persistence before the Alzheimer's Disease Research Semipostal Stamp was issued in 2017. Of the 500 million stamps printed, nearly 11 million have been sold as of April 2023, raising more than $1.4 million in funds for Alzheimer's research through the National Institutes of Health. (store.usps.com)

Volunteer however and wherever you can. Denny, caregiver for his wife Mary, was motivated by his faith to develop and offer a praise service for people with dementia at various care centers and memory cafes in his community.

Darrick volunteers with Healing Moments, leading programs when we began and now serving as treasurer. He volunteers this important service in remembrance of his great-grandmother Adele and his family's challenges of caring for her at home.

After her mother Ilene died, Coleen also volunteered with Healing Moments. She used her artistic talent and computer skills to design flyers, brochures, buttons, and power point slides.

Becky, in honor of her husband Mike, volunteers as a member of the Advisory Board for the new caregiver center in Dubuque, which opened in November 2022 thanks to endowment funds donated by a local philanthropist and caregiver, Jim, in honor of his wife, Marita.

Karen, who cared for her husband Paul, gives one of the best gifts imaginable to current caregivers. She volunteers a few hours a week to be with the loved ones with dementia while their caregivers attend support group meetings or educational programs. This gift is so important because the reason most often stated by caregivers for not attending these kinds of programs is that they can't leave their loved ones alone and don't have anyone to stay with them. Karen gives this gift in gratitude for the support she and Paul received.

Light the way . . . .

Lynda Everman shared with me that she began her activism and advocacy reluctantly, because speaking about her experience was so painful. People with Alzheimer's and their caregivers are ever-grateful to Lynda, and for all the teachers with lived experience who have gone before us, for their courage to overcome their fears and resistance and to do something. They didn't just survive the refiner's fire; they have thrived by transforming their pain into a passion for healing and change. In his poem, "Dry Salvages," T.S. Eliot speaks of a common human condition: "we have the experience but miss the meaning."[11]

Embarking on a quest to find meaning for the challenges in our lives, including those inherent in Alzheimer's, is one way we can deepen our humanity and enhance our spiritual lives. As we have learned from all of these caregivers—who did not miss the meaning—it is also a way to make a difference. "In some ways," writes Viktor Frankl, "suffering ceases to be suffering at the moment it finds meaning."[12] Steindl-Rast defines meaning through metaphor, "the light in which we see things." Our spirits naturally thirst for this light as we seek to accept, endure, and understand our difficult circumstances. Follow the light; quench the thirst; heal the wounds; make a difference. Each through our own unique graces.[13]

For Further Reading

Alterra, Aaron (Elliot Stanley Goldman). *The Caregiver: A Life with Alzheimer's*. Ithaca, NY: Cornell Paperbacks, 2007.

Angelica, Jade. "Alzheimer's Caring: How Faith Communities Can Serve People with Dementia and Their Families." *Huffington Post* (December 14, 2016), huffpost.com

Angelica, Jade. "Improvisation Can Help to Heal—Even Trauma, Even Alzheimer's," *Huffington Post* (June 23, 2017), huffpost.com

Angelica, Jade. *Meeting Alzheimer's: Learning to Communicate and Connect* (workshop from *Healing Moments*). The primary mission of Healing Moments' workshops and presentations is to improve the qualify of life for people with Alzheimer's and their loved ones by enlivening their hearts with hope and enhancing their belief that meaningful relationships remain possible. Additional goals include increasing caregiver knowledge, reducing caregiver stress, improving caregiver satisfaction, and decreasing conflict. Healing Moments' offerings include compassionate workshops and presentations for family and informal caregivers, conference presentations, services and presentations for faith communities, and educational workshops for pastors, parish nurses, and pastoral care team. All are available via Zoom. For more information, visit jadeangelica.com or contact Rev. Dr. Jade Angelica at jadeangelica@gmail.com.

Armstrong, Karen. *Twelve Steps to a Compassionate Life.* New York: Alfred A. Knopf, 2011.

Bredesen, Dale E. *The End of Alzheimer's: The First Protocol to Enhance Cognition and Reverse Decline at Any Age.* New York: Avery, 2020.

Chödrön, Pema. *When Things Fall Apart: Heart Advice for Difficult Times.* Boston: Shambala, 1997.

Coste, Joanne Koenig. *Learning to Speak Alzheimer's: A Groundbreaking Approach for Everyone Dealing with the Disease.* New York: Houghton Mifflin, 2003.

Doidge, Norman. *The Brain That Changes Itself: Stories of Personal Triumph from the Frontiers of Brain Science.* New York: Penguin Books, 2007.

Everman, Lynda, and Don Wendorf, Senior Editors. *Dementia-Friendly Worship: A Multifaith Handbook for Chaplains, Clergy, and Faith Communities.* Philadelphia: Jessica Kingsley Publishers, 2019.

Everman, Lynda, and Don Wendorf. *Stolen Memories: An Alzheimer's Stole Ministry & Tallit Initiative.* Eugene, OR: Wipf & Stock Publishers, 2019.

Genova, Lisa. *Remember: The Science of Memory & the Art of Forgetting.* New York: Harmony Books, 2021.

Genova, Lisa. *Still Alice.* New York: Simon & Schuster, 2009.

Good, Kathy. *My World Wore a Bow Tie: Care/Giving/Connections.* Cedar Rapids, IA: Family Caregivers Centers of Mercy, 2023.

Hoblitzelle, Olivia Ames. *Ten Thousand Joys and Ten Thousand Sorrows: A Couple's Journey Through Alzheimer's.* New York: Penguin Books, 2010.

Kleinman, Arthur. *The Soul of Care: The Moral Education of a Husband and a Doctor.* New York: Penguin Books, 2019.

Kleinman, Arthur. "On Caregiving." *Harvard Magazine* (July-August, 2010), harvardmagazine.com.

Kushner, Harold. *When Bad Things Happen to Good People.* New York: Anchor Books, 2004.

La Bey, Lori, and Scott Carlson. *Betty the Bald Chicken: Lessons in How to Care.* Burnsville, MN: Kirkhouse Publishers, 2023.

Leach, Michael, and Friends. *Soul Seeing: Light ★ Love ★ Forgiveness.* Maryknoll, NY: Orbis Books, 2018.

Levine, Stephen. *Unattended Sorrow: Recovering from Loss and Reviving the Heart.* Kutztown, PA: Rodale, 2005.

Lewis, Jacqueline J. *Fierce Love: A Bold Path to Ferocious Courage and Rule-Breaking Kindness That Can Heal the World.* New York: Harmony Books, 2021.

Madson, Patricia Ryan. *Improv Wisdom.* New York: Bell Tower, 2005.

McKim, Donald K., ed. *God Never Forgets: Faith, Hope, and Alzheimer's Disease.* Louisville: Westminster John Knox Press, 1997.

Nhat Hanh, Thich. *Being Peace.* Berkeley, CA: Parallax Press, 2005.

Post, Stephen G. *Dignity for Deeply Forgetful People: How Caregivers Can Meet the Challenges of Alzheimer's Disease.* Baltimore: The Johns Hopkins University Press, 2022.

Post, Stephen G. *The Moral Challenge of Alzheimer Disease: Ethical Issues from Diagnosis to Dying,* 2nd ed. Baltimore: The Johns Hopkins University Press, 2000.

Post, Stephen G., Jill Neimark, et al. *Why Good Things Happen to Good People: How to Live a Longer, Healthier, Happier Life by the Simple Act of Giving.* New York: Broadway Books, 2007.

Potts, Daniel, and Richard Morgan. *Treasure for Alzheimer's: Reflecting on experiences with the art of Lester Potts, Jr.* Tuscaloosa, AL: FAAN and Cognitive Dynamics Foundation, 2015. A catalog of Lester Potts's art is available at lesterslegacy.com.

Potts, Daniel, Lynda Everman, Steven Glazer, Richard Morgan, Max Wallack, eds. *Seasons of Caring: Meditations for Alzheimer's and Dementia Caregivers.* ClergyAgainstAlzheimer's Network, 2014.

Power, G. Allen. *Dementia Beyond Drugs: Changing the Culture of Care.* Baltimore: Health Professions Press, Inc., 2010.

Power, G. Allen. *Dementia Beyond Disease: Enhancing Well-being.* Baltimore: Health Professions, Inc., 2014.

Raia, Paul. "Habilitation Therapy: A New Star Scape." *Enhancing the Quality of Life in Advanced Dementia,* edited by Ladislav Volicer and Lisa Bloom-Charette. Philadelphia: Brunner/Mazel–Taylor Francis Group, 1999. nhqualitycampaign.org/files.

Rohr, Richard. *Falling Upward: A Spirituality for the Two Halves of Life.* San Francisco: Jossey-Bass, 2011.

Sabat, Steven. *Alzheimer's Disease and Dementia: What Everyone Needs to Know.* New York: Oxford University Press, 2017.

Shenk, David. *The Forgetting—Alzheimer's: Portrait of an Epidemic.* New York: Anchor Books, 2003.

Steindl-Rast, David. *Gratefulness, the Heart of Prayer: An Approach to Life in Fullness.* Mahwah, NJ: Paulist Press, 1984.

Taylor, Jill Bolte. *My Stroke of Insight: A Brain Scientist's Personal Journey.* New York: Plume, 2009.

Thibault, Jane Marie, and Richard L. Morgan. *No Act of Love Is Ever Wasted: The Spirituality of Caring for Persons with Dementia.* Nashville: Upper Room Books, 2009.

Veney, Loretta. *Being My Mom's Mom: A Journey Through Dementia from a Daughter's Perspective.* ANEW Press, 2019.

Wendorf, Don. *Caregiver Carols: A Musical, Emotional Memoir.* Scotts Valley, CA: Create Space Independent Publishing, 2014.

Notes

Introduction

1. *Marcus Borg, Meeting Jesus Again for the First Time: The Historical Jesus and the Heart of Contemporary Faith* (San Francisco: HarperCollins, 1995), 32–33, 42.

2. Wayne B. Arnason, *Singing the Living Tradition.* (Boston: Beacon Press, 1993), #698.

I In the Beginning

Epigraph: *Rainer Maria Rilke, "Gott spricht zu jedem . . . / God speaks to each of us . . . ,"* Rilke's Book of Hours: *Love Poems to God, translated by Anita Barrows and Joanna Macy* (New York: Riverhead Books, 1996).

1. Awakening

1. Richard Rohr, *Falling Upward: A Spirituality for the Two Halves of Life* (San Francisco: Jossey-Bass, 2011), 82–86. Rohr discusses what he describes as "the most problematic lines" of the New Testament, Luke 14:26: "Whoever comes to me and does not hate father and mother, wife and children, brothers and sisters, yes, and even life itself, cannot be my disciple" (NRSV). Rohr cites the lives of Buddha and Jesus as examples of leaving home and rejecting "business as usual."

2. Jacqui Lewis, *Fierce Love: A Bold Path to Ferocious Courage and Rule Breaking Kindness That Can Heal the World* (New York: Penguin, Random House, 2021), 39.

3. Lewis, 33.

4. David Shenk, *The Forgetting—Alzheimer's: Portrait of an Epidemic* (New York: Anchor Books, 2003), 258.

5. Alan Jones, *The Soul's Journey: Exploring the Three Passages of the Spiritual Life with Dante as a Guide* (San Francisco: Harper Collins, 1995), 6.

6. Jacqui Lewis, "Fierce Love: A Bold Path to Ferocious Courage and Rule-Breaking Kindness That Can Heal the World," 14th Annual Spiritual Care Conference (Wentworth-Douglass Hospital, October 18, 2022).

7. Lewis, *Fierce Love*, 209.

8. Lewis, "Fierce Love."

9. Lewis, *Fierce Love*, 209.

10. Lewis, "Fierce Love."

11. Lewis, *Fierce Love*, 60.

12. Lewis, Fierce Love, 12.

2. Accepting and Improvising

13. Joanne Koenig Coste, *Learning to Speak Alzheimer's: A Groundbreaking Approach for Everyone Dealing with the Disease* (New York: Houghton Mifflin, 2003), 32–34.

14. Paul Raia, "Habilitation Therapy: A New Starscape," *Enhancing the Quality of Life in Advanced Dementia*, edited by Ladislav Volcer and Lisa Bloom-Charette (Philadelphia: Brunner/Mazel-Taylor & Francis Group, 1999), 32–34. Dr. Raia's chapter can also be accessed at nhqualitycampaign.org.

15. Coste, 32–34. Joanne Koenig Coste and Paul Raia, vice president of Clinical Programs for the Alzheimer's Association, Massachusetts/New Hampshire Chapter, created a treatment plan for people with dementia called Habilitation Therapy. Coste defines *habilitation* as "an approach to caring for a person with progressive dementia that focuses on validating the patient's underlying emotions, maintaining dignity, creating

moments for success, and using all remaining skills" (204). "The literal meaning of habilitate is 'to clothe or to dress,' but [Coste uses] it in the sense of 'to make capable,' which is an older meaning of the word" (7–8). Raia describes the goal of habilitation therapy as "deceptively simple—to bring about a positive emotion and to maintain that emotional state throughout the day" (Raia, 23).

16. Raia, 22–23, 20. The six critical areas referred to by Raia and Coste as "domains" are the physical domain, the social domain, the functional domain, the communication domain, the perpetual domain, and the behavioral domain (Raia, 23–36).

17. Coste, 32–34. In this interaction, the aide met Mary in her improvised reality rather than attempting to correct her. Mary's feelings were noticed and validated, in this case loneliness and a longing for nurturing. The aide also averted a situation in which Mary could have felt a sense of failure. In taking this approach, the aide manifested the habilitation approach: know that communication is possible, live in the patient's world, and enrich the patient's life.

18. Coste, 6.

19. Keith Johnstone, *IMPRO: Improvisation and the Theatre* (New York : Routledge, 1992), 88.

20. Rohr, 142.

21. Katie Goodman, *Improvisation for the Spirit: Live a More Creative, Spontaneous, and Courageous Life Using the Tools of Improv Comedy* (Naperville, IL: SourceBooks, 2008), 131.

22. This is a strategy recommended by Michelle S. Bourgeois in "Unlocking the Silent Prison: Strategies for Communicating with Persons with Dementia, Memory Loss Conference at Southern Illinois University School of Medicine (November 8, 2011).

23. Tom Kitwood and Kathleen Bredin, "Towards a Theory of Dementia Care: Personhood and Well-being," *Ageing and Society* 12 (1992): 269–87. Kitwood and Bredin describe the following indicators of well-being in people with severe dementia:
- the assertion of will or desire, usually in the form of dissent despite various coaxings
- the ability to express a range of emotions

- initiation of social contact (for instance, a person with dementia has a small toy dog that he treasures and places it before another person with dementia to attract attention)
- affectional warmth (for instance, a woman wanders back and forth in the facility without much sociality, but when people say hello to her, she gives them a kiss on the cheek and continues her wandering)
- social sensitivity in the form of a smile or taking another's hand
- self-respect (for instance, a woman who has defecated on the floor in the sitting room attempts to clean up after herself)
- acceptance of other people with dementia (for instance, a fast wanderer takes the hand of a slow wanderer and leads him around)
- humor (for instance, when there is a technical problem with a video system, a person with severe dementia unexpectedly blurts out, "Try putting a shilling in the slot.")
- creativity and self-expression, often achieved through art, music, or therapy
- showing pleasure (for instance, smiling and laughing in an exercise event)
- helpfulness (for instance, a man provides a cushion for a woman seated on the hard floor)
- relaxation (for instance, a woman with dementia who has the habit of lying on the floor curled up tensely relaxes when led to the sofa)

3. Waiting and Preparing

24. Classes in improvisation are available in many areas of the country through comedy clubs, drama schools, and adult education centers. Programs designed for specifically teaching improvisation techniques to people caring for people with Alzheimer's are available worldwide through Healing Moments for Alzheimer's at www.jadeangelica.com.

25. Sandeep Jauhar, "When My Father Got Alzheimer's, I Had to Learn to Lie to Him," *New York Times*, nytimes.com (April 7, 2023).

26. Exodus 20: 1–17, *Holy Bible: New Revised Standard Version* (New York: Oxford UP, 1989).

27. Rukmini Chaitanya, lecture at Sivananda Ashram (May 21, 2023).

28. Raia, 32.

29. James Faust, quoted in Rammohan Rao, *Good Living Practices: The Best from Ayurveda, Yoga, and Modern Science for Achieving Optimal Health, Happiness, and Longevity* (n.p.: Kaivalya Wellness, 2020), 164.

30. Jauhar.

31. Jauhar.

32. Naomi Feil, "Preface," *V/F Validation: The Feil Method: How to Help Disoriented Old-Old* (Cleveland: Edward Feil Productions, 1982).

33. "Validation Therapy," A Train Education: Continuing Education for Health Care Providers, atrainceu.com.

34. Feil.

35. Loretta Veney, *Being My Mom's Mom: A Journey Through Dementia from a Daughter's Perspective* (Berkeley, CA: Anew Press, 2019), 58–60.

36. Adapted from "Elephant and the Blind Men," *Jainworld.com.*

II Into the Heart of Alzheimer's

Epigraph: Thomas Merton, *Conjectures of a Guilty Bystander* (New York: Image/Doubleday, 2009), 206.

4. Healing When There Is No Cure

1. Aaron Alterra, *The Caregiver: A Life with Alzheimer's* (Ithaca, NY: Cornell Paperbacks, 2007), 207. Elliot Stanley Goldman used a pseudonym, Aaron Alterra, when he first wrote this book, to protect the privacy of his wife and family.

2. David Shenk, *The Forgetting—Alzheimer's: Portrait of an Epidemic,* 12–14.

3. Shenk, 25.

4. Alzheimer's Association, "2024 Alzheimer's Disease: Facts and Figures," alz.org/media/documents/alzheimers-facts-and-figures.pdf. This report goes on to explain the following:

- One in nine people age 65 and older (10.9 percent) has Alzheimer's disease.
- About one-third of people age 85 and older (33.4 percent) have Alzheimer's disease.
- Only about half of those who would meet the diagnostic criteria for Alzheimer's disease and other dementias have received a diagnosis of dementia from a physician.

5. Zaven Khachaturian, quoted in Shenk, 65. Khachaturian is known as the "father of Alzheimer's research in the United States."

6. Alzheimer's Association.

7. Jeffrey Cummings, Dana P. Goldman, et al., "The costs of developing treatments for Alzheimer's disease: A retrospective exploration," *Alzheimer's & Dementia*, 18:3 (March 2022), alz-journals.onlinelibrary.wiley.com.

8. Pam Belluck, Sheila Kaplan, and Rebecca Robbins, "How An Unproven Alzheimer's Drug Got Approved," *New York Times*, nytimes.com (October 20, 2021).

9. Daniel Gilbert, "Alzheimer's Drug Shows Promise but Needs More Study for Safety, Researchers Say," *Washington Post*, washingtonpost.com (November, 29, 2022).

10. Rebecca Robbins and Pam Belluck, "Biogen Abandons Its Controversial Alzheimer's Drug Aduhelm," *New York Times* (January 31, 2024).

11. Dale Bredesen, *The End of Alzheimer's: The First Program to Prevent and Reverse Cognitive Decline* (New York: Avery, Penguin, Random House, 2020), 25–26. Bredesen claims to have discovered in his lab that amyloid plaques are a defense mechanism against inflammation, lack of nutrients, hormones, molecules out of balance, and exposure to toxic substance such as mold. Alzheimer's symptoms materialize when these threats become "chronic, multiple, unrelenting, and intense—so much so that the protective plaques cross the line into causing harm."

12.

12. Matthew Perrone, "FDA approves 2nd Alzheimer's drug that can modestly slow dementia," *PBS News Hour*, pbs.org (July 2, 2024).

13. Dale Bredesen, "Inventing the Future of Brain Health: A New Landmark Study" (webinar), *Awakening from Alzheimer's: Brain Health Breakthroughs* (November 11, 2022).

14. Bredesen, "Inventing the Future of Brain Health."

15. Hallie Levine, "Hispanics and Latinos and Alzheimer's Disease," *WebMD*, webmd.com (August 11, 2022). For more information about Hispanic Americans and Alzheimer's Disease, see Alzheimer's Association, alz.org/help-support/resources/Hispanics-and-alzheimers.

16. Dale Bredesen, Apollo Health, apollohealthco.com.

17. "The Finnish Geriatric Intervention Study to Prevent Cognitive Impairment and Disability (FINGER) trial is the first randomized control trial (RCT) showing that it is possible to prevent cognitive decline using a multidomain lifestyle intervention among older at-risk individuals" (Alzheimer's Association, "A Global Collaboration for Future Generations," *World Wide Fingers*, alz.org/wwfingers/overview. asp). Beginning in 2018, countries around the world, including the United States, planned to replicate the Finnish protocol.

18. Bredesen, Apollo Health. In his newest book, *The First Survivors of Alzheimer's*, Bredesen presents stories of seven individuals who reversed their cognitive decline using Bredesen's ReCODE protocol.

19. David Perlmutter, "The Biggest Breakthroughs from a Decade of Brain Health," *Awakening from Alzheimer's: Brain Health Breakthroughs* (webinar) (November 20, 2022).

20. Bredesen, Apollo Health.

21. Heather Sandison, *Awakening from Alzheimer's* (November 12, 2022), solcere.com. Multiple versions of Kirtan Kriya are available on YouTube. My favorite is Nina Mongendre's "Kirtan Kriya Meditation." You can find more information about research on Kirtan Kriya and its impact at the Alzheimer's Research & Prevention website, alzheimersprevention. org/research.

22. Daniel Lieberman, "The Evolution of Exercise" (webinar), Harvard University Alumni Association (October 20, 2022).

23. Kat Toups, "Reversing the Hidden Causes of Dementia," *Awakening from Alzheimer's*, op cit. (November 13, 2022), bayareawellness.net. Dr. Toups has a book in progress, *Dementia Demystified*.

24. T.S. Eliot, "Burnt Norton," *Four Quartets* (New York: Ecco, 2023).

25. Sandison.

26. Dale Bredesen, "Inventing the Future of Brain Health."

27. Paul Raia, "Habilitation Therapy: A New Starscape," *Enhancing the Quality of Life in Advanced Dementia*, edited by Ladislav Volcer and Lisa Bloom-Charette (Philadelphia: Brunner/Mazel-Taylor & Francis Group, 1999). In contrast, Raia's emphasis involves "active treatment of the symptoms... through a careful focus on the utilization of those capacities that remain, particularly the person's psychological capacity."

28. Alterra, 210.

29. Fred Reklau, "Theses on Healing (and Cure)," *Partners in Care: Medicine and Ministry Together* (Eugene, OR: Wipf and Stock, 2010), Appendix B.

30. Arthur Kleinman, "On Caregiving," *Harvard Magazine* (July-August 2010), 25.

31. Bredesen, "Inventing the Future of Brain Health."

32. Arthur Kleinman, Foreword, *The Caregiver: A Life with Alzheimer's*, by Aaron Alterra (Ithaca, NY: Cornell, 2007), xi.

33. Alterra, 209.

34. Kleinman, "On Caregiving," 29.

35. Venerable Tenzin Dasel, lecture at Sivananda Ashram, Paradise Island, Bahamas (March 10, 2023).

36. Kleinman, "On Caregiving," 29.

37. Michael Leach, "Soul seeing, like love, changes everything." *The National Catholic Reporter* (October 16, 2021), ncronline.org.

38. Michael Leach, "Know What Your Duty Is, Do It Without Hesitation," *Soul Seeing: Light*Love*Forgiveness* (Maryknoll, NY: Orbis Books, 2018), 6.

39. Leach, "Know What Your Duty Is," 8.

40. Kleinman, "On Caregiving," 29. Sallie McFague describes God as "the giver of life, as the power of being in all being," and invites her readers to consider that God can be imaged through the metaphor of mother and of father (Sallie McFague, "God as Mother," in *Weaving the Visions: New Patterns in Feminist Spirituality*, edited by Judith Plaskow and Carol P. Christ [New York: Harper Collins, 1989], 142.). McFague was not the first feminist to imagine God as mother. In the fourteenth century, Christian mystic Julian of Norwich publicly shared her "showings" from God. True to the feminist paradigm, Julian experienced God as relational: "I saw that God rejoices that he is our Father, and God rejoices that he is our Mother, and God rejoices that he is our true spouse, and that our soul is his beloved wife" (Julian of Norwich, *Showings*, translated by Edmund Colledge and James Walsh [Mahwah, NJ: Paulist Press, 1978], 279). Julian freely and often shared her experiences of both God and Christ as "our loving Mother" (Julian, 293). "The Creator of all things," Julian wrote, "created everything for love, and by the same love it is preserved, and always will be without end" (Julian, 190). "Parental love," according to McFague, "is the most powerful and intimate experience we have of giving love whose return is not calculated (though a return is appreciated): It is the gift of *life as such* to others. Parental love wills life … . Parental love nurtures what it has brought into existence, wanting growth and fulfillment for all" (Julian, 143). In the context of Alzheimer's care, if we apply McFague's premise that "God as Mother is parent to *all* species and wishes all to flourish" (McFague, 143), feminist caregivers will not allow this vulnerable population to be ignored, abused, or abandoned.

41. Keen, Sam. *To Love and Be Loved* (New York: Bantam, 1999), 115–116.

42. Erich Fromm, *The Art of Loving* (New York: Harper Perennial, 2006), 5.

43. Keen, 112. Adapted from Roman mythology as told by Martin Heidegger in *Being and Time* (New York: Harper & Row, 1962).

44. Keen, 119.

45. Kleinman, "On Caregiving," 29.

46. Arthur Kleinman, "The Art of Medicine," *The Lancet*, 378 (November 5, 2011): 1621.

47. Shenk, 222. Shenk describes the infant-like state that appears during the late stages of Alzheimer's disease: "can no longer walk without assistance, can no longer sit up without assistance, can no longer smile, can no longer hold up head... eyes lose their ability to focus... the return of infant reflexes."

48. Vaclav Havel, quoted in Stephen Sapp, "Hope: The Community Looks Forward," in *God Never Forgets: Faith, Hope, and Alzheimer's Disease*, edited by Donald K. McKim (Louisville: Westminster John Knox Press, 1997), 103.

49. Courtney Blanchard, "Chief Wadding Hangs Up Badge," *(Dubuque) Telegraph Herald* (March 10, 2009), A:1.

50. David Steindl-Rast, *The Grateful Heart* (Boulder, CO: Sounds True Recordings, 1992), audiocassette.

51. Angela L. Smith and Jennifer Harkness, "Spirituality and Meaning: A Qualitative Inquiry with Caregivers of Alzheimer's Disease," *Journal of Family Psychotherapy* 13:1–2 (2002), 88, 90.

52. Julian of Norwich, *"Showings,"* translated by Edmund Colledge and James Walsh (Mahwah, NJ: Paulist Press, 1978), 279.

53. William Blake, quoted in Keen, 106.

54. Pierre Teilhard de Chardin, *The Divine Milieu* (New York: Perennial Classics, 2001), 56.

5. The Value and Beauty of Every Person

54. Kurt Ullrich, "With Alzheimer's, Watch Keeps Ticking," *(Dubuque) Telegraph Herald* (September 16, 2010).

55. "As the number of people with Alzheimer's disease and other dementias grows, spending for their care will increase dramatically. For people with these conditions, aggregate payments for health care, long-term care and hospice are projected to increase from $345 billion in 2023 (this represents an increase of $142 billion since 2013) to just

under $1 trillion in 2050 (in 2023 dollars). Medicare and Medicaid cover about 70 percent of the costs of care. (Alzheimer's Association, "2023 Alzheimer's Disease: Facts and Figures," *Alzheimer's & Dementia*, 19:4 [2023], 66, 84).

56. Stephen Sapp, "Memory: The Community Looks Backward," and "Hope: The Community Looks Forward," in *God Never Forgets: Faith, Hope, and Alzheimer's Disease*, edited by Donald K. McKim (Louisville: Westminster John Knox Press, 1997).

57. Ezekiel 12:2, *Holy Bible: New Revised Standard Version* (Oxford University Press, 1989).

58. Sue Bender, *Everyday Sacred: A Woman's Journey Home* (New York: HarperCollins, 1996), 22.

59. James Ellor, "Celebrating the Human Spirit," *God Never Forgets: Faith, Hope, and Alzheimer's Disease*, edited by Donald K. McKim (Louisville: Westminster John Knox Press, 1997), 20.

60. John Dominic Crossan, quoted in Burton Mack, *A Myth of Innocence* (Minneapolis: Fortress Press, 1988), 142–143. Crossan is an Irish-American religious scholar and former Catholic priest known for co-founding the Jesus Seminar.

61. "The True Meaning of Nasrudin," *Idries Shah Foundation*, idriesshahfoundation.org/nasrudin.

62. Antoine de Saint-Exupéry, *The Little Prince*, translated by Katherine Wood (New York: Harcourt, Brace & World, 1943), 70.

63. Pat Robertson, quoted on *World News Tonight*, ABC (September 15, 2011). The context for this remark was Robertson's statement that spouses of people with Alzheimer's could divorce them without sin. He also stated that he presumed the spouse with Alzheimer's was receiving appropriate custodial care. He acknowledged that this is a complicated question and best responded to by ethicists.

64. Robert Stern, appearing on *World News Tonight*, ABC (September 15, 2011).

65. Augustine of Hippo, quoted in *A Treasury of Traditional Wisdom*, edited by Whitall N. Perry (San Francisco: Harper & Row, 1986), 819.

66. Sol Rogers, submitted to Helpline of the Massachusetts/New Hampshire chapter of the Alzheimer's Association (April 30, 2008).

67. Marissa Payne, "Elizabeth Hoskins, former Waypoint Services leader, dies at 73," *(Cedar Rapids) Gazette* (February 2, 2022).

68. Jacobi Feckers, "Caregiving Lessons from Liz" (eulogy delivered on February 26, 2022).

69. Adapted from Jade Angelica, "Yes, Virginia, There Is a Santa Claus," *Journal of Pastoral Care & Counseling* 65: 2 (2011), 10:1–2.

70. Olivia Ames Hoblitzelle, *Ten Thousand Joys and Ten Thousand Sorrows: A Couple's Journey Through Alzheimer's* (New York: Penguin, 2010), 125.

6. Redefining Self

71. David Shenk, *The Forgetting—Alzheimer's: Portrait of an Epidemic* (New York: Anchor, 2003), 13.

72. Richard Rohr, *True Self/False Self* (Cincinnati: St. Anthony Messenger Press, 2003), audiocassettes. Rohr claims Descartes was just being "consistent," since the West defines itself by "thinking." "After a while," Rohr continues, "we think we are our thinking, and this is the hardest thing to disassociate from.... You cannot experience your deepest level of being or consciousness or the True Self... through your head."

73. Antonio Damasio, *Descartes' Error: Emotion, Reason, and the Human Brain* (New York: Penguin, 2005).

74. Citing the language used by D. H. J. Davis ("Dementia: Sociological and Philosophical Constructions," *Social Science and Medicine*, 58: 369–78), Stephan Millet writes, "If we take a view that people with dementia are in the process of losing their 'self' then the end result of the process of loss is a non-person, an ontological null point .... Moving away from a view of dementia in which the self is disintegrating has the potential to provide some solace to family carers" ("Self and Embodiment: A Biophenomenological Approach to Dementia," *Dementia* [June 15, 2011]: 1, 12). The premise of Where Two Worlds Touch echoes Davis's conclusion: Helping caregivers to "let go

of the idea of the person with dementia as an ontological unit in decay, and understand that their loved one is, in effect, continuing the process of creating a life-world through the changed perceptions that come with dementia" (12).

75. Judith Plaskow and Carol P. Christ write, "The notion of self as relational is prominent in feminist thinking." They explain that twentieth-century feminists challenge Descartes's position "that selfhood is to be found in the rational self-reflection of the isolated ego." Feminist thinkers are "united in their insistence that the self is essentially embodied, passionate, relational and communal .... They affirm that knowledge arises from the body-mind continuum, which includes passions and feelings as well as thinking. They assert that the self cannot exist apart from relationship. And they insist that identity is found in community" ("Self in Relation," *Weaving the Visions: New Patterns in Feminist Spirituality* [New York: HarperCollins, 1989], 173). Feminist Beverly Wildung Harrison writes, "If we begin, as feminists must, with 'our bodies, ourselves,' we recognize that all our knowledge ... is body-mediated knowledge. All knowledge is rooted in our sensuality. We know and value the world, if we know and value it, through our ability to touch, to hear, to see. Perception is foundational to conception. Ideas are dependent on our sensuality. Feeling is the basic bodily ingredient that mediates our connectedness to the world. All power, including intellectual power, is rooted in feeling" ("The Power of Anger in the Work of Love," in Plaskow and Christ, 218).

76. Robert Stern, quoted in Neil Munshi, "A Healing Touch," *Boston Globe*, August 10, 2008.

77. Damasio, xix.

78. Justin S. Feinstein, et al., "Sustained Experience of Emotion after Loss of Memory in Patients with Amnesia," *Proceedings of the National Academy of Sciences of the United States of America*, 107: 17 (April 27, 2010): 7674–79.

79. Paul Raia, "Habilitation Therapy: A New Starscape," *Enhancing the Quality of Life in Advanced Dementia*, edited by Ladislav Volcer and Lisa Bloom-Charette (London: Routledge, 1999), 31.

80. Damasio, xix.

81. Damasio, xi.

82. Steven Sabat and Rom Harre, "The Construction and Deconstruction of Self in Alzheimer's Disease," *Aging and Society* 12 (1992): 443–61.

83. Michelle S. Bourgeois, "Unlocking the Silent Prison: Strategies for Communicating with Persons with Dementia," Memory Loss Conference at Southern Illinois University School of Medicine (November 8, 2011). Bourgeois is a professor of speech pathology at Ohio State University. Her book, *Memory Books and Other Graphic Cueing Systems: Practical Communication and Memory Aids for Adults with Dementia*, offers helpful guidance for maintaining speech and communicative engagement in people with dementia.

84. "Dale Tip #6: A Person's Name Is the Sweetest Sound," dalecarnegieboston.tumblr.com.

85. "AD [Alzheimer's Disease] patients are whole individuals and can still surprise us with their ability to communicate .... Most people suffering from AD retain their capacity to understand simple language, as well as their ability to follow clear and concise instructions" (Pierre Parenteau, "Communication with Alzheimer's Patients: A Matter of Time, Caring and Contact," *Canadian Alzheimer Disease Review* [November 2000], 7).

86. Luke 11:5–8, *The Holy Bible: New Revised Standard Version* (Oxford University Press, 1989).

87. G. Allen Power, *Dementia beyond Drugs: Changing the Culture of Care* (Baltimore: Health Professions Press, 2010), 3.

88. Ram Dass and Mirabai Bush, *Walking Each Other Home* (Louisville, CO: Sounds True, 2022), audiocassette.

89. Teresa of Avila, *Interior Castle*, translated and edited by E. Allison Peers (Mineola, NY: Dover Publications, 2007): 150, 146.

90. *The Bhagavad-Gita: Krishna's Counsel in Time of War*, translated by Barbara Stoler Miller (New York: Bantam Books, 1986), 32.

91. In his book *Dementia Reconsidered: The Person Comes First* (London: Open University Press, 1997), Tom Kitwood writes, "Even when cognitive impairment is very severe, an I-Thou form of meeting and relating is often possible" (2). He is referring to Martin Buber's book *I and Thou*.

92. *Bhagavad-Gita*, 58.

93. Steven Sabat and Rom Harre, "The Construction and Deconstruction of Self in Alzheimer's Disease," *Aging and Society* 12 (1992): 443–61.

94. Teresa, 49. Arthur Kleinman quotes Emmanuel Levinas, a twentieth-century French philosopher and Talmudic commentator, as another voice with feminist undertones of relationality challenging his countryman Descartes. According to Kleinman, Levinas "insists that the ethical must always precede the epistemological or ontological in human relationships. How we know and what our being is about take second place to the affirmation of the other and responses to the other's suffering" (Arthur Kleinman, Foreword, *The Caregiver: A Life with Alzheimer's* by Aaron Alterra [Ithaca, N.Y.: Cornell Paperbacks, 2007], xi).

95. Sam Keen, *To Love and Be Loved* (New York: Bantam, 1999), 3.

96. Stephan Millett, "Self and Embodiment: A Biophenomenological Approach to Dementia," *Dementia* (June 15, 2011), 12.

97. Olivia Hoblitzelle, *Ten Thousand Joys and Ten Thousand Sorrows: A Couple's Journey Through Alzheimer's* (New York: Penguin, 2010), 60. In her discussion of "the grace of diminishment," Hoblitzelle summarizes and paraphrases Teilhard de Chardin.

98. Desiderius Erasmus, quoted in Kelly Conkling Schneider, *Prayer of the Heart: A Journey Through the Heart with Visual Prayer* (New York: Morehouse Publishing, 2006), 24. This quotation is often credited to psychologist Carl Jung.

99. Supporting this type of connection, Maurice Friedman writes, "Only when one really listens—when one becomes personally aware of the 'signs of address' that address one not only in the words of but

in the very meeting with the other—does one attain to that sphere of the 'between' that Buber holds to be the 'really real'" (introduction to Martin Buber, *Between Man and Man* [New York: Collier Books, 1965]: xv).

100. Stephan Millett, "Self and Embodiment: A Biophenomenological Approach to Dementia," *Dementia* (June 15, 2011): 12.

101. Stephen G. Post, *Dignity for Deeply Forgetful People: How Caregivers Can Meet the Challenges of Alzheimer's Caregiving* (Baltimore: Johns Hopkins University Press, 2022), 3.

102. Post, 3. *Namaste* is a Sanskrit word originating in the ancient Hindu tradition and is most commonly translated as "I bow to you," acknowledging the Divine within everyone; including people with Alzheimer's and dementia.

103. Post, 3.

7. Into Our Hands

104. James Ellor, "Celebrating the Human Spirit," God Never Forgets: Faith, Hope, and Alzheimer's Disease, edited by Donald K. McKim (Louisville, KY: Westminster John Knox Press, 1997).

105. Keith Johnstone, *IMPRO: Improvisation and the Theatre* (New York: Routledge, 1992), 100.

106. Arthur Kleinman, "On Caregiving," *Harvard Magazine* (July–August 2010), 25. For those who don't feel willing or able to actively care for their parent, spouse, relative, or friend (for any number of reasons), one option is to care about them by choosing a qualified, caring, professional guardian and/or conservator.

107. Ellor, 17.

108. "Brooke Astor Trial Verdict Latest in Long Family Drama," *20/20*, ABC (October 8, 2009); "Elder Abuse Is Not Limited Just to Rich Like Brooke Astor," *Patriot-News* (November 4, 2009), PennLive.com.

109. The attitude that elder abuse cases are family matters and should be resolved within the family is disheartening and reminiscent of antiquated social service attitudes from twenty-five years ago regarding child abuse allegations.

110. James Ellor, "Love, Wisdom, and Justice: Transcendent Caring," *God Never Forgets: Faith, Hope, and Alzheimer's Disease*, edited by Donald K. McKim (Louisville, KY: Westminster John Knox Press, 1997), 59.

111. National Center on Elder Abuse. "Research, Statistics, and Data," ncea.acl.gov.

112. Stephen Post, The Moral Challenge of Alzheimer's Disease: Ethical Issues from Diagnosis to Dying (Baltimore: Johns Hopkins UP, 2000), 26.

113. E. T. Lucas, "Elder Abuse and Its Recognition Among Health Service Professionals," *The Elderly in America* (New York: Garland, 119), 118.

114. National Center on Elder Abuse, "Research, Statistics, and Data."

115. Post, 26.

116. Lois Moorman and Sally Petrone, "Elder Abuse and Neglect Laws: Protecting Older Adults," Memory Loss Conference at Southern Illinois University School of Medicine (November 7, 2011).

117. As Sam Keen explored the sacred relationship between love and care, he noted that in our society, care is most often defined in burdensome ways. Based on this understanding, Keen noticed that we rely more and more on "caring professionals," whom he refers to as "care-sellers" (116). Although his observations are stunningly accurate, applying this term to the professionals who care for the vulnerable population of people with Alzheimer's causes me to shudder.

118. See Helga Niesz, "Nursing Home 'Green Houses,'" State of Connecticut General Assembly, cga.ct.gov, for information about the "Green House" approach to elder care in nursing homes. See "Nursing Homes Create Home-Like, Resident-Focused Environment and Culture, Leading to Better Quality and Financial Performance, Higher Resident Satisfaction, and Lower Staff Turnover," Agency for Healthcare Research and Quality, U.S. Department of Health and Human Services

(innovations.ahrq.gov), for information about "neighborhood" designs in long-term care centers.

119. Marcus Borg translates Luke 6:36 as: "Be compassionate as God is compassionate" (replacing *merciful*, the word in the New Revised Standard Version of the Bible, with *compassionate*). According to Borg, "Compassion is not only the fruit of transformation, but the sign/mark/test of authentic Christian transformation" ("Redeeming Christian Language," lecture at Wartburg Theological Seminary (October 15, 2009).

120. Simone de Beauvoir, quoted in David Keck, *Forgetting Whose We Are: Alzheimer's Disease and the Love of God* (Nashville: Abington, 1996), 16.

121. Marty Richards, *Caresharing: A Reciprocal Approach to Caregiving and Care Receiving in the Complexities of Aging, Illness or Disability* (Woodstock, VT: Sky Light Paths, 2009), 44.

122. Clara Vila-Castelar, et al., "A cultural approach to dementia—insights from US Latino and other minoritized groups," *Nature Reviews/Neurology*, 18 (May 2022): 307, 309.

123. Lisa Barnes, "Alzheimer's disease in African American Individuals: Increased incidence or not enough data?" *Nature Reviews/Neurology* (December 6, 2021), nature.com.

124. "What Are the Signs of Alzheimer's Disease?" National Institute on Aging, nia.nih.gov.

125. Vila-Castelar, et al., 307.

126. Daisy Duarte, interviewed by Jason Resendez, "The Economic Impact of Alzheimer's on Latinos," March 16, 2021, youtube.com.

127. Vila-Castelar, et al., 307.

III Spirit-Inspired Caring

Epigraph: Myra Scovel, "The Wind of the Spirit," in *The Weight of a Leaf* (Philadelphia: Westminster Press, 1970).

8. Points of Surrender

1. Marcus Borg, *Meeting Jesus Again for the First Time: The Historical Jesus and the Heart of Contemporary Faith* (San Francisco: HarperCollins, 1995): 125–126. Jesus scholar Marcus Borg analyzes the Hebrew Bible story of exile and return in the context of an iconic journey story for humanity. "As a life of being separated from that to which one belongs," he writes, "exile is often marked with grief." He cites Psalm 137:1: "By the rivers of Babylon, there we sat down and wept when we remembered Zion." Borg also indicates, again from Psalm 137, that "the experience of exile can also generate intense anger" (139). For biblical descriptions of the exile, see Isaiah 40–55 (for the good news of the return), Psalm 137, and the Book of Lamentations, "which describes the suffering, despair, and angst of the generation living after the destruction of Jerusalem and the temple" (138).

2. Borg, 127.

3. Keen, 116.

4. Shams al-Din Hafiz, "Absolutely Clear," *The Subject Tonight Is Love: Sixty Wild and Sweet Poems of Hafiz*, translated by Daniel Ladinsky (London: Penguin, 2002).

5. Janet Ramsey, "Spiritual Resilience and Aging," Tri-State Forum at Wartburg Theological Seminary (October 12, 2012).

6. James Gordon, *Manifesto for a New Medicine* (Reading, MA: Perseus, 1996), 104. Carolyn Myss takes Gordon's thought a step further. She concludes that, even during difficult times, we are so afraid of change that we link our energy with the "saboteur archetype" and go into denial. Therefore, we don't actually allow ourselves to know just how *not* well things are going (Carolyn Myss, with Michael Toms, *Healing with Spirit* [Carlsbad, CA: Hay House Audio, 1997]). The early Christian father Evagrius Ponticus described this archetype as temptations "experienced at the hand of the demons" (quoted in Anselm Gruen, *Heaven Begins within You: Wisdom from the Desert Fathers* [New York: Crossroad, 1999], 60). St. Ignatius referred to the saboteur archetype as "the enemy," whose tactic is "to put before [people] illusory gratifications, prompting them to imagine sensual delights and

pleasures, the better to hold them and make them grow in their vices and sins" (Jules Toner, *Spirit of Light or Darkness? A Casebook for Studying Discernment of Spirits* [St. Louis: The Institute of Jesuit Sources, 1995], 5.)

7. Viktor Frankl, *Man's Search for Meaning* (New York: Pocket, 1984), 135–36.

8. Kayli Reese, "Statewide Iowa report, local nursing home administrators cite staffing as top challenge," *(Dubuque) Telegraph Herald* (March 8, 2023), telegraphherald.com.

9. Alzheimer's Association, "2023 Alzheimer's Disease: Facts and Figures," *Alzheimer's & Dementia*, 19:4 (2023), alz-journals.onlinelibrary.wiley.com.

10. Robert Erlewine, "The Legacy of Abraham Joshua Heschel," *Tikkun* (September 20, 2011).

11. Richard Rohr, *The Spirituality of Imperfection* (Cincinnati: St. Anthony Messenger Press, 1997), audiocassette. Rohr paraphrases Abraham Joshua Heschel.

12. Marty Richards, *Caresharing: A Reciprocal Approach to Caregiving and Care Receiving in the Complexities of Aging, Illness or Disability* (Woodstock, VT: Sky Light Paths, 2009), 83–117.

9. The Dance of Yes and No

13. Deuteronomy 30:19, *Holy Bible: New Revised Standard Version* (New York: Oxford UP, 1989).

14. Richard J. Foster, Introduction, *Testament of Devotion* by Thomas R. Kelly (New York: Harper, 1941), vii–x.

15. Maurice Friedman, *Martin Buber: The Life of Dialogue* (Chicago: University of Chicago Press, 1976), 139–140.

16. Martin Buber, *I and Thou*, translated by Ronald Gregor Smith (New York: Collier, 1987), 11.

17. Matthew 15:21–28 (NRSV).

18. David V. Powers et al., "Coping and Depression in Alzheimer's Caregivers: Longitudinal Evidence of Stability," Journal of Gerontology: Psychological Sciences 57B:3 (2002), 206.

19. Stephen Pattison, *Shame: Theory, Therapy, Theology* (New York: Cambridge University Press, 2000), 53.

20. J. E. Earl Thompson, Jr., "Pastoral and Clinical Implications of Shame," lecture at Andover Newton Theological School (October 5, 2010). Dr. Thompson summarizes the extensive work on shame by sociologist Thomas Scheff and psychotherapist Suzanne Retzinger, both of whom were influenced by Helen Block Lewis, one of the first psychoanalysts to write about shame. Beverly Wildung Harrison writes, "It is within the power of human love to build up dignity and self-respect in each other or to tear each other down. We are better at the latter than the former. However, literally through acts of love directed to us, we become self-respecting and other-regarding people, and we cannot be one without the other. If we lack self-respect, we also become the sorts of people who can neither see nor hear each other" ("The Power of Anger in the Work of Love," *Weaving the Visions: New Patterns in Feminist Spirituality*, edited by Judith Plaskow and Carol P. Christ [New York: HarperCollins, 1989], 218).

21. Martin Buber, *I and Thou*, translated by Ronald Gregor Smith (New York: Collier, 1987), 11.

22. Tom Kitwood and Kathleen Bredin, "Towards a Theory of Dementia Care: Personhood and Well-being," *Ageing and Society* 12 (1992): 283.

10. The Sacrament of the Present Moment

23. Buber, *I and Thou*, translated by Ronald Gregor Smith (New York: Collier, 1987), 4.

24. Martin Buber, *Encounter: Autobiographical Fragments* (LaSalle, IL: Open Court, 1967): 3.

25. Buber, *Encounter*, 38.

NOTES

26. Gerald May, *The Awakened Heart: Opening Yourself to the Love You Need* (New York: HarperCollins, 1993), 3.

27. Richard Rohr, *Just This – Daily Meditation: Be Awake* (Albuquerque, NM: Center for Action and Contemplation).

28. Thomas Merton, *The Asian Journal*, edited by Naomi Burton et al. (New York: New Directions, 1973), 308.

29. Martin Buber, "Replies to My Critics," *The Philosophy of Martin Buber,* edited by P. A. Schilpp and M. Friedman (LaSalle, IL: Open Court, 1967), 693.

30. G. Allen Power, *Dementia Beyond Drugs: Changing the Culture of Care* (Baltimore: Health Professions Press, 2010), 196–97.

31. Pierre Parenteau, "Communication with Alzheimer Patients: A Matter of Time, Caring and Contact," *The Canadian Alzheimer Disease Review* (November 2000), 6.

32. Henry Miller, *Big Sur and the Oranges of Hieronymus Bosch* (New York: New Directions Publishing Corp., 1957).

33. Jane Marie Thibault and Richard Morgan, *No Act of Love Is Ever Wasted: The Spirituality of Caring for Persons with Dementia* (Nashville, TN: Upper Room Books, 2009), 29.

34. Jill Bolte Taylor, *My Stroke of Insight: A Brain Scientist's Personal Journey* (New York: Plume, 2009), 35.

35. Taylor, 41.

36. The following resources about the spiritual benefits of meditation and prayer and being present in the moment were informative and inspiring companions on my journey.

In the Buddhist tradition:

- Pema Chödrön, *Awakening Compassion: Meditation Practice for Difficult Times* (Louisville, CO: Sounds True, 1995), 6 audiocassettes with booklet.
- Tara Bennett-Goleman, *Emotional Alchemy: How the Mind Can Heal the Heart* (Rochester, NY: Audio Renaissance, 2001), 2 audiocassettes.
- Thich Nhat Hanh, *The Miracle of Mindfulness: A Manual on Meditation,* translated by Mobi Ho (Boston: Beacon Press, 1987).

In the Christian tradition:
- Thomas Keating, *Open Mind, Open Heart: The Contemplative Dimension of the Gospel* (New York: Continuum, 2005).

New Age teachings:
- Eckhart Tolle, *The Power of Now: A Guide to Spiritual Enlightenment* (Novato, CA: New World Library, 2004).

37. The following resources about the health benefits of meditation were helpful, healing companions on my journey:
- Herbert Benson, with Miriam Z. Klipper, *The Relaxation Response* (New York: Avon, 1976).
- Dean Ornish, *Love & Survival: 8 Pathways to Intimacy and Health* (New York: Harper Perennial, 1999).
- Jon Kabat-Zinn, *Full Catastrophe Living: Using the Wisdom of Your Body and Mind to Face Stress, Pain, and Illness* (New York: Delta, 1991).

38. Harvard Mahoney Neuroscience Institute, "Growing the Brain through Meditation," *On the Brain*, 12:3 (Fall 2006).

39. *Mindfulness* is defined by Buddhist teacher Thich Nhat Hanh as "the energy to be here and to witness deeply everything that happens in the present moment, aware of what is going on within and without" (*Living Buddha, Living Christ* [New York: Riverhead Books, 1995], 204).

40. Hiakajo Roshi, quoted in Pema Sherpa & Brendan Barca, "Eat When you Eat, Sleep When You Sleep," *The Mindful Minute*, LinkedIn. com.

41. Pema Chödrön, *When Things Fall Apart: Heart Advice for Difficult Times* (Boston: Shambala, 1997), 16.

11. Gifts from the Alzheimer's Journey

42. Mary Oliver, "Uses of Sorrow." *Thirst* (Boston: Beacon Press, 2006).

43. Helen Keller, "Optimism," *The World I Live In and Optimism: A Collection of Essays* (Mineola, NY, 2010), 89.

44. Viktor Frankl, *Man's Search for Meaning* (New York: Washington Square Press, 1985), 121.

45. Durga Leela, *Yoga of Recovery* (Singing Dragon/Kingsley Publishers: London, 2022), 134–35.

46. Loretta Ann Woodward Veney, *Being My Mom's Mom: A Journey through Dementia from a Daughter's Perspective* (Berkeley, CA: aNewPress, 2019), 100.

47. David Steindl-Rast, *The Grateful Heart* (Louisville, CO: Sounds True Recordings, 1992).

48. Jane Thibault and Richard Morgan, *No Act of Love Is Ever Wasted: The Spirituality of Caring for Persons with Dementia* (Nashville, TN: Upper Room Books, 2009), 15.

49. Harold Kushner, *When Bad Things Happen to Good People* (New York: Anchor Books, 2004), 45–46.

50. Stephen Mitchell, *The Book of Job* (New York: Harper Perennial, 1992), xvi.

51. Mitchell, xix, xxvii.

52. Kushner, 50–51.

53. Mitchell, xxi.

54. Steindl-Rast, *The Grateful Heart*.

55. David Steindl-Rast, *Gratefulness, the Heart of Prayer: An Approach to Life in Fullness* (Mahwah, NJ: Paulist Press, 1984): 182.

56. Steindl-Rast, *Gratefulness*, 175–76.

57. Thich Nhat Hanh, "Walking Meditation," in *Engaged Buddhist Reader*, edited by Arnold Kotler (Berkeley: Parallax Press, 1996): 46.

58. At the "Map Through the Maze" dementia conference in Massachusetts in May 2012, author and presenter Joanne Koenig Coste shared the importance of waiting for people with dementia to find their words. In an early-stage support group Coste leads for people with dementia, one of the male participants was asked how he was. He replied with a labored stutter, "I'm f-f-f-f-f… " "You're fine," another man jumped in. But the first man's face turned red, and he continued to try to speak, "No, f-f-f-f-f…" With patience facilitated by Coste, the man finally spoke his truth, which wasn't "fine" but "frustrated." This was an exceedingly important difference! Some "experts" will

encourage caregivers to complete sentences and fill in the blank with words we think people with dementia mean in order to relieve the stress of word finding and to take attention away from their failing abilities. But in this situation, I agree with Coste: Being patient and waiting for people with dementia to bring forward their own words will lead to more satisfying communication and connection.

59. Steindl-Rast, 176.

60. "Mother Marianne Cope and the Sisters of St. Francis," National Park Service, www.nps.gov/kala/historyculture/marianne.htm.

61. Robert Louis Stevenson, "To Mother Maryanne," *Songs of Travel and Other Verses*, Project Gutenberg, gutenberg.org.

62. C. Robert Mesle, *Process Theology: A Basic Introduction* (St. Louis: Chalice Press, 1993): 75–79.

63. Mesle outlines three aspects of a process theology of liberation:
- God has a relational character and experiences the joy and suffering of humanity. God suffers with those who experience [pain and loss] and seeks to actualize all positive and beautiful potentials.
- God seeks the actualization of the greater good.
- God exercises relational power and not unilateral control. God cannot instantly end evil [or suffering]. God works in relational ways to help guide people to freedom [and healing].

64. Mesle, 79.

IV Believing in Relationship

Epigraph: Libbie Deverich Stoddard, "How Shall I?"

1. Paul Raia, "Habilitation Therapy: A New Starscape," in *Enhancing the Quality of Life in Advanced Dementia*, edited by Ladislav Volcer and Lisa Bloom-Charette (London: Routledge, 1999).

2. N.R. Kleinfield, "Alzheimer's in the News: A Behind the Scenes Special Report: More Than Death, Fearing a Muddled Mind," *New York Times* (November 11, 2002), nytimes.com.

12. Emotional Memory

3. Louise M. Eder, "Heart Memories," Kansas City Alzheimer's Disease and Related Disorders Association newsletter (Spring 1984).

4. Raia, 23.

5. Raia, 31.

6. Colleen Carroll Campbell, "Alzheimer's Kills Memories, Not Emotions," *St. Louis Post-Dispatch* (April 22, 2010), colleen-campbell. com.

7. Lisa Genova, "Just Say Yes-And," blogs.alz.org.

8. Raia, 33.

9. Campbell.

10. Daniel Tranel, interview (October 25, 2011). Tranel changed the actual names and locations of the people involved to protect their privacy.

11. Norman Doidge explains, "The hippocampus turns our short-term explicit memories into long-term explicit memories for people, places, and things—the memories to which we have conscious access .... Explicit memory consciously recollects specific facts, events, and episodes. It is the memory we use when we describe and make explicit what we did on the weekend, and with whom, and for how long. It helps us to organize our memories by time and place" (*The Brain That Changes Itself: Stories of Personal Triumph from the Frontier of Brain Science* [New York: Penguin Books, 2007], 229). Doidge compares the explicit memory system, which is supported by language, and the "procedural or implicit" memory system. Procedural/implicit memory is well developed by the time a child is twenty-six months old and will remain functional for people with Alzheimer's long after cognition and verbal language skills decline. He writes, "Procedural/implicit memory functions when we learn a procedure or group of automatic actions occurring outside our focused attention, in which words are not generally required. Our nonverbal interactions with people and many of our emotional memories are part of our procedural memory system" (228). Doidge cites the work of E. R. Kandel, who says,

"During the first 2–3 years of life, when an infant's interaction with its mother is particularly important, the infant relies primarily on its procedural memory systems" (E. R.Kandel, "Biology and the Future of Psychoanalysis: A New Intellectual Framework for Psychiatry Revisited," *American Journal of Psychiatry*, 156:4 [1999], 505–24). Similarly, people in the later stages of Alzheimer's disease will be relying on and using their remaining capacities for experiencing procedural/ implicit memories.

12. Justin S. Feinstein, Melissa Duff, and Daniel Tranel, "Sustained Experience of Emotion after Loss of Memory in Patients with Amnesia," *PNAS/ Proceedings of the National Academy of Sciences of the United States of America*, 107:17 (April 27, 2010): 7674.

13. Pam Belluck, "Giving Alzheimer's Patients Their Way, Even Chocolate," *The New York Times* (December 31, 2010), nytimes.com.

14. Justin S. Feinstein et al., 7674.

15. Alaine Reschke-Hernandez, Amy Belfi, Edmarie Guzman-Velez, and Daniel Tranel, "Hooked on a Feeling: Influence of Brief Exposure to Familiar Music on Feelings of Emotions in Individuals with Alzheimer's Disease," *Journal of Alzheimer's Disease* 78 (2020), 1020.

16. Justin Feinstein, quoted in Belluck.

17. Feinstein, quoted in Belluck.

18. John Riehl, "Alzheimer's patients can still feel the emotion long after the memories have vanished." *Iowa Now*, (Iowa City, IA: University of Iowa, September, 24, 2014), now.uiowa.edu.

19. Alaine E. Rescheke-Hernandez, Amy M. Belfi, Edmarie Guzman-Velez, and Daniel Tranel, "Hooked on a Feeling: Influence of Brief Exposure to Familiar Music on Feelings of Emotion in Individuals with Alzheimer's Disease." *Journal of Alzheimer's Disease* 78 (2020), 1019–31.

20. U.S. Food & Drug Administration, "FDA Approves First Drug to Treat Agitation Symptoms Due to Alzheimer's Disease," news release (May 11, 2023), fda.gov.

21. MedlinePlus, "Brexpiprazole," medlineplus.gov.

22. Naomi Feil and Gladys Wilson, "Memory Bridge," youtube.com.

23. Riehl.

24. Kelsey Spalding-Wilson, Edmarie Guzman-Velez, Jade Angelica, et al., "A novel two-day intervention reduces stress in caregivers of people with dementia,'" *Alzheimer's & Dementia: Transactional Research and Clinical Interventions*, 4 (2018), 450.

25. Spalding-Wilson, et al., 458.

26. Stephen G. Post, *Dignity for Deeply Forgetful People: How Caregivers Can Meet the Challenges of Alzheimer's Disease* (Baltimore: John's Hopkins University Press, 2022), 88.

27. Raia, 22.

28. Joseph Campbell, interview by Bill Moyers, *The Power of Myth*, PBS (1988).

29. A currently popular anti-psychotic drug, Abilify, is advertised on television as a compliment to anti-depressant medication. The advertisement contains a warning that Abilify may cause death for elderly patients with dementia.

30. Feinstein, 76–78.

13. Time Enough

31. Rabindranath Tagore, "Fireflies," *Poetry Chaikhana: Sacred Poetry from Around the World*, poetry-chaikhana.com.

32. Dietrich Bonhoeffer, *Letters and Papers from Prison* (New York: Touchstone, 1997), 3.

33. Abraham Joshua Heschel, *The Sabbath* (New York: Farrar, Straus and Giroux, 1975), 3, 6, 29.

34. Sherri Edwards, "My Mother's Unlikely Gift of Dementia," *Huffington Post* (December 8, 2011), huffingtonpost.com.

35. Stephen Post, *The Moral Challenge of Alzheimer's Disease: Ethical Issues from Diagnosis to Dying* (Baltimore: The Johns Hopkins University Press, 2000), 1.

36. Coleen attended college part-time for six years; during these same years, she worked full-time, parented her two sons, and cared for her

mom on a regular basis. Coleen completed her BA in business one year before her mom died.

37. David Shenk supports Mary Anne's awareness that the losses associated with Alzheimer's disease could be worse for the caregiver than the afflicted person: "Still, caregivers must try to understand both the frustrations and the unexpected benefits of having an unraveling mind. What they may at first presume to be a uniformly awful experience for the victims can sometimes perhaps be peculiarly satisfying and even enriching—a final intellectual and esthetic adventure.... Alzheimer's keeps things new. The Alzheimer's mind is constantly flooded with new stimuli; everything is always in the moment, a rich, resonant, overwhelming feeling.... Ever-freshness, then, may be considered an Alzheimer's consolation prize. This may be a particularly difficult idea for caregivers to swallow ... they must suffer through the oppressive repetition.... in the often deadening, disheartening world of Alzheimer's care, caregivers wake up thousands of days in a row facing the same tourist wanting to take exactly the same tour" (*The Forgetting—Alzheimer's: Portrait of an Epidemic* [New York: Anchor Books, 2003], 194–195).

38. Myra Scovel, "The Wind of the Spirit," in *The Weight of a Leaf* (Philadelphia: The Westminster Press, 1970), 45.

39. Carl is paraphrasing 2 Corinthians 7:2 (NRSV).

14. The Last Word

40. Rainer Maria Rilke, *Letters to a Young Poet*, translated by M. D. Herter Norton (New York: W. W. Norton, 1962), 35.

41. Joanne Koenig Coste, *Learning to Speak Alzheimer's: A Groundbreaking Approach for Everyone Dealing with the Disease* (New York: Houghton Mifflin, 2003), 7.

42. Stephan Millett, "Self and Embodiment: A Biophenomenological Approach to Dementia," *Dementia* (June 15, 2011), 12. Millet writes, "People with dementia are ... 'driven by meaning'—but without committing to cognition-reliant definitions of selfhood and intentionality."

43. Stephen Levine, *Unattended Sorrow: Recovering from Loss and Reviving the Heart* (Emmaus, PA: Rodale Books, 2005), 192.

44. Stephen Levine and Ondrea Levine, *Who Dies? An Investigation of Conscious Living and Conscious Dying* (New York: Anchor Books, 1989), 163.

45. Levine and Levine, 163.

46. Levine, 204.

47. G. Allen Power, *Dementia Beyond Drugs: Changing the Culture of Care* (Baltimore: Health Professions Press, 2010), 196–197; Pierre Parenteau, "Communication with Alzheimer Patients: A Matter of Time, Caring and Contact," *The Canadian Alzheimer Disease Review* (November 2000), 6; Millett, 12; Levine, 74.

48. Joan Chittister, *The Rule of Benedict: A Spirituality for the 21st Century* (New York: Crossroad Publishing Company, 2014), 3. The first rule of St. Benedict is based on these lines: "My child, be attentive to my words; incline your ear to my sayings. Do not let them escape from your sight; keep them within your heart" (Proverbs 4:20–21, *Holy Bible: New Revised Standard Version* [New York: Oxford UP, 1989]).

49. Levine and Levine, 163.

50. Doidge describes the right-hemisphere nonverbal capacities of the developing brain between the ages of ten months and twenty-six months as similar to those of a person in the later stages of Alzheimer's: "During the first two years of life, the mother principally communicates nonverbally with her right hemisphere to reach her infant's right hemisphere .... The right hemisphere generally processes nonverbal communication; it allows us to recognize faces and read facial expressions, and it connects us to other people. It, thus, processes the nonverbal visual cues exchanged between a mother and her baby. It also processes the musical component of speech, or tone, by which we convey emotion" (226).

51. Levine, 76.

52. Levine, 74.

53. Levine and Levine, 164.

54. Levine, 196.

55. Jill Bolte Taylor, who suffered and recovered from a stroke, writes, "I shifted from the doing-consciousness of my left brain to the being-consciousness of my right brain . . . . I stopped thinking in language and shifted to taking new pictures of what was going on in the present moment . . . . All I could perceive was right here, right now, and it was beautiful . . . . The now offline intellectual mind of my left hemisphere no longer inhibited my innate awareness that I was the miraculous power of life . . . . in the absence of my left hemisphere's negative judgment, I perceived myself as perfect, whole, and beautiful just the way I was . . . . Although I could not understand the words they spoke, I could read volumes from their facial expression and body language. I paid very close attention to how energy dynamics affected me. I realized that some people brought me energy while others took it away" (*My Stroke of Insight: A Brain Scientist's Personal Journey* [New York: Plume, 2009], 71–77).

56. Raia cites Abraham Maslow's *Toward a Psychology of Being* (New York: John Wiley & Sons, 1968) as a basis of habilitation therapy. In addition, Raia applies Maslow's humanistic perspective to people with Alzheimer's and dementia (22).

57. Mark 14:33–34 (*Holy Bible: NRSV*).

58. Jane Thibault and Richard Morgan, *No Act of Love Is Ever Wasted: The Spirituality of Caring for Persons with Dementia* (Nashville: Upper Room Books, 2009), 111.

V Looking Back, Walking On

Epigraph: Adapted from Dag Hammarskjold quote in Stephen Sapp, "Hope: The Community Looks Forward," in *God Never Forgets: Faith, Hope, and Alzheimer's Disease*, edited by Donald K. McKim (Louisville: Westminster John Knox Press, 1997), 103.

1. David Steindl-Rast, *The Grateful Heart* (Louisville, CO: Sounds True Recordings, 1992).

2. Richard Rohr et al., *Loving the Two Halves of Life* (Albuquerque, NM: Center for Action and Contemplation, 2011), compact discs.

NOTES

15. Forgetting, Forgiving, Reconciling

3. Dennis Linn et al., *Don't Forgive Too Soon: Extending the Two Hands That Heal* (Mahwah, NJ: Paulist Press, 1997); Marie M. Fortune, "Forgiveness: The Last Step," *Violence Against Women and Children: A Christian Theological Sourcebook*, edited by Carol J. Adams and Marie M. Fortune (New York: Continuum, 1995), 201–6.

4. Marie M. Fortune, "Forgiveness: The Last Step," *Violence Against Women and Children: A Christian Theological Sourcebook*, edited by Carol J. Adams and Marie M. Fortune (New York: Continuum, 1995), 204; Ellen Bass and Laura Davis, *The Courage to Heal: A Guide for Women Survivors of Child Sexual Abuse* (New York: HarperCollins, 1994), 162.

5. Robert L. Browning and Roy A. Reed cite the *process model of forgiveness* developed by Robert D. Enright, indicating that there are several challenging steps:

  1. Experience negative psychological consequences of the injury.
  2. Recognize a need for resolution.
  3. Decide between justice and mercy as a strategy.
  4. Identify your forgiveness motive.
  5. Make a decision to forgive.
  6. Execute internal forgiveness strategies.
  7. Execute behavioral reconciliation strategies, culminating in release (*Forgiveness, Reconciliation and Moral Courage: Motives and Designs for Ministry in a Troubled World* [Grand Rapids, MI: Eerdmans, 2004], 65–9).

  Professor J. Earl Thompson, Jr., quotes Enright as he writes about step 5 in the above model of forgiveness. The decision to forgive is "a moral choice based in a long and arduous process of struggle and suffering. Forgiveness is not cheap. It costs the injured dearly in emotional and spiritual pain" ("Steps Toward Forgiveness [A Process of Forgiveness]: Insights from Robert D. Enright and Terry Hargrave, Modified by Professor Thompson," lecture at Andover Newton Theological School, November 9, 2010).

6. Solomon Schimmel, *Wounds Not Healed by Time: The Power of Repentance and Forgiveness* (New York: Oxford University Press, 2002), 122, 85. Citing Mishnah, Bava Kamma 8:7, Schimmel states, "The

Mishnah and other rabbinic sources emphasize that the victim must forgive the offender who has appropriately repented."

7. Everett L. Worthington, Jr., *Forgiving and Reconciling: Bridges to Wholeness and Hope* (Downers Grove, IL: InterVarsity Press, 2003), 31–41.

8. Schimmel, 137.

9. Jacqui Lewis. *Fierce Love: A Bold Path to Ferocious Courage and Rule-Breaking Kindness That Can Heal the World* (New York: Penguin Random House, 2021), 13.

10. Naomi Feil, *Validation: The Feil Method: How to Help Disoriented Old-Old* (Cleveland: Edward Feil Productions, 1982), 17.

11. Browning and Reed, 49.

12. J. Earl Thompson, Jr., "Forgiveness—Everett L. Worthington, Jr. and Terry Hargrave," lecture at Andover Newton Theological School (November 16, 2010). Using the forgiveness work of Hargrave as a springboard, Professor Thompson begins the discussion of reconciliation, which is essentially "a rebirth of the relationship" brought forth by the restoration of trust in relationships that have been fractured—*if* the restoration is safe and possible."

13. Janet Ramsey, "Forgiveness and Healing," lecture at Tri-State Forum, Wartburg Theological Seminary (April 15, 2010).

14. J. Earl Thompson, Jr., "Steps Toward Forgiveness (A Process of Forgiveness): Insights from Robert D. Enright and Terry Hargrave, Modified by Professor Thompson," lecture at Andover Newton Theological School (November 9, 2010). This Biblical reference to a "Refiner's Fire" is from Malachi 2:17–3:60. It is possible for an injured person to discover fresh meaning for one's self and perhaps even a new purpose in life as a result of suffering and engaging in the process of forgiveness. This insight "speaks to the idea that life is loss and paradoxically gain. Being injured and experiencing numerous losses can lead us into deeper maturity and greater clarity of purpose and direction if we can turn loose of our bitterness and resentment."

15. Bass and Davis, 162.

16. Ramsey.

17. Schimmel, 123.

18. Ellen Bass and Laura Davis, *The Courage to Heal: A Guide for Women Survivors of Child Sexual Abuse* (New York: HarperCollins, 1994), 162.

19. Ramsey. Dr. Judith Lewis Herman supports Ramsey's position that forgiveness is not a human achievement. Herman indicates that revenge fantasies and forgiveness fantasies are an "attempt at empowerment" for victims of abuse. "The survivor imagines that she can transcend her rage [through forgiveness] and erase the impact of the trauma through a wild, defiant act of love. But it is not possible to exorcise the trauma through either hatred or love. Like revenge, the fantasy of forgiveness often becomes a cruel torture because it is out of reach for most ordinary human beings" (*Trauma and Recovery: The Aftermath of Violence—From Domestic Abuse to Political Terror* [New York: Basic Books, 1992], 89–90).

20. Bass and Davis write, "Feeling compassion for another human being feels good. It often arises out of the fact that you are feeling compassionate toward yourself, or because you have begun to view a particular family member in a different way" (162). Enright's model of forgiveness also acknowledges the importance of empathy, suggesting that the injured person must take the offender seriously and seek to understand who she is, and how she perceives and senses the world. Professor Thompson acknowledges, along with Bass, Worthington, and Enright, that "empathy is incredibly difficult for us under any circumstances" (J. Earl Thompson, Jr., lecture [November 9, 2010]).

21. Worthington, 95–112. Worthington proposes a five-step process of forgiveness, which he names R-E-A-C-H:
    Recall the hurt.
    Empathize with the person who injured us.
    Conceptualize forgiveness as an **A**ltruistic gift.
    Commit to forgive.
    Hold onto forgiveness.

22. Browning and Reed, 55.

23. Thompson.

24. Martin Buber, *I and Thou*, translated by Ronald Gregor Smith (New York: Collier, 1987), 18.

16. Nourishing Compassion

25. George Odell, "We Need One Another," *Singing the Living Tradition* (Boston: Unitarian Universalist Association, 1993), #468.

26. Karen Armstrong, *Twelve Steps to a Compassionate Life* (New York: Knopf, 2010), 19.

27. Christine Louis de Canonville, "Narcissism and Inadequate Mirroring," Narcissistic Behavior, narcissisticbehavior.net

28. Jacqui Lewis, *Fierce Love: A Bold Path to Ferocious Courage and Rule-Breaking Kindness That Can Heal the World* (New York: Penguin Random House, 2021), 13, 41.

29. Canonville.

30. Danielle Maxon, "Mirroring Your Child's Intense Emotions: 4 Easy Steps," blog (April 7, 2016), daniellemaxon.com.

31. David Shenk, *The Forgetting—Alzheimer's: Portrait of an Epidemic* (New York: Anchor, 2003), 225–226.

32. Jacinta Jimenez, "Compassion vs. Empathy: Understanding the Difference," Betterup (July 16, 2021), Betterup, betterup.com.

33. Danusha Laméris, "Small Kindnesses," *Bonfire Opera.* (University of Pittsburgh Press, 2020).

34. Stephen G. Post, *Dignity for Deeply Forgetful People: How Caregivers Can Meet the Challenges of Alzheimer's Disease* (Baltimore: Johns Hopkins University, 2023), 17.

35. Armstrong, 116.

36. Armstrong, 6

37. Post, 161.

38. Sam Keen, *To Love and Be Loved* (New York: Bantam, 1999), 116.

39. Jeffrey Bishop, "A Call to Cure, A Call to Care," lecture at Joy of Caring Conference, Clarke University (August 17, 2013).

40. Bishop.

41. According to Bishop, the depersonalization of patients by the conventional medical system, particularly those who can't be cured and are dying, is the basis for burnout of health care providers.

42. Armstrong, 8.

43. Pema Chödrön, *Start Where You Are: A Guide to Compassionate Living* (Boston: Shambala, 1994), x.

44. Armstrong, 9.

45. Richard Rohr, *True Self/False Self* (audiocassettes) (Cincinnati: St. Anthony Messenger Press, 2003).

46. Marcus Borg, *Meeting Jesus Again for the First Time: The Historical Jesus and the Heart of Contemporary Faith* (San Francisco: HarperCollins, 1995), 47.

47. Borg, 48–49. Borg also writes, "For Jesus, this is what God is like …. According to Jesus, compassion is to be the central quality of a life faithful to God the compassionate one."

48. Bishop.

49. Rohr.

50. Through her actions, Julie was manifesting the goal of habilitation therapy. She was helping Mom to begin her day in a positive emotional state.

51. Mary Vineyard, *11ᵗʰ Sunday in Ordinary Time 6/17/12, reflections on scripture readings: Ezk 17:22–24, Ps 92, 2 Cor 5:6–10, Mk 4:26–34* (email).

52. Armstrong, 9–11. Armstrong identifies the four elements of love from the Buddhist tradition as *maîtri* ("loving kindness"), the desire to bring happiness to all sentient beings; *karuna* ("compassion"), the resolve to liberate all creatures from their pain; *mudita* ("sympathetic joy"), which takes delight in the happiness of others; and *upkesha* ("even-mindedness"), an equanimity that enables us to love all beings equally and impartially.

53. Armstrong, 21–22.

54. Borg, 49.

55. David J. Fleming, *Draw Me Into Your Friendship: The Spiritual Exercises—A Literal Translation and Contemporary Reading* (St. Louis: Institute of Jesuit Sources, 1996).

56. Naomi Shihab Nye, "Kindness," *Words Under the Words: Selected Poems* (Portland, OR: Far Corner Books, 1995).

57. Martha Beck, *Finding Your Own North Star: Claiming the Life You Were Meant to Live* (Sounds True, June 1, 2005), compact disc.

17. Re-imagining Survival

58. Cooper Worth, "County Tops State Average in Alzheimer's Rate," *(Dubuque) Telegraph Herald* (July 26, 2023).

59. Marcus Borg, *Meeting Jesus Again for the First Time: The Historical Jesus and the Heart of Contemporary Faith* (San Francisco: HarperCollins, 1995), 69–95.

60. Pema Chödrön, *When Things Fall Apart: Heart Advice for Difficult Times* (Boston: Shambala, 1997), 143.

61. Borg, 70.

62. Borg, 69.

63. 2 Corinthians 4:18, *Holy Bible: New Revised Standard Version* (New York: Oxford UP, 1989).

18. Companionship on the Journey

65. Sopurkh Singh, presentation at the Sivananda Ashram Yoga Retreat in Nassau, Bahamas (December 27, 2022).

Resources for Caregivers

Epigraph: Richard Wagamese, *Embers: One Ojibway's Meditations* (Toronto: Douglas & McIntyre, 2013), 58.

1. Reinhold Niebuhr, The Essential Reinhold Niebuhr: Selected Essays and Addresses (Binghamton, NY: Vail-Ballou Press, 1986), 251.

2. Meister Eckhart, Sermon 27, The Complete Mystical Works of Meister Eckhart, translated by Maurice O'C. Walshe (New York: Herder & Herder, 2009), 173.

3. David Steindl-Rast, The Grateful Heart (Boulder, CO: Sounds True Recordings, 1992), audiocassette.

4. Adapted from Dag Hammarskjold quote in Stephen Sapp, "Hope: The Community Looks Forward," in *God Never Forgets: Faith, Hope, and Alzheimer's Disease*, edited by Donald K. McKim (Louisville: Westminster John Knox Press, 1997), 103.

5. At a workshop at the Omega Institute in Reinbeck, New York, in 1998, led by the Vietnamese Buddhist teacher Thich Nhat Hanh, I learned a simple meditation mantra: "Breathing in I calm myself, breathing out I smile."

Caregivers Making a Difference and Finding Meaning

6. Stephen Post, *The Moral Challenge of Alzheimer's Disease: Ethical Issues from Diagnosis to Dying,* Second Edition (Baltimore: The Johns Hopkins Press, 2000), 2.

7. Lisa Genova, Preface and "The First Decade" timeline, *Still Alice*, 10th anniversary edition (New York: Gallery Books, 2019).

8. Kathy Good. *My World Wore a Bow Tie* (Cedar Rapids, IA: Family Caregivers Center of Mercy, 2023), 11, 6, 84, 85.

9. Alzheimer's Speaks, "About Our Founder," alzheimersspeaks.com.

10. Good.

11. T.S. Eliot, "Dry Salvages," *The Four Quartets*, davidgorman.com

12. Viktor E. Frankl, *Man's Search for Meaning* (New York: Washington Square Press, 1984), 135.

13. David Steindl-Rast, *Gratefulness, the Heart of Prayer: An Approach to Life in Fullness* (Mahwah, NJ: Paulist Press, 1984).